ORAL DIAGNOSIS

SECOND EDITION

ORAL DIAGNOSIS

Donald A. Kerr, D.D.S., M.S.

*Professor and Head, Department
of Oral Pathology, University
of Michigan School of Dentistry,
Ann Arbor, Mich.*

Major M. Ash, Jr., D.D.S., M.S.

*Professor of Dentistry (Oral
Pathology and Periodontia),
University of Michigan School
of Dentistry, Ann Arbor, Mich.*

H. Dean Millard, D.D.S., M.S.

*Associate Professor of Dentistry
(Oral Diagnosis) and Director
of Department of Oral
Diagnosis, University of
Michigan School of Dentistry,
Ann Arbor, Mich.*

With 246 illustrations

THE C. V. MOSBY COMPANY

Saint Louis   1965

Not until diagnosis becomes the foundation on which the whole structure of dentistry is built can it lay claim to be a learned profession or an important branch of the great art and science of healing.

—Leroy M. S. Miner
J.A.D.A., Jan., 1937

Preface to second edition

The gratifying acceptance of the first edition of *Oral Diagnosis* indicates that the field of oral diagnosis is rapidly being recognized as an important discipline in the teaching and practice of dentistry.

The preparation of this second edition has involved the hazard of incorporating material that might detract from the goal of presenting the basic principles of taking a history, examination procedures, and formulating a diagnosis. The challenge to incorporate more material on disease entities has resulted in many new illustrations. It is hoped that these additions will enhance the presentation of the subject matter.

The temptation to change the orderly presentation of the subject matter could not be justified on the basis of critical analysis. The general organization of the book follows the actual procedures expected in the evaluation of patients. For this reason it did not appear logical to subdivide chapters for the sake of brevity or to indulge in change merely for change's sake.

The temptation to include the details of disease usually found in textbooks of oral medicine and oral pathology was avoided because it is apparent that the details of oral diagnosis are sufficiently comprehensive to benefit its status as a separate subject. Efforts have been made to make this second edition as detailed and temporal as methods of publication permit while keeping in mind the needs of students and practitioners of dentistry.

Donald A. Kerr
Major M. Ash, Jr.
H. Dean Millard

Preface to first edition

The fundamentals of the interview, clinical examination, diagnosis, and the rationale for the employment of therapeutic measures have been described in curriculum outlines as Oral Diagnosis. In many courses and textbooks of oral diagnosis, descriptions of disease, radiographic methods, laboratory procedures, specific therapies, special examination methods, and the study of oral pathology and dental medicine have seriously encroached upon the teaching of the principles of obtaining a history, undertaking a physical examination, and formulating a diagnosis. The plan of this book is to avoid these distractions by presenting only the principles of oral diagnosis.

In many school clinics where each phase of dentistry is departmentalized, the teaching of the subject matter of oral diagnosis is limited to the material considered to be important to each department, thereby permitting the omission of the principles of diagnosis common to all phases of dentistry. The manner of presentation of the subject of oral diagnosis in this book will serve to illustrate those elements of diagnosis which should be covered in a formal course in oral diagnosis.

The old classic approach for presenting and teaching oral diagnosis, with the emphasis on specific diseases, is inadequate, for the dentist cannot be expected to recognize and treat diseases unless the basic mechanisms are understood. The dentist is faced not only with the problem of recognizing signs and symptoms of many diseases of the mouth and body, but also with the intelligent and skillful treatment of disease based on physical as well as biologic principles. The functional approach to the recognition and treatment of disorders of the mouth employs physiologic principles for the solution of these problems of disease. The student seeking only the diagnosis or name for a set of signs and symptoms rather than the nature of the disease may place too much emphasis on the terminology and subsequently be treating the diagnosis rather than the disease as it exists.

The chapter on radiographic interpretation has been written with the assumption that methods for taking and processing radiographs have been covered adequately elsewhere. Rather than detract from the principles of radiographic interpretation which have been presented here, detailed lists of all possible abnormalities usually but incorrectly found in a textbook of this nature have not been included. The principles presented are based on physiologic foundation; it is only from this base line that significant deviations from the range of normal can be understood in relation to the examination of a patient.

This is not a reference book of signs and symptoms of oral disease; the principles of oral diagnosis set forth provide the fundamentals for the selective use of reference material that may be found in textbooks of oral pathology, oral medicine, and radiography. The reference lists are not intended to be comprehensive; however, they do include papers and reviews which, in themselves, contain extensive references.

Interviewing a patient correctly is an art developed by experience; its principles are based on a mental discipline or outline that permits the examiner to cover a certain minimum field of information that may in itself call attention to the significant items in the patient's past history. This discipline of procedure may at the time facilitate the interview and establish rapport with the patient. Thus the establishment of a proper discipline of history taking can be considered fundamental to obtaining subjective information that will call attention to the departure of a patient from good health. The foundation needed for performing a physical examination is a knowledge of the normal physiologic and anatomic state of the body and its variations, the correct utilization of a procedure to adequately gather the particulars about a patient, and a knowledge of the relationship between the examination and the mechanisms of disease.

While this book is primarily concerned with the principles of diagnosis, it is also concerned with the actual procedures. Sufficient specific methods have been given in illustrating the principles to establish the necessary guideposts for the solution of practical problems. No rigid pattern of diagnostic procedure is suggested, since methods may vary from school clinic to dental office and from patient to patient, whereas the principles of oral diagnosis remain the same.

The procedures utilized by the student must be detailed and comprehensive in all cases to establish a discipline utilizing the principles of oral diagnosis. The practitioner who knows the fundamentals of oral diagnosis may, in many cases, reduce the details of the objective technics to a great degree and to a relative brevity without sacrificing the essentials necessary for a complete diagnosis. In a few cases where a more detailed evaluation of the patient is necessary than office time will allow, a complete case study may be made either after office hours or during a special appointment with the patient. One of the objectives of this book is to teach the principles of objective technics that may be used both in the dental school clinic and in the office of the practitioner.

Elaborate details of laboratory procedures and special studies of only occasional value have been omitted. There has been a tendency for the student and the practitioner to rely heavily upon knowledge gained from special laboratory and clinical procedures for the solution of clinical problems. It is not our purpose here to stress or deplore the use of these special examinations; rather it is to teach their limitations and their proper use in the practice of dentistry.

The concept of teaching principles of oral diagnosis as presented here is inductive rather than deductive in nature. In *deductive* instruction the student is taught many facts from which he is expected to single out the particular facts needed and then correctly apply them in order to deduce a diagnosis; in *inductive* instruction the student is taught to begin with the gathering of particular findings and to work toward an inductive conclusion. To repeat, it is not the objective here to teach oral diagnosis by elaborating on descriptions of disease in terms of physical signs or to teach technics of oral diagnosis by emphasizing technics for the discovery of physical signs; rather the objective is to teach the synthesis of both the technics of oral diagnosis and the mechanisms of disease to the end that the student will utilize inductive processes for the proper formulation of a diagnosis and treatment plan.

In order to carry out these principles of teaching, this textbook will follow the following outline: (1) presentation of the principles for the gathering of information about a patient; (2) relation of the information to the normal state of the body and to the mechanisms of disease; (3) presentation of the principles for the formulation of a diagnosis; and (4) utilization of the information gathered to make a treatment plan for the patient.

We want to express our sincere appreciation to those who, by their willing assistance, contributed a great deal to the preparation of this text: Mr. Edward Crandall, photographer at the School of Dentistry, who prepared our photographs; Miss Rose Grace Faucher, librarian at the School of Dentistry, who helped us obtain references; Dr. Gerald T. Charbeneau, Assistant Professor of Operative Dentistry, who aided in the preparation of operative charts; Miss Betty Sundbeck, secretary, who contributed many hours of secretarial assistance; Mr. Thomas Anderson, dental class of 1959, who prepared the line drawings; and Mr. Albert G. Richards, of the Radiography Department, who made radiographs available for our use.

Donald A. Kerr
Major M. Ash, Jr.
H. Dean Millard

Contents

CHAPTER 1

Introduction, 17

Scope of Oral Diagnosis, 17
Changing Scope of Dentistry, 19
Types of Examinations, 21
    Periodic Health-Maintenance Examination, 21
    Screening Examination, 26
    Emergency or Incomplete Examination, 33
Summary, 34
Significance of Questions in Health Questionnaire, 36

CHAPTER 2

Signs and symptoms, 48

Cardinal Manifestations of Disease, 50
    Pain, 51
    Headache, 56
    Weakness, 56
    Dyspnea, 57
    Other Cardiovascular Manifestations, 58
    Alteration of Weight, 59
    Lesions, 60

CHAPTER 3

Case history, 75

Approach to the Patient, 77
Plan of History Taking, 77
    Chief Complaint(s), Symptom(s), 79
    Present Illness, 83
    Past History, 84

Family History, 96
Personal and Social History, 96
Systems Review, 96

CHAPTER 4

Clinical examination—general, 113

Principles, 113
Clinical Examination of the Patient—General, 119
   General Survey, 119
   Head, 124
   Skin, 135
   Neck, 145
   Jaws, 156

CHAPTER 5

Clinical examination—oral, 159

Clinical Examination of the Mouth, 160
   General Appraisal, 160
   Lips, 163
   Labial and Buccal Mucosa, 171
   Palate, 185
   Oropharynx, 194
   Floor of the Mouth, 196
   Tongue, 200
   Gingiva, 211
   Teeth, 245
   Occlusion, 269
   Edentulous Mouth, 299
   Partially Edentulous Mouth, 306

CHAPTER 6

Radiographic examination, 313

Interpretation of Normal Radiographs, 314
   Normal Landmarks—Periapical Radiographs, 315
Method of Radiographic Examination, 320
Radiographs of the Complete Mouth, 320
   Lamina Dura—Continuity and Thickness, 320
   Periodontal Spaces—Variations in Width, 324
   Level of the Alveolar Crest in Relation to the Cementoenamel Junction, 325
   Periapical Radiolucency, 328
   Pathologic Conditions of the Teeth, 329
   Pathologic Conditions of the Jaws, 336
      Osseous Radiolucencies, 337
      Osseous Radiopacities, 343
      Combination of Osseous Radiolucency and Radiopacity, 346
   Other Dental Findings, 348
Posterior Bite-wing Radiographs, 350
   Lamina Dura Continuity, 350

Alveolar Crest Level, 350
Crown Shape and Formative Defects, 351
Pulp Size and Pulpal Calcification, 352
Existing Restorations, 352
Location of Calculus, 352
Location of Carious Lesions, 352
Supplemental Radiographs, 353
Special Radiographic Procedures, 356
Radiographs for Children, 356
Radiation Hazards, 356
Illustrative Case, 358
Comment, 361

CHAPTER 7

Supplementary examination aids, 363

Bacteriologic Studies, 366
Blood Studies, 370
Hematologic Diagnosis Associated With Anemia and Polycythemia, 371
Hematologic Diagnosis Associated With Bleeding, 372
Hematologic Diagnosis Associated With Infections, 375
Hematologic Diagnosis Associated With Lymph Node Enlargement, 376
Hematologic Diagnosis Associated With Leukemias, 376
Hematologic Diagnosis Associated With Chemotherapy, 377
Serologic Tests, 378
Urine Studies, 382
Contact Sensitivity Tests, 383
Biopsy, 383
Exfoliative Cytology, 389
Pulp Vitality Tests, 391
Study Casts, 403
Articulation of Casts, 403
Use of Surveyor, 411
Disclosing Solution, 412

CHAPTER 8

Diagnosis and treatment planning, 415

Diagnosis, 415
Collecting the Facts, 417
Analysis of the Facts, 418
Synthesis of Examination Facts and of Descriptive Features of Disease, 421
Making the Diagnosis, 422
Diagnosis of Neoplasms, 423
Prognosis, 425
Treatment Planning, 425
Rationale and Outline for a Treatment Plan, 425
Systemic Treatment, 426
Preparatory Treatment, 429
Corrective Treatment, 431
Periodic Recall Examinations and Maintenance Treatment, 431
Principles for Outlining a Treatment Plan, 432
Illustrative case, 436

ORAL DIAGNOSIS

CHAPTER 1

Introduction

Oral diagnosis as a subject consists of the fundamentals of the interview, principles and procedures of clinical examinations, methods of identifying oral disease, and the rationale for oral therapy. Oral diagnosis may also be defined as the identification of oral disease by interviewing, examining, and synthesizing the descriptive features of diseases and the facts obtained from the examination and interview. Finally, oral diagnosis is a systematic method of identifying oral disease.

SCOPE OF ORAL DIAGNOSIS

The basis for modern therapy is diagnosis. This concept of diagnosis presupposes that the disease be identified first and then eliminated. The procedure by which the information needed to make a diagnosis is obtained is directly related to the success of a diagnosis since the diagnosis itself is based on a favorable interview and examination of the patient.

Probably the most important concept that a student must learn, whether in school or out, is the importance of an efficient discipline for collecting the material necessary to make a diagnosis. It is sometimes thought by students and by some teachers that much of the information gathered about patients in a dental school clinic is unnecessary and far removed from the practical aspects of a dental office. At times a student is impressed by the apparent ability of a teacher or practitioner to arrive at a diagnosis rather quickly. Such a quick diagnosis does not necessarily represent snap judgment but reflects the examiner's ability to reduce the history to a minimum while at the same time covering the necessary field of inquiry and examination. A history that is brief but good represents the product of adequate training and practice in the subject of oral diagnosis; it does not represent any special innate ability of the clinician to "pull a diagnosis out of thin air." This is especially true in dealing with pain and soft tissue lesions in the oral region.

In addition to being able to reduce the detail of a history to a great degree, a "busy" general practitioner has very few new complete histories to take because much of the time is spent in caring for those individuals who have been his patients for years. In view of these considerations, objections to teaching a procedure which in itself may seem too detailed for practical application in a dental office appear to be unjustified.

Since most students can learn in school only a small part of what they need to know about diagnosis, and since much of what is learned is forgotten, it is necessary that they be taught a systematic approach to diagnosis that is simple enough to learn yet so rational as to be difficult to forget. It should supply the foundation that best fits the student not only to start practicing dentistry, but also to improve continually his diagnostic ability.

Only a few observations will lead to original descriptions of disease. However, in order to describe the wide variations in disease that exist and to apply facts and ideas to new situations, a practitioner must be able to grasp broad principles and use a method of thought and action that will enable him to meet such a variety of situations. The Hippocratic method of systematic observation and description is the foundation of oral diagnosis. Practice in observation and description is necessary even though the approach is logical and systematic. Sound reasoning is hard to attain, but training and practice in a rational discipline of thinking promote this faculty.

The first principle of oral diagnosis is to observe and describe deviations from normal. It is the accurate and pointed description that enables a student to utilize reference material to the greatest advantage. It is impossible for a student or general practitioner to recognize all the various diseases that exist; nor is it expected that searching through voluminous reference books for an identical picture of the clinical manifestation of a disease will improve anything but an ability to "thumb" through reference books. It is true that this form of diagnosis brings fair results in matching clinical and textbook pictures, but it can never lead to a system of diagnosis which is not dependent on trial and error. Further, the practitioner who is thoroughly trained in observation is apt to contribute to the scope of information already known about disease. Thus matching clinical with textbook pictures, either mentally or with the reference book at hand, is not a method of diagnosis to be desired. Not only does it consume valuable time, but all too often the patient's abnormality does not exactly match anything in the reference material because of the wide range of expression that any disease may present. This does not mean that reference books are not valuable in diagnosis; it does mean that they should be used efficiently and when necessary to substantiate a diagnosis. Thus the diagnostician should have a basic knowledge of disease and at least know where to look to verify his clinical impression of a disease without leafing through a reference book in hope of finding a "picture" that will "match" the one that presents the diagnostic problem.

The diagnostician must recognize that disease exists and must be able to describe it and to classify it within certain limits, viz., type of lesion, tissue involved, etiologic agent, or whether it represents a developmental disturbance. A diagnosis is not always apparent, but the acute observer pays attention to details and is systematic in his approach to the problem. "Spot" diagnoses that impress students usually are based on rapid, almost subconscious, but thorough observations. However, all too often an attempt is made to arrive at a diagnosis without first considering all the items which may have a bearing on the diagnosis. If the facts are first collected by a definite procedure, little will be left to doubt regarding the rationale of the diagnosis.

CHANGING SCOPE OF DENTISTRY

The study and practice of dentistry today must take into consideration not only changes in management of disease, but also changes in its prevention. The rise of more effective control of dental caries by fluoridation, diet, and therapeutic dentifrices presents a whole set of new problems for which the dentist is responsible. The dental practitioner is confronted with a changing set of demands upon his services and skill not only because of the changes in therapy, but also because of the increasing number of persons in the older age groups. Because of the remarkable control which has been established over acute and communicable diseases and the decrease in infant mortality, people are living to an older age.

While the main effort of the dentist today is directed toward the restoration of carious teeth, the changing scene of dental practice would indicate that the prevention and early detection of periodontal disease will play an important role in the future. Traditionally, people have come to the dentist with the complaint of a toothache; now it appears that in the near future the patient will come to the dentist for a periodic examination in the hope of preventing dental disease. With this change in pace the dentist is faced not only with the treatment of oral disease, but also with the examination of patients who are ostensibly well. This is especially true of children whose parents are concerned with their welfare and desire them to be examined at periodic intervals to be sure that all is progressing normally. If this trend continues, it is to be expected that this demand for periodic examination will be carried over into adult life. The changing pattern of dental care does not mean that the restoration of carious teeth will be a minor part of dental practice but means that in the future more time will have to be spent in the prevention of oral disease. In order to carry out the early detection of disease effectively, it will be necessary for the examiner not only to attend properly to signs when they first appear, but also to give repeated examinations before symptoms and signs develop. The dental practitioner who is geared to the changing scene must be interested in the health as well as the illnesses of his patients, and he must be adequately prepared in the technics of clinical examination. This means that he must develop not only his ability to carry out the technical aspects of restorative procedures, but also his acuity in the powers of observation.

The dental profession has done exceedingly well in educating the public about oral health, and this advice to the public has either implied or explicitly suggested that to consult one's dentist regularly will maintain his health and prevent disease. It is not by chance that industry and large universities are particularly demanding of preventive medicine and dentistry. These demands are not simply altruistic, since the prevention of disease pays off in terms of healthier workers, less loss of valuable personnel because of sickness, and less absenteeism. There can be no doubt that periodic examination of the mouth by the general practitioner who is prepared to thoroughly examine his patients will do much toward the prevention of disease. The accumulating body of information being gathered from surveys of ostensibly well people indicates that a high percentage of diseases are present which clearly could have been prevented.

There are several obstacles to the practice of preventive dentistry even though everyone knows that prevention of disease is a worthy aim. The changes in man brought about by his living to an older age and by changes in his environment have resulted in a relative increase in some diseases and a relative decrease in others. These changes usually occur faster than the dentist and his scientific collaborators can provide therapeutic measures to control them. Thus, while inroads are being made in the prevention of dental caries in children, a larger population is reaching the age at which disease of the supporting structure becomes paramount. The lapse of time before scientific knowledge can be widely and effectively applied is well known. For example, chlorination of drinking water was not effectively utilized for many generations after its discovery even though its effectiveness in the prevention of disease was known. There can be no question that fluoridation will be impeded by the same lack of interest on the part of the dental profession and the public.

Another obstacle to the practice of preventive dentistry is exemplified by the lack of interest in the periodic examination of the ostensibly well patient; the tendency of the majority of patients is to wait and pay only for delayed therapy. People are far more ready to pay for the treatment of oral disease than they are to pay for preventive services. Some of this enigma has developed because of the availability of relatively cheap over-the-counter medications, such as certain tooth pastes which are widely proclaimed in advertising media to prevent all kinds of oral disease. To the prospective patient this alternative appears to be far less unpleasant in terms of cost and time than making and keeping an appointment with a dentist.

Another obstacle to the practice of preventive dentistry lies in our formal dental education, in which little or no stress is laid upon the prevention of disease. This state of affairs may be aptly defined by paraphrasing Vines: the academic blunder of the divorce of preventive from clinical dentistry and its forced marriage to public health dentistry has lead to the subsequent relegation of the unhappy pair to the isolation of a faintly depressed specialism. For this mistake there is much to answer; through it, generations of dentists have been trained in the belief that preventive dentistry is inseparably linked with fluoridation, special city and county pedodontic clinics, and the supervision of campaigns to make dental health a national habit.

It is hoped that the present trend in dental education to institute courses in preventive medicine and oral diagnosis will do much to place these fields of endeavor into their proper perspective. The place of oral diagnosis in preventive dentistry can be readily appreciated since the prevention of disease is based upon a thorough examination of the ostensibly well patient. Thus the disciplines of an examination as taught in oral diagnosis must be directed not only to the examination and diagnosis of obvious disease, but also to an examination which will stress the normal development of children and the range of normal in the adult. With this concept in mind, it is to be expected that the dental practitioner will broaden his interest in the diagnosis and care of disease and encourage his patients in the maintenance of good health.

Many practitioners integrate an appreciable amount of preventive dentistry into their practice; however, many find it difficult to spend any time in the examination of the well patient for the prevention of disease since the benefits of this type of examination are usually much less prompt, less obvious, and less appreciated. Many individuals without obvious symptoms of disease benefit from a thorough examination because previously known but neglected conditions may be re-evaluated. It must be emphasized that the examination of the supposedly healthy mouth must be thorough and careful, since the early detection of disease demands that minute and inconspicuous deviations from the normal be carefully evaluated. There can be no doubt that there is a greater likelihood of a favorable eventual outcome from a disease when it is discovered in relatively early stages. This is true not only for neoplasms but also for dental caries, periodontal disease, malocclusion, and other abnormalities in the mouth and adjacent structures.

TYPES OF EXAMINATIONS

From a practical standpoint it appears that at least three types of examination procedures should be employed in a general practice: (1) a thorough and *complete* examination, utilizing all the skills of interviewing, physical examination, and supplementary diagnostic aids; (2) a *screening* type of examination, utilizing a dental modification of the Cornell Medical Index Health Questionnaire, a brief clinical examination of the teeth and supporting structures and mouth, and limited x-ray examination utilizing posterior bite-wing radiographs; and (3) the emergency or *limited* type of examination necessary for the diagnosis and management of acute and emergency conditions.

The latter two forms of examination represent a practical compromise with a more complete form of examination; however, they should be used only when indicated. From the standpoint of being indicated, the routine examination of the teeth with a pulp tester in those patients complaining of toothaches hardly seems less indicated than a bite-wing radiographic examination of the teeth when the patient complains of the same symptom. It is apparent that the findings which may be found in both forms of examination are sufficient to constitute an indication for their performance. While the complete testing of the teeth (by a pulp tester or by thermal tests) is considered to be a part of a more complete examination than a screening examination, this arbitrary assignment of examination procedures to a particular form of examination is not sufficient justification for the exclusion of one or the other, since both forms may be indicated in any particular instance. A thorough and complete examination should include all the commonly accepted diagnostic and examination procedures.

Periodic Health-Maintenance Examinations

A periodic health-maintenance examination must necessarily be initiated by a complete and thorough examination of the patient; the results are then used in subsequent examinations to measure what deviations might have occurred during the interval. When health-maintenance examinations are repeated on the same individuals after varying intervals of time, significant changes are likely to be encountered. Many factors such as age, sex, and initial examination findings influence the interval of time between examinations. While the ideal time interval between thorough examinations of supposedly healthy individuals free of disease would appear to be from six months to a year, it is apparent that certain individuals might be able to go as long as two years between thorough periodic health-maintenance examinations. In such instances the use of a screening type of examination in the interval between complete examinations should be considered. A thorough examination should include the following (see also Chapters 3 and 4 for details).

OUTLINE OF EXAMINATION

1. Case history
   Patient's chief complaint, present illness, past history, and systems review
2. Clinical examination
   (a) General appraisal of the patient
   (b) Detailed oral examination
   (c) Supplementary examinations and special tests when indicated
3. Diagnosis
   (a) Summary of the nature of the abnormality, its etiology and significance
   (b) Prognosis
4. Treatment plan
   (a) Ideal
   (b) Alternate

The extent of the screening examination will depend largely upon the yield of positive findings which may be expected from a particular examination procedure and its relationship to the cost of testing in terms of time, patience, and expense. The examination for acute and emergency conditions will depend upon the nature of the disease and whether or not the disease is local or systemic in origin. Obviously the localization, examination, and diagnosis of a toothache will utilize those examination procedures necessary to make a diagnosis in order that prompt therapeutic measures may be instituted. In certain instances it is conceivable that acute or emergency conditions may require an examination as thorough as any that can be devised. At other times a screening type of examination may be necessary to rule out contraindications for the particular type of therapy which is to be used in the treatment of patients with acute or emergency conditions. Thus while certain basic forms of examination procedures might be outlined for differing purposes, it must be recognized that from a practical standpoint the diagnosis of any disease, regardless of its nature, may require the most extensive form of examination. The vast majority of patients who have a thorough examination will be found to have some type of periodontal disease of which they are totally unaware. The high prevalence of incipient periodontal disease and incipient caries found during a health-maintenance examination alone justifies the performance of this type of examination.

An analysis of the complete dental examinations carried out at the University

Health Service of the University of Michigan as a part of the periodic health appraisal program of the faculty reveals that the yield for a complete examination is significantly high. As a part of a total health appraisal program, its value to the patient warrants the small amount of time required to carry it out. The findings from the history of those examined reflect its value (Table 1).

Table 1

History of rheumatic fever	8%
Sensitivity to drugs used in dental therapy	14%
Past history of significant systemic disease	12%
History of periodontal therapy	14%
History of necrotizing gingivitis	5%

The frequency of rheumatic fever, sensitivity to drugs, and systemic disorders such as hypertension and diabetes mellitus emphasizes the necessity of obtaining this information before beginning treatment.

The findings presented in Table 2 are of significance in view of the fact that 60 per cent of those examined visited their own dentist at periodic intervals of six months or one year, and 32 per cent visited their dentist regularly at greater than one-year intervals. Only a small percentage showed complete lack of oral health and dental care.

Table 2

Simple gingivitis	11%
Necrotizing gingivitis—acute, subacute, and recurrent	4%
Periodontitis—incipient	
Unknown to patient	7%
Periodontitis—moderate	
Known to patient	5%
Unknown to patient	14%
Periodontitis—advanced	
Known to patient	7%
Unknown to patient	5%
Dental caries (% of individuals having incipient to moderate carious lesions)	80%
Advanced dental caries	9%

The findings from radiographic examination of the teeth and periodontium show the need for complete mouth radiographs, as well as posterior bite-wings, periodically. The findings in 261 patients examined in a one-year period are given in Table 3.

These findings indicate that even patients who are obviously well cared for need periodic complete and thorough dental examinations. The prevalence of disease might well be expected to be considerably higher in a general population

Table 3

Nonvital teeth (not including those endodontically treated)	27
Periapical radiolucencies	36
Retained root tips	5
Impactions	11
Radicular cysts	3

group who are not so interested in oral health as the faculty members of a university. Thus a complete and thorough examination of a general population group should show even a greater yield of disease than the results of the survey given here.

It is obvious that the clinical examination and radiographic examination are probably responsible for the discovery of more asymptomatic phases of disease than is the case history. While the interview of the patient appears to be of relatively less value in preventive dentistry than in emergency and acute disease, the value of a history which is taken in the examination of ostensibly well people should not be underestimated, since the diagnosis of many important disorders depends upon the history obtained from the patient. This does suggest, however, that where circumstances do not permit extensive history taking by the dentist, the use of a questionnaire type of history to be completed by the patient should be used, provided the dentist elaborates on the positive and significant negative answers to the questions on the questionnaire. The type of questions and the number of questions included in a health questionnaire will depend upon the yield in a form of positive findings. In order that the questionnaire not be too extensive and filled with questions whose yield does not present statistically proved evidence of their value, only those questions which may be expected to effectively uncover the cardinal manifestations of the most common forms of disease should be used. The accompanying health questionnaire is utilized for the purpose of supplementing the case history. It is basically a systems review and is not intended to determine the patient's complaints nor describe his disease. It is a practical method of evaluating a patient's general health and serves to alert the examiner's attention to a departure from good health which may have a bearing on the presence and treatment of oral disease.

A health questionnaire should obtain certain vital statistics about the patient such as the name, age, height, weight, occupation, marital status, and the name of the patient's physician. Introductory statements should be made relative to how the questionnaire is to be answered, and some reassurance should be given on the questionnaire that the answers to the questions will be held confidential. It can be further stated that the questions contained in the questionnaire all have some direct or indirect bearing on the diagnosis of the patient's condition and may be significant in providing treatment for him comfortably and safely. The questions in a health questionnaire should be so stated that only the affirmative answers require further interview for the purpose of obtaining details. The significance of affirmative answers to the questions in the questionnaire may be found at the end of the chapter.

HEALTH QUESTIONNAIRE

Name _____ Sex _____ Age _____
Address _____
Telephone _____ Height _____ Weight _____
Date _____ Occupation _____ Marital status _____
Name of physician _____

Directions

If your answer is YES to the question asked, put a circle around "Yes."

If your answer is NO to the question asked, put a circle around "No."

Answer all questions. You may comment on answers which require explanation by writing in the space between questions.

Answers to the following questions are for our records only and will be considered confidential.

1. Do you think that your teeth are affecting your general health in any way?   Yes   No
2. Are you dissatisfied with the appearance of your teeth?   Yes   No
3. Are you worried about receiving dental treatment?   Yes   No
4. Do you have difficulty in chewing your food?   Yes   No
5. Are you being treated for any condition by a physician now?   Yes   No
6. Are you taking any medicines now?   Yes   No
7. Have you been examined by your physician within the last year?   Yes   No
8. Has there been any change in your general health in the last year?   Yes   No
9. Have you lost weight without dieting in recent months?   Yes   No
10. Have you ever been seriously ill?   Yes   No
11. Have you ever been hospitalized?   Yes   No
12. Have you ever had a major operation?   Yes   No
13. Have you ever had a blood transfusion?   Yes   No
14. Have you had any of the following diseases:
     Rheumatic fever   Yes   No   Tuberculosis   Yes   No
     Inflammatory rheumatism   Yes   No   Venereal disease   Yes   No
     Jaundice (yellow skin and   Heart attack   Yes   No
     eyes)   Yes   No   Stroke   Yes   No
     Diabetes (sugar disease)   Yes   No
     High blood pressure   Yes   No
15. Have you ever been told by a physician that you have a heart murmur?   Yes   No
16. Do you ever have asthma or hay fever? (Underline which one.)   Yes   No
17. Do you ever have hives or skin rash?   Yes   No
18. Have you ever experienced an unusual reaction to any of the following drugs:
     Aspirin   Yes   No   Sulfonamides (sulfa)   Yes   No
     Penicillin   Yes   No   Barbiturates (sleeping pills)   Yes   No
     Iodine   Yes   No   Other medicines   Yes   No
19. Have you ever experienced an unusual reaction to a dental anesthetic?   Yes   No
20. Do you bleed for a long time when you cut yourself?   Yes   No
21. Have you ever had any injury to your face or jaws?   Yes   No
22. Have you ever had surgery or x-ray treatment for a tumor, growth, or other condition in your mouth or on your lips?   Yes   No
23. Do you have frequent, severe headaches?   Yes   No
24. Do you have any complaints regarding your eyes?   Yes   No
25. Do you have any ear trouble?   Yes   No
26. Do you have frequent colds?   Yes   No
27. Do you have sinus trouble?   Yes   No
28. Do you have nosebleeds?   Yes   No
29. Do you have frequent sore throats?   Yes   No

Continued on next page.

30. Are you a mouth breather?	Yes	No
31. Do you have any sensitive teeth?	Yes	No
32. Have you had a toothache recently?	Yes	No
33. Do you have bleeding gums?	Yes	No
34. Do you have frequent canker sores or cold sores?	Yes	No
35. Have you ever had a severe sore mouth?	Yes	No
36. Is it difficult for you to open your mouth as wide as you would like?	Yes	No
37. Does your jaw click when you chew?	Yes	No
38. Do you have any chest pain on exertion?	Yes	No
39. Are you ever short of breath on mild exertion?	Yes	No
40. Do your ankles swell?	Yes	No
41. Do you have a persistent cough?	Yes	No
42. Do you ever cough blood?	Yes	No
43. Has your appetite changed recently?	Yes	No
44. Are there any foods you cannot eat?	Yes	No
45. Do you have any difficulty swallowing?	Yes	No
46. Do you have frequent indigestion?	Yes	No
47. Do you vomit frequently?	Yes	No
48. Do you have kidney trouble?	Yes	No
49. Do you urinate more than six times a day?	Yes	No
50. Are you thirsty much of the time?	Yes	No
51. Have you ever had painful and swollen joints?	Yes	No
52. Do you have any numb or prickling areas on your skin?	Yes	No
53. Do you ever have fits or convulsions?	Yes	No
54. Do you have a tendency to faint?	Yes	No
55. Do you bruise easily?	Yes	No
56. Do you have any blood disorder such as anemia (thin blood)?	Yes	No
57. Does hot weather bother you more than it does other people you know?	Yes	No
58. Are you excessively nervous?	Yes	No
59. Do you get tired easily?	Yes	No
60. (Women) Are you pregnant at the present time?	Yes	No

Patient's signature _____

Screening Examination

A screening examination is one which attempts to compromise between a thorough and complete examination and a less extensive examination because of the practical aspects of reduced time, costs, and skill involved in a shorter type of examination. The degree of compromise of course depends upon the decrease in potential yield in the form of positive findings that the examiner wishes to allow. While the yield from a screening type of examination and a more thorough complete type of examination may be the same in some instances, both the dentist and physician should be aware of their potential difference. Obviously the yield of certain forms of screening examinations directed toward a particular lesion or disease may compare favorably with that of a more extensive examination, since the procedures used may be the same. For example, the use of posterior bite-wing radiographs for the detection of carious lesions is used both in the complete examination and the screening examination. The posterior bite-wing radiographic examination may be expected to yield about 75 per cent or more of the carious lesions present; however, a more complete examination utilizing periapical radiographs and a sharp explorer and mouth mirror may raise the yield to 100 per cent. Thus the yield from bite-wing radiographs compares somewhat favorably with the extensive form of examination in yield of carious lesions. It must be remembered that other lesions of the supporting structures and of the apices of the teeth may show additional disease that would not be indicated by posterior bite-wing radiographs. Thus the examiner must take into consideration those factors for which he is screening, the efficiency of the screening procedure, and the scope of the screening process. The scope of the screening examination must necessarily be determined by the examiner with regard to time available, number of patients to be screened, purpose of the screening, facilities available, economic considerations, skill of the examiner, and desires of the patient. The following screening examination outline is presented as one form of this type of examination which might be used routinely to yield a fairly high percentage of potential positive findings either in the office of a general practitioner or a dental clinic.

OUTLINE OF A SCREENING EXAMINATION

1. Chief complaint—an ostensibly well patient may or may not have a significant complaint, but the chance to express one should be given
2. Health questionnaire
3. Posterior bite-wing radiographs
4. Gross appraisal for decay, missing and filled teeth
5. General appraisal of the gingiva for alteration of color and form
6. Gross appraisal of the soft tissues for the presence of lesions
7. Brief appraisal of oral hygiene
8. Brief appraisal of occlusion

This form of general screening examination may be expected to yield a significant amount of disease in unselected patients and will provide a certain degree of coverage in a health-maintenance examination. As has been previously stated, this form of examination may well be utilized to bridge the gap between more extensive and thorough examinations and thus is more successfully used as an adjunct to an initial thorough periodic health-maintenance examination. This form of examination may also be used as a precursor to a more thorough examination. In fact, it may well serve to point out the necessity for a more thorough examination. Probably the minimum type of screening examination includes posterior bite-wing radiographs and a series of questions to reveal whether or not a patient has or has had some type of disease which contraindicates a proposed dental treatment. Such questions as "Are you now under the care of a physicians?" "Have you ever had rheumatic fever?" "Do you have difficulty with bleeding?" and "Are you sensitive to any drug such as penicillin, iodine, etc.?" are representative of the type which may be used. More often than not a brief type of screening examination is carried out by a simple study of posterior bite-wing radiographs. Further examination is solely for the purpose of confirming clinically the presence of carious lesions which are manifest in the radiographs. It is evident that there is as much variation in the contents of a screening examination as there is in a more thorough and complete type of examination. Irrespective of the type of examination used, there can be no doubt that the more detailed the examination, the greater will be the yield of positive findings from the performance of the examination. Generally the omission of any portion of the thorough examination in favor of a screening examination will compromise any examiner's effectiveness, but the adverse effect on the yield of the examination is necessarily dependent upon the scope and demand on the examination. In respect to the shorter screening type of examination, the following general rules should apply: *No patient should be given a short or screening type of examination unless there is an awareness of its limitations.* Awareness includes both that of the examiner and the patient. When patients are told of having chronic destructive periodontal disease which has been present for many years, they will complain, all too often, of having had many examinations in the past without being told of this condition. This dilemma can be avoided by a thorough examination of the mouth, including an analysis of the supporting structures of the teeth, and by telling the patient of potential and existing disease. The responsibility of the examiner lies not only in the discovery of carious lesions which he may expect and treat, but also in the discovery of any latent or other disease in the mouth requiring treatment or referral; this is what a patient should receive when coming to a dentist for an examination. When anything less than a thorough examination has been made, the patient should be told. There is a place for a screening type of examination in the general practitioner's office, but it is not meant to exclude or take the place of a more thorough and complete examination of the mouth as it relates to the rest of the body. As previously mentioned, a screening type of examination may be used.

USE OF SCREENING EXAMINATION

1. To indicate gross disease in broad surveys
2. To indicate the necessity for a complete and thorough examination where screening of ostensibly well patients is being undertaken
3. To allow practical extension of the interval of time between thorough periodic health-maintenance examinations
4. To take the place of a thorough type of examination when time, cost, and skill prevent its use

Role of the Hygienist in "Screening".—A health history may be defined as the answers to a few questions concerning a patient's dental and systemic health or a detailed account of all the data that may have a bearing on the present health of the patient. Utilizing the first definition and the principles of a screening examination, the hygienist may be effective in a screening procedure. A brief health history obtained by the hygienist may be instrumental in instituting precautionary measures for the good of the patient and the hygienist.

It is realized that the hygienist does not have the legal obligation of the dentist, nor is she trained to diagnose diseases of the mouth; however, it is reasonable to assume that by obtaining a brief history she may cover a certain minimum field of information that may in itself point out that disease exists. It will also allow her to make a more efficient referral to the dentist for consultation.

In those instances in which a patient is being seen for periodic prophylaxis by the hygienist, it is apparent that referral to the original history will facilitate care of the patient; however, it must not be overlooked that changes in the patient's health, both systemic and oral, may occur. The hygienist should be alert to these possibilities and call them to the attention of the dentist. An interim history to cover those contingencies should be considered as a routine part of the patient's care.

Whenever a patient is being given a prophylaxis for the first time by the hygienist to facilitate later examination by the dentist, it is imperative that the hygienist be alert not only for the signs of disease, but also for significant items of the patient's history that may have a bearing upon the treatment which is to be rendered.

The questionnaire below may be used by the dentist for patients requiring emergency treatment and by hygienists under the supervision of a dentist for patients requiring dental prophylaxis. The questions may be asked verbally by the hygienist before treatment or be answered by the patient on a self-examination questionnaire while in the waiting room. In either event, the questions and answers should be made a part of the patient's permanent record. A more detailed questionnaire is not necessary since the question about the patient being under a physician's care should reveal those patients having such diseases as diabetes, epilepsy, blood dyscrasias, and chronic infectious diseases.

HEALTH QUESTIONNAIRE

Name _____ Sex _____ Age _____
Address _____
Telephone _____ Height _____ Weight _____
Date _____ Occupation _____

Directions

If your answer is YES to the question asked, put a circle around "Yes."
If your answer is NO to the question asked, put a circle around "No."

1. Are you under a physician's care now?   Yes   No
2. Do you bleed for a long time when you have cut yourself?   Yes   No
3. Have you ever had rheumatic fever, inflammatory rheumatism, or growing pains?   Yes   No
4. Have you ever been told by a physician that you have a heart murmur?   Yes   No
5. Have you ever experienced an unusual reaction to iodine or other drugs?   Yes   No
6. Do you have a condition in your mouth which is causing you pain or discomfort?   Yes   No
7. Is there additional information about your general health which should be known?   Yes   No

The general health of a patient is of significance to the hygienist and to the dentist under whose supervision she is working. Many times ill health may directly affect the tissues of the mouth or the ability and inclination of a patient to carry out home-care instructions. It is not suggested that the hygienist obtain an extensive history of the patient's general health. If the patient's interim health history is not up to date or the patient is being seen for the first time, screening questions should be asked about the patient being under the care of a physician at the present time and about having a history of recent serious illness. It is assumed that the hygienist will make use of any history that the dentist has previously taken and will inform him of any interim changes that she believes may be present either as the result of answers to the screening questions or because of changes that she has observed.

The fact that a patient may be under a physician's care is of extreme importance. An affirmative answer to the question as to whether or not a patient is under the care of a physician may imply treatment of many diseases. Such diseases as epilepsy, diabetes mellitus, cardiac disease, and blood dyscrasias are of such a nature that treatment should not be instituted without the dentist first having evaluated the patient. It is not necessary that a disease express itself in the oral cavity by *signs* that can be observed by the hygienist. It is therefore very important that a health history be accomplished for screening purposes before treatment begins to uncover any *symptoms* of disease that may exist.

While blood dyscrasias are rare diseases, they are of considerable importance because patients with such disorders occasionally come to a dental office for the treatment of gingival enlargement and bleeding. Since many patients present with gingival enlargement and bleeding, it is obvious that simple screening questions will not aid in detecting the patients with blood dyscrasias. However, many times these patients are aware of a blood disorder but are not aware of the serious consequences that may result from a prophylaxis. It is this group of individuals that can be screened by the use of a brief health history that includes a question related to the presence of a blood disorder. A positive history of a blood dyscrasia warrants a consultation with the dentist. The presence of gingival enlargement, ulcerative lesions, and gingival bleeding requires that the patient be evaluated by the dentist.

Hemophilia is a hereditary disease which is manifested clinically in the male. Small lacerations such as may be caused by scaling may result in the death of a patient with this disease. Fortunately most patients with hemophilia are aware of the disease and the serious consequences of small cuts. Occasionally a patient may presume that a hygienist knows that he has the disease; the use of the question relating to blood disorders and bleeding should prevent unfortunate accidents from scaling procedures.

Prevention of subacute bacterial endocarditis is of prime importance. It should be emphasized that preventive measures prior to the scaling procedure should be considered whenever a history of rheumatic fever, heart murmur, or congenital heart disease is found. Further, no scaling procedures should be started before the patient is asked if he has had rheumatic fever, a heart murmur, or congenital heart disease. Thus, before a hygienist commences treatment, she should avail herself of a history taken previously by the dentist or simply ask the patient about these conditions. If there is an affirmative answer or if there is any question about the answer, the dentist should be consulted so preventive measures may be taken. In some instances the patient may have to be referred by the dentist to a physician for evaluation. The hygienist working in close cooperation with the dentist has the opportunity possibly to save lives that otherwise might be jeopardized by subacute bacterial endocarditis following scaling procedures.

"Drugs" as used in the questionnaire refers to those therapeutic substances used by the hygienist as cleansing compounds, obtunding agents, and bacteriostatic preparations—in short, any substance used by the hygienist to facilitate prophylaxis and promote healing following dental prophylaxis.

"Unusual reaction" as used in the questionnaire means an altered reactivity of the tissues to a foreign substance as a result of previous contact with it. It is well known that some persons develop symptoms from contact with substances which are quite harmless to most individuals. These reactions differ from the usual toxic effects of the drugs.

The skin or mucous membrane may become sensitized by contact with a particular agent which in itself is not usually harmful. Repeated contact with such a substance leads to the development of lesions usually characterized by erythema and vesiculation. Almost everyone is familiar with dermatitis that may result from mascara, material used in dress shields, fur dyes, shoe dyes, and repeated contact with certain detergents. Less familiar are those reactions caused by repeated contact with drugs used in the mouth. Since the drugs used by the hygienist are limited in number, the probability of a sensitivity reaction occuring is not great. However, an alertness to the possibility of its occurrence will be a factor in preventing an unfavorable reaction from the drugs that are used. Thus the responsibility of the hygienist is to prevent possible hypersensitive reactions from drugs she may use by determining in advance whether or not a patient is sensitive or allergic to any of the drugs she expects to use. When lesions are already present, possibly due to drug hypersensitivity, it is the responsibility of the dentist to make the diagnosis. Recognition of a wide variety of drug reactions demands considerable experience and training in history taking and diagnostic procedures which often fall into the province of a competent allergist.

The mechanism by which these sensitizing reactions occur is not well understood, but it is generally believed that many are the result of immune reactions. Immune reactions are those produced by the interaction of an allergen, a foreign substance, with an immune body produced by the body in response to the foreign substance.

Practically any chemically active substance that is soluble in water or lipids can penetrate the epidermis or mucous membrane and occasionally cause sensitization. Other reactions due to unusual susceptibility to known toxic or pharmacologic actions of the drugs or to mechanical effects are not dependent upon an antibody mechanism.

Drugs used by the hygienist which may give rise to allergic or hypersensitive reactions are tooth pastes, volatile oils, tannic acid, aspirin, and iodine.

Iodine as used in iodine lotion or in some disclosing solutions is one of the drugs most frequently used by hygienists. Reactions to iodine may result from contact with the mucous membrane or its ingestion in small amounts in sensitized individuals. Since this drug has been in wide use, most individuals who are sensitive to it are aware of the untoward reactions resulting from its use. Therefore a hygienist need only ask the patient about this possibility before using iodine in any form. In some instances a very small amount applied locally or ingested at the time of topical application may produce severe local and/or systemic reactions.

When tooth paste, oil of wintergreen, and iodine are used in polishing compounds, it is possible that an individual may be sensitive to any of the ingredients. Thus before using polishing compounds it may be well to inquire into the possibility of each ingredient causing a sensitivity reaction. In general, a rather broad question may serve to screen against the possibility of a sensitivity reaction to any drug. For example, patients may be asked if they are allergic or sensitive to *any* drugs. If further details seem necessary, specific reference to a particular drug like iodine may be made.

Of primary concern to a patient are conditions in the mouth that cause pain or discomfort. To proceed with a prophylaxis when the patient has symptoms and possibly signs of disease in the mouth is overlooking the basic principles of a health service. A question to the patient concerning any pain or discomfort in the mouth not only tells the patient that his welfare is considered, but also may call attention to the presence of disease in the mouth that would have gone unnoticed.

A health history as utilized by the hygienist is of value in the ways listed below.

VALUE OF HYGIENIST'S EXAMINATION

1. Serves to discover complaints about the oral structures that might otherwise go unnoticed
2. Calls attention to the patient's general health, which may have a direct relationship to dental procedures
3. Facilitates the recognition of disease such as rheumatic fever which may predispose to subacute bacterial endocarditis following dental procedures, including scaling of the teeth
4. Indicates when prophylactic or precautionary measures are necessary for the safeguard of the patient and the hygienist
5. Establishes a sound basis for referral of an abnormal condition to the dentist
6. Serves to discover any unusual reactions that the patient may have to drugs

These considerations are all related to the health of the patient and are directly concerned with prophylaxis. The utilization of subjective information within certain limits by the hygienist is to be encouraged. All objective information (signs of disease) obtained by the hygienist should be augmented by subjective information (symptoms of disease) for a better understanding of disease. An understanding of disease permits the hygienist to refer the patient to the dentist for evaluation, diagnosis, and treatment.

The dentist is dependent upon the hygienist for assistance in maintaining the oral health of his patients. In many instances the hygienists may be considered to play an integral part in the detection of disease. By the use of a health history and through the use of her ability to observe abnormalities, the hygienist can render a valuable service not only in the maintenance of oral hygiene, but also in the screening and referral of patients who may need services outside those rendered by the hygienist. This concept of the use of a health history and the hygienist's part in the rendering of a health service does not imply that the hygienist have an extensive knowledge for the purpose of diagnosis. It only suggests that she can fulfill her obligation to the dentist and the patient by an efficient method of recognizing the presence of disease. This serves to extend the scope of oral diagnosis by utilization of qualified assistants within their proper limits.

The yield of information presented in Table 4 is the result of the evaluation of 500 consecutive health questionnaires. The questionnaire (sample of which is given on p. 29) was given to each patient in the Dental Hygiene Clinic at The University of Michigan by a student hygienist and was evaluated by a dentist for "yes" answers before prophylaxis was commenced.

Table 4. *Distribution of affirmative answers to hygienist's questionnaire*

Question 1	12.0%
Question 2	1 0%
Question 3	6.0%
Question 4	5.0%
Question 5	0.5%
Question 6	8.0%
Question 7	4.0%

The reasons for positive answers to Question 1 include pregnancy, diabetes, arthritis, thyroid disease, kidney disease, coronary disease, jaundice, and others. The "yes" answers to Question 7 include such reasons as pregnancy, heart disease, asthma, diabetes mellitus, arthritis, and others. Of special significance to the dentist is the number of "yes" answers to Question 6 concerning any condition in the mouth causing pain or discomfort. Complaints include cavities, calculus, toothache, third molars (pericoronitis), sore mouth (herpetic stomatitis and necrotizing gingivitis), focal hyperkeratosis, bleeding gums, periodontal abscesses, receding gums, and sharp edges of teeth. It is obvious that the dental hygienist is in no position to evaluate contraindications for therapy as a result of an affirmative answer to any of the questions. The use of such a questionnaire serves to orient the dentist to the necessity for premedication or special therapy and allows the patient to inform the dentist of complaints which might be overlooked.

Emergency or Incomplete Examination

An emergency type of examination is limited to those procedures which obviously appear related to the complaint of the patient. The history and examination of the complaint are initially sharply limited to the signs and symptoms of the disease and its causative agent. In certain instances the problem may be broad enough in scope to tax the ingenuity of the examiner and demand all his diagnostic acumen.

The simplest form of emergency examination may consist only of having the patient open the mouth and the examiner observing the disease, e.g., a fractured tooth. The history will consist solely of the time of occurrence, the manner in which the accident occurred, the presence or absence of associated signs and symptoms, and the presence or absence of systemic disease of immediate importance to therapy. The clinical examination would consist of an inspection of the fracture to determine involvement of the pulp and testing of the pulp to determine its vitality. The radiographic examination would include periapical radiographs to determine the possibility of root fracture, bone fracture, and apical involvement.

This type of examination is minimal and for obvious reasons cannot be utilized for a screening or periodic health examination. For expediency the emphasis is placed upon the evaluation of acute and known complaints and their relief. In those instances in which the diagnosis may not be easily obtained, this type of examination may well serve to provide the examiner with sufficient information to institute treatment of the symptoms. Once again it should be pointed out that this type of examination does not take the place of a more thorough examination, and the relief of a symptom itself, without due regard for the determination of the cause and its eradication, cannot be considered as a logical approach to therapy. This does not mean that the relief of symptoms does not have a place in the practice of dentistry. All too often the location of the offending tooth causing severe pain cannot be immediately determined and the treatment of the symptoms becomes of primary concern to the dentist. In the emergency type of examination the dentist has no routine or set pattern of procedures; the circumstances that exist will determine the trend of the examination. The success of the emergency examination is directly related to the ability of the examiner to effectively utilize the basic principles of oral diagnosis (interviewing, clinical examination, and formulation of a diagnosis).

SUMMARY

It is not our intent to list all the possible diseases and their cardinal manifestations. The objectives of this book are to (1) present an outline for the systematic collection of subjective information alluding to the cardinal manifestations of disease; (2) give the actual procedure for determining the presence of cardinal manifestations of disease; (3) show by illustrative cases how to make a differential diagnosis; and (4) show how a clinical history, examination, and diagnosis are utilized in the practice of dentistry. The pertinent content of preclinical sciences will be integrated with clinical dentistry. No attempt will be made to incorporate all of the physiologic bases for disorders of structure and psychology since such material can be found elsewhere.

When cardinal manifestations of disease exist in a patient, the dentist should be aware of their basic mechanisms for the purpose of establishing a basis for initiating further diagnostic and therapeutic procedures. While taking the clinical history, the examiner may find that a patient has one of the cardinal manifestations of disease such as pain. Before appropriate measures for its relief can be instituted it is necessary that he be aware of the physiologic basis for pain and know its causes. For example, he may know that certain manifestations of pain may be related to angina of effort, but he may not know that this condition is due to arteriosclerosis which in some manner sensitizes the coronary arteries to the effects of increased demands on the heart and reacts by spasms of the coronary arteries at a time when increased myocardial circulation is required. A spasm of the coronary artery produces myocardial hypoxia, which causes the pain. The examiner will have established that the precipitating cause of the pain is effort and in a general way is related to heart disease. However, he can in no way establish a rational basis for treatment unless he is aware that the basic cause of the pain is arteriosclerosis and that the functional cause is a spasm of the coronary arteries. In this particular instance the basic cause of the pain is not treatable; however, in other instances the cause of pain may be of primary consideration. In this and in some other cases, pain must be treated by removal of the precipitating cause or by treatment of the functional cause of the disease.

Another example where the concept involved in the proper evaluation and treatment of disease may be readily appreciated concerns the diagnosis of pain associated with dysfunction of the temporomandibular joint. The examiner may determine from the clinical history that the patient is in distress when functional movements of the temporomandibular joint are made. If he is unaware of the underlying basic pathologic disturbances responsible for the production of pain in the region of the joint, he may be satisfied to treat only the symptom or the precipitating cause of the symptom. In this case the precipitating cause would be the movement of the jaw. Thus his treatment might be directed toward palliation of pain by injection of hydrocortisone or sclerosing solution into the joint or even by surgical removal of the disc. Or he may attempt to treat the precipitating cause by complete immobilization of the mandible by wiring or by reducing the function of the mandible by Hawley retainers or splints. Such treatment implies a lack of knowledge of the functional ultimate cause of the pain—occlusal trauma. This does not imply that all pain associated with the temporomandibular joint has its origin in occlusal trauma. Though this is probably the most frequent cause of pain in the temporomandibular joint, other conditions may also produce pain in this area. These will be discussed in more detail elsewhere.

The practical approach to oral diagnosis requires that the diagnostician utilize a systematic method for determining the subjective manifestations of disease. This is best initiated by the proper taking of a case history. The facts gathered in a case history should orient the examiner's thinking to the basic mechanisms responsible for the symptoms which have been elicited in the case history, and this orientation should direct the examiner to certain areas of emphasis in the general appraisal of the patient. This step-by-step discipline will expedite the examination and serve to gain the patient's confidence. The use of such a procedure allows the complete evaluation of all the possible ramifications that disease may present. Even when the procedure is reduced to a minimum for the simplest and most obvious cases, it will assure the examiner that he has not overlooked some significant and latent aspect of the patient's complaint.

This book provides a method of approach to the diagnosis of disease. In presenting a systematized discipline, certain premises must be adhered to. It will be noted that, aside from any illustrative cases presented to show the procedures for arriving at a diagnosis, many of the photographs depict the normal and deviations within the range of normal. This is done for two reasons: (1) an appreciation for the normal is necessary before abnormal states can be detected and (2) the illustration for the procedures of a clinical examination will not be subject to distraction by emphasis on pathologic states.

A section of illustrative cases is presented to bring out those analytic processes which are necessary for the final diagnosis of abnormal conditions. In general, those cases involving the most common diagnostic problems are presented. Inasmuch as this is not a textbook of dental medicine or oral pathology, no claim to complete coverage of all the diseases or their descriptions is made. The systematic procedure for making a diagnosis which is presented herein will serve to make more efficient the use of descriptions of disease that may be obtained in textbooks and other reference material on dental medicine and oral pathology. Stated simply, the objective of this book is to answer the question of how a diagnosis is made. It is assumed that the reader has already acquired the fundamentals of the basic sciences and has had some training in the clinical sciences.

SIGNIFICANCE OF QUESTIONS IN HEALTH QUESTIONNAIRE

Below are the same questions which are found in the sample questionnaire on page 25 with the significance of each question stated briefly. More detailed information relating to each of the subjects will be found in Chapter 3, *Case History*.

1. **Do you think that your teeth are affecting your general health in any way?** This question establishes the relationship between general and oral health. Also, it tends to bring to light any notions that the patient may have that the condition of his mouth is influencing another health problem of a more generalized nature, such as rheumatism or indigestion.

2. **Are you dissatisfied with the appearance of your teeth?** Often esthetic considerations are paramount in the patient's mind. This question gives him an opportunity to express his concern about the appearance of his teeth.

3. **Are you worried about receiving dental treatment?** This question provides the patient with an opportunity to admit that he is apprehensive about receiving dental treatment. It also gives the dentist an opportunity to identify individuals who require sedation prior to a dental appointment.

4. **Do you have difficulty in chewing your food?** The patient's appraisal of the functional status of his mouth may be evaluated here. Quite frequently the patient is able to point to a specific situation which has reduced his functional effectiveness.

5. **Are you being treated for any condition by a physician now?** The influence of medical treatment on the practice of dentistry is significant from the standpoint of the diagnosis of the condition for which the patient is under treatment and because of the reactions and side effects produced by the many new drugs that are continually being introduced into the practice of medicine. It is imperative that the dentist have a fundamental knowledge of systemic illnesses and of some of the methods of treatment which are employed currently in medical practice, particularly those that involve treatment with drugs. The influence of certain dental procedures on patients who have systemic illnesses is well established, and the hazards that are encountered in connection with some of the drugs being employed in medical treatment are well known. If the patient is unaware of his systemic condition but is aware that he is receiving a form of medical

treatment, a written statement from his physician is appropriate prior to instituting dental treatment.

6. **Are you taking any medicines now?** This question is closely related to the previous question and is intended to determine specifically what drugs a patient is taking. If the patient does not know the name of the drug, it is possible to identify the drug either by calling the physician or the pharmacist or by referring to the proper publication which illustrates most of the drugs according to the manufacturer's identification.

7. **Have you been examined by your physician within the last year?** Individuals who have been examined within the past year should be questioned about the reason for seeking medical examination. If the patient is in the habit of receiving annual examinations, it provides an opportunity to establish on the dental record that the patient is in good general health, or it provides an opportunity to bring to light important findings from the medical examination.

8. **Has there been any change in your general health in the last year?** An affirmative answer to this question may indicate an improvement in general health or the onset of a significant illness. In either event, it is of interest, if not always of importance, to the dentist to be aware of the general condition of his patient. Many times a patient will give a subjective appraisal of his general health in answering this question affirmatively and will not base the affirmative answer on a professional diagnosis. In such cases, it is advisable to recommend a physical examination by a physician rather than to give advice to a patient relative to his general health.

9. **Have you lost weight without dieting in recent months?** There are numerous illnesses that are accompanied by weight loss, particularly in their more advanced stages. Characteristically, diabetes is accompanied by weight loss if the disease goes undetected. In the case of diabetes, the affirmative answers to Questions 9 and 50 would be of significance. Other illnesses which are accompanied by a weight loss are tuberculosis, cancer, and the blood dyscrasias. Unexplained rapid weight loss of ten pounds or more should always be investigated.

10. **Have you ever been seriously ill?** It is difficult to define the term "seriously ill" used in this question, but it may be explained as referring to an illness which has required hospitalization for more than one week or which has been life-threatening. In any event, the purpose of this question is to point to illnesses in the individual's past history which are indicative of permanent impairment of health. Impairment of health may require that special precautions be taken during dental treatment. In some instances, the illnesses described by a patient as serious may be recurrent or chronic in nature.

11. **Have you ever been hospitalized?** The responses of an affirmative nature to this question commonly will be the result of tonsillectomy, adenoidectomy, and childbirth. The question is asked to determine the possible history of an illness which may be defined as serious, resulting in hospitalization of the patient. When the question is answered affirmatively, it is necessary to inquire further as to the cause and length of time of hospitalization and whether or not there was any important event, such as serious reaction to a drug, that took place during the hospitalization.

12. **Have you ever had a major operation?** The purpose of this question is not to have the patient enumerate his scars and their history. If answered affirmatively, this question should be followed by questions on what procedure was carried out, whether local or general anesthesia was used, how well the procedure was tolerated, whether or not healing was uneventful and, if not, what complications occurred, and if any drug allergies or idiosyncrasies were encountered. It may be significant to know that an individual has had a major operation for a malignant neoplasm prior to planning treatment.

13. **Have you ever had a blood transfusion?** Most blood transfusions are given as part of supportive care during major surgery; however, an affirmative answer to this question may uncover repeated blood transfusions which are being received in the treatment of a blood dyscrasia.

14. **Have you had any of the following diseases?**

Rheumatic fever: The importance of a history of rheumatic fever or rheumatic heart disease is well known. The special precautions that must be taken are clearly indicated whenever dental procedures which produce bleeding are to be carried out. This is especially true of the extraction of teeth and scaling of teeth. The dental profession may not have a true appreciation of the hazard of subacute bacterial endocarditis, because in most instances the disease does not develop for two or more weeks following the production of a bacteremia. The connection between subacute bacterial endocarditis and a dental procedure may be quite remote and yet quite significant.

Inflammatory rheumatism: Inflammatory rheumatism is a term which was used for a number of years to indicate rheumatic fever. Today it may be interpreted by patients as indicating rheumatoid arthritis or even what the layman refers to as rheumatism.

Jaundice (yellow skin and eyes): The significance of a history of jaundice is twofold, particularly when the disease causing jaundice is recent. If jaundice is precipitated by hepatocellular disease or cirrhosis, it is particularly significant to the dentist because of the possibility of reduced prothrombin production, with a resultant hemorrhagic tendency.

When a history of viral hepatitis is given, the dentist should protect himself from encountering the blood of his patient directly, since the disease may be transmitted through infected blood. Special precaution must be taken against transmission of the disease by improperly sterilized syringes or other instruments.

Diabetes (sugar disease): Diabetes is classified as adult and juvenile. The blood sugar level tends to be better controlled in patients in the adult diabetic group than in juvenile diabetic patients, in whom the level shows tendencies for fluctuation to the point that insulin shock is not an infrequent occurrence. In general, diabetic patients are more susceptible to infection than nondiabetic patients. In addition, infection has a great influence on the insulin requirements of the diabetic individual. It is entirely possible for a diabetic patient to slip into diabetic coma while receiving daily doses of insulin if he has an infection. Another consideration in diabetes is the timing of the dental appointment. It is advisable to take diabetic patients soon after a meal, unless, of course, use of a general anesthetic is anticipated. The timing of dental appointments shortly after meals tends to avoid the possibility of insulin shock. It is advisable to have a source of sugar on hand, since most diabetic patients can feel the onset of insulin shock and may have time to receive sugar by mouth to elevate the blood sugar level and prevent insulin shock.

High blood pressure: High blood pressure is an important consideration in dentistry, particularly in the use of vasoconstrictors. In general, it is believed that vasoconstrictors in the quantity contained in dental anesthetics are of no great significance in individuals with hypertension. On the other hand, the apprehension that the individual is subjected to prior to a dental appointment and during dental procedures may be of great significance. It has been shown that proper sedation for individuals with hypertension prior to stressful dental procedures reduces greatly the degree of increase in blood pressure related to apprehension.

Tuberculosis: If a patient gives a history of tuberculosis, he should also give a history of receiving a checkup every six months. If this is not the case, the dentist is justified in deferring treatment of the patient until it has been verified by x-ray films and by other means that his disease is inactive.

Venereal disease: A history of venereal disease is probably more easily obtained on a questionnaire than by interview and may be of significance in some instances in which clinical findings suggest a possibility either of gonococcal temporomandibular joint arthritis or lesions of secondary or tertiary syphilis in the oral cavity. Whenever a history of venereal disease is obtained, the possibility of reinfection should be considered even though medical treatment has been received for the disease at one time or another.

Heart attack: Heart attacks today are commonly treated by the use of anticoagulant drugs. The drugs which are taken by mouth reduce the production of prothrombin. The prothrombin level is usually controlled by monthly determinations of prothrombin time. It is important to know whether or not this test is done by means of the Quick method or other methods, since the values may differ significantly and may therefore influence the interpretation of the laboratory test. Many individuals today are being maintained on anticoagulants for an indefinite period. Such individuals may not consider themselves as taking a medication or being treated by their physician, since the therapy that they are receiving has become longstanding and routine.

Stroke: The history of stroke can be important in the same respect as the history of heart attack, since anticoagulant drugs also are used in the treatment of cerebrovascular accident. The paralysis associated with stroke frequently is also important with particular reference to insertion and removal of dental appliances and the maintenance of adequate oral hygiene.

15. **Have you ever been told by a physician that you have a heart murmur?** The concern of the dentist is in determining whether or not a heart murmur is functional or organic in nature. So-called functional heart murmurs may be disregarded as far as premedication for the prevention of bacterial endocarditis is concerned. Since organic heart murmurs are based on a defect in the endocardium which renders the affected individuals susceptible to subacute bacterial endocarditis, premedication is indicated prior to extractions, scaling of teeth, and other procedures which interrupt tissue continuity.

16. **Do you ever have asthma or hay fever? (Underline which one.)** This question is intended to reveal a history of allergy to pollens, dusts, and animal danders. It is important to note that the individuals who give a history of asthma are more likely to experience a severe asthmatic reaction to aspirin than are non-asthmatic patients.

17. **Do you ever have hives or skin rash?** In general, hives or skin rash is associated with food and drug allergies. The reactions are nonspecific, and in many cases a thorough search of ingested foods or chemical agents is necessary to determine the allergen.

18. **Have you ever experienced an unusual reaction to any of the following drugs?** This question should identify persons who have had serious reactions to one or more drugs. In all probability if any drug is given to enough individuals, an allergic manifestation or idiosyncrasy will develop in one of them.

Aspirin: Aspirin is a widely used drug that produces a great many allergic reactions, including a severe asthmatic reaction. This reaction is usually nonreversible and may be precipitated by as little as five grains of aspirin. Aspirin also may produce generalized urticaria as well as angioedema.

Penicillin: Penicillin, another widely used drug, is a notorious allergen. The reactions to penicillin range from mild skin rash to a fatal anaphylactoid type of reaction. Any suggestion in the history of a previous allergic reaction to penicillin contraindicates the future use of the drug, no matter how mild the reaction might have been, since successive allergic reactions to drugs tend to increase in severity.

Iodine: Iodine is not a potent sensitizer, but in some individuals it is capable of producing a skin rash. The topical use of iodine in dentistry precipitates few allergic reactions.

Sulfonamides (sulfa): The sulfonamide drugs are a group of drugs which in the past have been known to produce a wide variety of untoward reactions, both allergic and toxic. The allergic reactions attributed to sulfonamide drugs vary as widely as do allergic reactions to penicillin. A number of sulfa drugs are still prescribed for the treatment of urinary tract infections. Sulfonamides are available in combination with antibiotics for treatment of other infections.

Barbiturates (sleeping pills): Barbiturates can precipitate dermatitis medicamentosa. They have been known to produce stomatitis medicamentosa also. It is interesting to note that cross-sensitivities among the various barbiturates do not exist with any frequency, so that it is possible to prescribe an alternate barbiturate if the patient develops a sensitivity to the one initially prescribed.

Other medicines: The entry "other medicines" is included in Question 18 so that the patient may include drugs to which he has had an unusual reaction that are not listed on the questionnaire.

19. **Have you ever experienced an unusual reaction to a dental anesthetic?** Most unusual reactions to the local anesthetics that are used in dentistry are mild syncope and occur on a psychogenic basis rather than on an allergic basis. However, true allergies and idiosyncrasies to dental anesthetics do exist. Procaine seems to be a more potent sensitizer than lidocaine. Cross-reactions occur in the drugs related to procaine, rendering a person sensitized to procaine also sen-

sitized to butacaine and Monocaine. Frequently the psychogenic reactions to dental anesthetics can be avoided by proper sedation of the patient prior to dental appointments and by use of a reassuring approach. It is extremely important to recognize a history of true allergic reaction or idiosyncrasy to a dental anesthetic in order to avoid an uncomfortable or even serious experience.

20. **Do you bleed for a long time when you cut yourself?** Questions 55 and 56 are related to Question 20. These questions are an attempt to disclose a history of a hemorrhagic disease. If there is a possibility that a patient may bleed excessively, a further detailed history should be obtained, along with the appropriate laboratory studies to reveal whether or not a hemorrhagic diathesis exists.

21. **Have you ever had any injury to your face or jaws?** Injuries to the face or to the jaws in the history may be related to delayed manifestations involving the temporomandibular joint or previously injured teeth. Acute traumatic temporomandibular joint arthritis often can be related to injuries to the jaws in which the temporomandibular joints were involved through severe stresses placed on the joint region. It is not unusual for teeth to become devitalized and remain asymptomatic following injuries to the face or jaws. Injuries to the teeth may result from automobile accidents or other traumatic incidents which the patient may not relate to the oral or facial region because of more serious injury to other parts of the body.

22. **Have you ever had surgery or x-ray treatment for a tumor, growth, or other condition in your mouth or on your lips?** A history of surgery for a tumor in the oral region, particularly a malignant one, may modify the approach to the clinical examination in that it requires particular attention to the possibility of metastases to the regional lymph nodes and also the possibility of recurrence at the primary site. Irradiation therapy for tumors in the oral region presents certain hazards in dental treatment, particularly where surgical procedures are indicated. It is well known that irradiation therapy involving bone reduces the vitality of bone through reduction in vascularity. Osteoradionecrosis may result from trauma to previously irradiated bone. Dental extractions are strictly contraindicated from irradiated bone.

•   •   •

From this point on in the questionnaire, the questions are intended to elicit symptoms which may indicate disease processes in the various systems of the body. These questions comprise a part of the history referred to as the systems review.

•   •   •

23. **Do you have frequent, severe headaches?** Most of the headaches about which individuals complain are the result of tension. True histamine and migraine headaches occur less frequently. Hypertension may be the basis of recurrent, severe headaches. Most headaches caused by tension are frontal in location. Histamine and migraine headaches are extremely severe and blinding types of headaches, whereas hypertensive headaches tend to be occipital in location. It is possible that a unilateral headache, particularly in the temporal region, may be

related to temporomandibular joint disease or to muscular spasm in the muscles of mastication.

24. **Do you have any complaints regarding your eyes?** The most common complaint registered is the necessity for wearing glasses. Of significance to the dentist is the patient with glaucoma, since the use of antisialogogues is contraindicated in such patients, Antisialogogues tend to further increase intraocular pressure, which is already elevated in glaucoma. Occasionally an ophthalmologist will refer a patient to the dentist for examination to rule out foci of infection associated with the teeth as a possible source of an inflammatory process in the eye. It is unusual to find any relationship between dental foci of infection and inflammatory processes of the eye, but the ophthalmologist wishes to rule out all possibilities in his search for a causative factor.

25. **Do you have any ear trouble?** Because of the proximity of the temporomandibular joint to the ear, complaints originating in the temporomandibular joint may be attributed to a disease process in the ear. An otologist may ask for dental consultation to rule out the possibility of dental or temporomandibular joint disease in a patient who complains of pain in the ear without evidence of an inflammatory process involving the middle or outer ear.

26. **Do you have frequent colds?** Frequent colds can be described as more than three or four during one winter. A continuous cold during the winter is suggestive of allergy to house dust or of vasomotor rhinitis.

27. **Do you have sinus trouble?** A history of acute sinusitis is rather significant in some individuals because it is possible for a toothache to develop in the teeth which approximate the maxillary sinus. Teeth with roots close to an infected sinus may become sensitive to biting pressure. In general, chronic sinus problems do not affect the adjacent teeth in any way, nor do the teeth contribute to chronic disease processes in the maxillary sinuses.

28. **Do you have nosebleeds?** Nosebleeds may result from frequent trauma to the nasal mucosa. Another local cause of nosebleeds is a nasopharyngeal tumor which has invaded a blood vessel. More generalized causes of nosebleed are hypertension and blood dyscrasias. Nosebleeds in an adult patient, if they are more than a simple show of blood occurring when the individual blows his nose, should be investigated thoroughly to determine the cause of bleeding.

29. **Do you have frequent sore throats?** Frequent sore throats are often the result of habitual mouth breathing. Frequent sore throats may be seen in individuals with enlarged tonsils and adenoids. Tongue thrusting habits have been attributed to frequent sore throats in children, since the child can swallow more comfortably if the tongue is thrust forward during the act of swallowing.

30. **Are you a mouth breather?** Mouth breathers many times complain of a dry mouth. They are also susceptible to periodontal disease in the anterior part of the mouth resulting from the irritation of continual drying of the gingival tissues. It is entirely possible that a mouth breathing habit may be the result of nasal congestion which may be corrected by medication. On the other hand, the correction of a mouth breathing habit may necessitate surgical intervention to clear nasal obstructions.

31. **Do you have any sensitive teeth?** A positive response to this question

should be followed by additional questions such as "To what are your teeth sensitive? Heat, cold, or biting pressure?" The placement of a new, large metal restoration may elicit one or all three of these types of sensitivity; however, in the absence of the of the placement of a new restoration, sensitivity to cold suggests hyperemia of the dental pulp and the possibility that the situation is reversible. Sensitivity to heat suggests an irreversible process in the dental pulp, whereas sensitivity to biting pressure suggests an involvement of the periodontal membrane either as the result of trauma to the tooth in question or as the result of periapical inflammation secondary to a devital pulp. The complaint of sensitive teeth should be pursued until the cause of the complaint is determined.

32. **Have you had a toothache recently?** This question is related to the previous question and is included in the questionnaire to identify painful areas in the patient's mouth which have occurred in the recent past and which might not be recalled unless the patient is reminded.

33. **Do you have bleeding gums?** If the patient answers this question affirmatively, he should be asked whether the bleeding is spontaneous at any time or whether it is necessary for him to stimulate bleeding, for example, through use of a toothbrush. If spontaneous hemorrhage is experienced by the patient, it is necessary to determine whether or not the gingival tissues are painful. On clinical examination, it is necessary to look for evidence of necrotizing ulcerative gingivitis, and in the absence of these findings, blood dyscrasias should be suspected. Many laymen feel that it is normal for the gingiva to bleed to some extent when the teeth are brushed, and it is the tendency for many dentists to ignore gingival bleeding on toothbrushing as evidence of periodontal disease. Nevertheless, under normal conditions the gingival tissues should not bleed when the teeth are brushed nor during any other procedure related to the maintenance of oral hygiene.

34. **Do you have frequent canker sores or cold sores?** Canker sores or cold sores may be defined as frequent if they occur more than four to six times a year. Frequently recurring lesions which can be identified as those produced by the herpes simplex virus may be a source of constant oral discomfort for the patient. The determination of whether or not to treat lesions resulting from the herpes simplex virus must be based on the severity of the discomfort and the degree of incapacitation they produce. Infrequently recurring herpetic lesions can be treated on a local basis. The injection of immune serum globulin has proved to be a satisfactory method of delaying recurrence of frequently recurring herpetic lesions.

35. **Have you ever had a severe sore mouth?** An affirmative answer to this question leads to more specific questions to determine the number of times that a sore mouth has been experienced, to a detailed description of what is meant by a severe sore mouth, and to a consideration of the possible diagnosis or causative agent. A variety of disease processes may result in a severe sore mouth, such as primary herpetic gingivostomatitis, Vincent's infection, erythema multiforme, stomatitis medicamentosa, and others.

36. **Is it difficult for you to open your mouth as wide as you would like?** This question is an attempt to discover any functional limitations in the

movement of the mandible. An affirmative answer to this question should be followed by a question about the progressive or static character of the limitation of opening of the mouth. It is also important to note whether the limitation of mandibular movement is of recent onset or is long standing and whether or not movement is restricted because of pain or mechanical obstruction.

37. **Does your jaw click when you chew?** An affirmative answer to this question suggests altered relationship in the components of the temporomandibular joint during functional movements of the mandible. It should be determined during what excursion or in what position of the mandible the noise occurs in the temporomandibular joint region. It should be further determined whether or not pain is experienced in relation to clicking in the temporomandibular joint.

38. **Do you have any chest pain on exertion?** Chest pain (angina pectoris) on exertion suggests insufficiency of blood supply to the myocardium. If an affirmative answer to the question is obtained and the patient has not sought medical advice for the complaint, he should be urged to see his physician at an early date. Nitroglycerin is given routinely for control of anginal pain. The administration of nitroglycerin sublingually just prior to a stressful dental procedure may prevent the patient from experiencing angina pectoris during the procedure.

39. **Are you ever short of breath on mild exertion?** The patient who complains of shortness of breath may do so for a number of reasons, one of the most important of which is cardiac failure. An overweight individual with a normally functioning heart often becomes short of breath on mild exertion. Cardiac insufficiency or heart failure is further indicated if the patient is unable to sleep all night in a recumbent position or if he must prop himself up with several pillows to breathe more easily.

40. **Do your ankles swell?** Dependent edema frequently occurs in patients with heart failure and in those with chronic nephritis. The relationship of this question to Question 39 is apparent, and a combination of affirmative answers to these two questions should stimulate the dentist to consider a medical consultation for his patient to rule out heart failure.

41. **Do you have a persistent cough?** A persistent cough may be the result of chronic irritation from smoking, carcinoma of the lung, tuberculosis, or bronchiectasis. A chronic cough that is productive of sputum suggests the presence of an inflammatory process with the production of an exudate. A chronic nonproductive cough is suggestive of bronchogenic neoplasm.

42. **Do you ever cough blood?** Hemoptysis may be the result of tuberculosis, bronchiectasis, or lung cancer. The most common cause of hemoptysis in the United States is bronchiectasis, whereas the most common cause of hemoptysis in the world is tuberculosis.

43. **Has your appetite changed recently?** A sharp increase in appetite may be suggestive of hyperthyroidism or diabetes. A marked decrease in appetite may be suggestive of hepatitis, gastrointestinal cancer, and several other generalized disease processes.

44. **Are there any foods you cannot eat?** Individuals will most commonly

avoid certain foods because of peptic ulcer, gall bladder disease, or allergy to certain foods.

45. **Do you have any difficulty swallowing?** Difficulty in swallowing may be related to anxiety, globus hystericus, pharyngeal carcinoma, or cardiospasm.

46. **Do you have frequent indigestion?** The most common causes of indigestion are peptic ulcer and gall bladder disease.

47. **Do you vomit frequently?** Frequent vomiting may be the result of functional disease, hiatus hernia, or esophageal diverticulum. It is important to determine whether or not actual stomach contents are regurgitated into the mouth. Persons who vomit frequently may show evidence of the decalcifying effect of hydrochloric acid on the enamel of the teeth.

48. **Do you have kidney trouble?** Chronic renal disease often results in anemia at some point in the course of the disease. In patients with advanced chronic renal disease, compensatory hyperparathyroidism may occur with mobilization of calcium from bone, including the bones of the jaws.

49. **Do you urinate more than six times a day?** Increased frequency of urination may be the result of functional disease, renal disease, prostatic hypertrophy, or diabetes. The increased frequency of urination related to diabetes is also accompanied by an increase in thirst.

50. **Are you thirsty much of the time?** An affirmative answer to this question accompanied by an affirmative answer to Question 49 is strongly suggestive of diabetes. The suspicion of diabetes is even stronger if there has been a recent loss of weight and an increase in appetite.

51. **Have you ever had painful and swollen joints?** If this question is answered affirmatively, it should be determined whether or not the patient is referring to single or multiple painful and swollen joints. Most often the involvement of a single joint with pain and swelling is the result of trauma. Pain and swelling in multiple joints may be the result of rheumatic fever, rheumatoid arthritis, or osteoarthritis. The involvement of the temporomandibular joint in the generalized arthritides must always be considered.

52. **Do you have any numb or prickling areas on your skin?** Anesthesias and paresthesias of unexplained origin may be the result of injury to the nerve trunk or possibly a tumor located more centrally which interferes with the transmission of nerve impulses along a nerve trunk. When areas of anesthesia and paresthesia are localized to the facial region, it is important to outline the area of involvement in an effort to determine the distribution of the nerve which is being affected. If explanations are not possible on a local basis, it may be necessary to refer patients with the complaint of paresthesia or anesthesia to a neurologist for more extensive investigation of the defect in transmission of nerve impulses. It is not unusual for anesthesia and paresthesia to result from the extraction of mandibular molar teeth when the roots are closely related to the mandibular canal. In most instances, the anesthesia or paresthesia disappears in a matter of a few days or weeks after the extraction site is healed.

53. **Do you ever have fits or convulsions?** The purpose of this question is to identify the individual with epilepsy so that special care may be taken in his management during dental appointments. It is entirely possible for an epileptic

patient to experience a seizure in spite of the fact that he has received his daily medication when he is placed under the additional stress of a visit to the dental office. Consultation with the patient's physician is helpful in determining if increased dosages of the anticonvulsive drugs are advisable during the period in which the individual is receiving dental care.

54. **Do you have a tendency to faint?** The main purpose in this question is to identify the individual who has a tendency to experience syncope reaction following the administration of local anesthetics in the oral region. It is entirely possible that individuals who experience petit mal seizures may describe them as a tendency to faint without any relationship to stressful procedures or time of day.

55. **Do you bruise easily?** This question has already been related to Question 20. The purpose in listing a history of bruising easily is to determine whether or not unusual capillary fragility exists. In many instances, mature women will answer this question affirmatively without actually having an exceptional degree of capillary fragility.

56. **Do you have any blood disorder such as anemia (thin blood)?** It is well known that persons with anemia experience more difficulty during stressful procedures and may be more susceptible to shock than normal patients when additional loss of blood occurs during a surgical procedure. This question is also directed at revealing any other blood dyscrasias that might exist.

57. **Does hot weather bother you more than it does other people you know?** Individuals with hyperthyroidism complain about the heat and prefer a lower room temperature than that thought comfortable by other members of their family. It is important to recognize the patient with hyperthyroidism to avoid surgical procedures and to encourage them to seek prompt treatment. Surgical procedures may precipitate thyroid storm in the hyperthyroid individual.

58. **Are you excessively nervous?** Excess of "nervousness" may be simply the result of the current "age of anxiety." Increase in thyroid activity produces increased "nervousness." In the former cause, "nervousness" may be controlled by sedation; in the latter, medical consultation is imperative.

59. **Do you get tired easily?** Ease of tiring may be the result of advancing age, insufficient rest, or decrease in thyroid function, as well as a host of other generalized diseases. The onset of leukemia or infectious mononucleosis may be accompanied by ease of tiring.

60. **(Women) Are you pregnant at the present time?** The importance of being aware of early pregnancy is important in the recognition of gingival changes associated with pregnancy and commonly referred to as pregnancy gingivitis. It is also important to avoid exposing the patient to x-rays and stressful procedures during the first trimester of pregnancy if it is at all possible. The quantity of x-rays used for exposing dental films is not harmful to the pregnant patient or the developing embryo. Most dental procedures are not stressful enough to cause difficulty during early pregnancy; nevertheless, the first trimester of pregnancy is the period during which abortion is most likely to occur. An attempt may be made months later by a patient who has received exposure to dental x-rays to relate the exposure to a congenital anomaly in the infant.

REFERENCES

Ash, M. M., Hard, D., and Tondrowski, V. F.: The Role of the Hygienist in the Detection of Disease, J.A.D.A. **59**:546-548, 1959.

Barr, J. H.: Trends in the Development of Courses in Oral Diagnosis, J. D. Educ. **18**:25-29, 1954.

Bodecker, C. F.: Oral Diagnosis, J. D. Educ. **8**:244-256, 1944.

Brodman, K., Erdman, A. J., Jr., Lorge, I., and Wolff, H. G.: The Cornell Medical Index: An Adjunct to Medical Interview, J.A.M.A. **140**:530-534, 1949.

Easton, G. S.: The Place of Systemic Studies in Undergraduate Instruction in Oral Diagnosis, J. D. Educ. **18**:40-45, 1954.

Editorial: The Dentist and the Medical Patient, J.A.D.A. **56**:253-254, 1958.

Hubbard, J. P. (editor): The Early Detection and Prevention of Disease, New York, 1957, The Blakiston Division, McGraw-Hill Book Co., Inc.

Levin, M. L.: Detection of Chronic Disease, J.A.M.A. **146**:1397-1401, 1951.

Millard, H. D., and Tupper, C. J.: The Role of Oral Diagnosis in Periodic Health Appraisal Examinations, Oral Surg., Oral Med., & Oral Path. **121**:1273-1278, 1959.

Muhler, J. C., Hine, M. K., and Day, H. G.: Preventive Dentistry, St. Louis, 1954, The C. V. Mosby Co.

Petrie, L. M., Bowdoin, C. D., and McLoughlin, C. J.: Voluntary Multiple Health Tests, J.A.M.A. **148**:1022-1024, 1952.

Vines, H. W. C.: To Make Preventive Medicine a Clinical Reality, We Must Overcome Our Obsession With Beds, Mod. Hosp. **81**:51-54, 106-108, 1953.

Ziskin, D. E., Burket, L. W., and Blevins, G. C.: Teaching Oral Diagnosis to Dental Students, J. D. Educ. **10**:61-82, 1945.

Signs and symptoms

It is obvious to almost everyone commencing the study of oral diagnosis that several of the symptoms of one disease are also the symptoms of some other disease. Many diseases have numerous symptoms in common because the external conditions are actually secondary or nonspecific reactions. These conditions are the result of biologic variations from individual to individual, variations within the same individual, and variations in the causative agents. Thus the manifestations of disease are many and varied.

Applied symptomatology of disease may be considered to be the descriptive knowledge of the subjective and objective manifestations of disease necessary to carry out the process of oral diagnosis. Lest the examiner become confused with the wide variety of symptoms that may be presented to him during the examination, it is necessary that some useful grouping of manifestations of disease be utilized.

The cardinal signs of inflammation as one group are an example of a symptomatologic classification which aids in identifying tissue alteration and disease. Manifestations of disease may also be classified on an anatomic or system basis whereby symptoms are grouped according to the part of the body or system involved. Symptomatology may also be based on morphologic alteration of the tissues which gives rise to characteristic types of lesions; these are divided into so-called elementary or *primary* lesions and *secondary* lesions which occur consecutively in consequence to the primary lesions. It must be remembered, however, that all classifications are artificial and are made by emphasizing certain differences and neglecting certain resemblances. The examiner should not let any arbitrary division of symptoms detract from the evaluation of the whole individual, since the process of analyzing and interpreting symptoms cannot be based on the description of an isolated symptom relative to a classification but must be based upon the orientation of the symptoms not only to the classification, but also to the whole body as a physiologic and psychologic unit. The most common classification in symptomatology is the division of symptoms into objective and subjective manifestations of disease.

Subjective symptoms are those which may be discerned by the patient and are obtained by inquiry during the case history. In most instances the subjective symptoms are the ones which bring the patient to the dentist. In some instances the symptoms will present the picture that will largely establish the diagnosis regardless of the outcome of the clinical and/or laboratory examinations. The subjective symptoms usually determine the line of inquiry that the examiner must take to determine the various causes for the symptoms. While subjective symptoms may be related entirely to local disturbances of the mouth, they may also be expressions of general or systemic disease. Thus, the examiner must be aware not only of subjective manifestations of disease of the mouth, but also of subjective symptoms outside this area that will complete the pattern or clinical picture of the patient's departure from good health. The subjective oral manifestations of disease, or complaints of the patient referable to the mouth, are various types of pain, alteration of taste, foul breath, inability to masticate food, esthetic and psychogenic complaints, dryness of the mouth, swelling, speech problems, and a sense of an unclean mouth. Obviously these same symptoms will rarely be described in the same way by all patients. Not infrequently patients will present without obvious subjective symptoms of disease because of their adaptation to the distress or discomfort or because of indifferent effects on the body or its functions. Today, with periodic dental examinations being made on presumably well people, the dentist has an additional obligation to seek out those manifestations of latent disease or potential sources of disability.

Objective symptoms or signs of disease are those which produce functional and structural changes which may be seen by the naked eye of the patient and/or the examiner. Generally, alteration of structure and function may be manifested by changes in shape, size, color, form, density, number, position, and relationships. The clinical evaluation of the alterations of form and structure is carried out by inspection, palpation, percussion, and auscultation. While these technics are used in examination of the entire body, their application varies with the part of the body being investigated. Thus examination of the mucous membrane entails chiefly inspection and palpation, whereas examination of the teeth, jaws, and temporomandibular joint entails inspection, palpation, percussion, and auscultation. Radiographic examination may be considered as an extension of the visual examination.

From the foregoing it may be readily seen that subjective manifestations of disease are elicited by inquiry and that objective manifestations of disease are found by clinical examination. The basis for modern therapy is diagnosis; this proposes that the cause of the disease be identified and eliminated. While this is a modern approach to treatment, it is not always feasible, since many situations will arise in which the relief of symptoms becomes an important adjunct in caring for the patient. The relief of symptoms is important to the patient and may provide positive benefits in the treatment of the disease provided that the symptom relief does not interfere with the diagnosis of the disease. For example, it is necessary to make a differential diagnosis between herpetic gingivostomatitis and acute necrotizing ulcerative gingivitis, but the basis for therapy is not directed toward elimination of the disease in both instances. Inasmuch as herpetic gingivostomatitis is a self-limiting disease, therapy is generally directed toward relief of symptoms associated with this condition. The symptomatic relief of acute necrotizing ulcerative gingivitis is contraindicated since the cause of the disease or predisposing factors in the causation of the disease have not been eliminated. Symptomatic relief in the treatment of acute necrotizing gingivitis should be considered only as an adjunct to formal therapy. Symptomatic treatment of patients following gingivectomy, endodontics, oral surgery, and operative dental procedures is advocated only when the cause of the symptoms has been taken into proper consideration. Therefore, the examiner should institute symptomatic therapy only after he has identified the cause of the symptoms. Thus, he should evaluate the symptoms of a patient in terms of the previous treatment of the patient and what complication or unfavorable sequela may have arisen as the result of such treatment.

CARDINAL MANIFESTATIONS OF DISEASE

Just as the cardinal signs of inflammation are heat, redness, swelling, and pain, the cardinal manifestations of systemic disease are pain, weakness, shortness of breath, circulatory disturbances, indigestion, jaundice, polyuria, oliguria, edema, alteration of weight, anemia, bleeding, and lymphadenopathy. In rendering a health service the dental practitioner has a professional, legal, and moral obligation to learn as much as possible about the health of his patient before beginning treatment, since the knowledge gained may be a basic consideration in the clinical examination and in the determination of treatment. The emphasis on the clinical manifestations of systemic disease should be directed toward the correlation of signs and symptoms of disease in all areas of the body that may be related or possibly related to oral disease. The purpose of the evaluation of the clinical manifestations of systemic disease is not to establish a medical diagnosis but to make an evaluation of the health of the patient that will allow the examiner (1) to consider the presence of systemic disease and its relation to dental treatment; (2) to take prophylactic or precautionary measures for the good of the examiner and the patient; (3) to determine the best treatment possible in the presence of systemic disease; (4) to establish a sound basis for medical consultation when indicated; and (5) to give the dentist a better idea of what to expect in the way of prognosis.

It is obvious that the indications for the evaluation of the cardinal manifestations of systemic disease will depend upon the character of the disease and the therapeutic procedures which are to be instituted. Since the relationship of oral disease to systemic disease is not always obvious, nor is the need for systemic evaluation always apparent, the oral examination of any patient should include a basic screening discipline to uncover any systemic disease that may be present. The proper rationale for oral therapy demands that the examiner (1) consider the constitutional status of the patient (with emphasis on nutrition, metabolism, and hormonal balance) and (2) recognize systemic disease which may modify the therapeutic procedures (rheumatic or congenital heart insufficiencies, blood dyscrasias, and contagious diseases). The recognition of the clinical manifestations of systemic disease should not be considered as usurping the province of the physician. It is not intended that the dental practitioner be as proficient as a physician in the recognition of all the signs and symptoms of systemic disease but rather that he be proficient in the recognition of systemic disease that might have a bearing on oral diagnosis and therapy.

The following presentation of the cardinal manifestations of systemic disease is not intended to be all inclusive, since coverage of this material may be found in textbooks of internal medicine and oral medicine.

Pain

Pain is a specific sensory experience mediated through nerve structures which are separate from those which mediate other sensations such as touch, pressure, heat, and cold. Pain cannot be considered as being desirable; however, it is an important warning of the presence of noxious stimuli, although pain itself does not appear to be essential to a suitable biologic adjustment since many persons without ability to experience pain are able to adjust themselves to their environment. Pain may produce a protective adaptive reaction to noxious stimulation which causes significant impairment of bodily function or actual tissue damage. Adaptive or protective reactions may become especially significant when an individual reacts to any stimulus that has been previously associated with dangerous situations or injuries. These reactions to symbols of danger are the same as those which might be expected from actual tissue damage but are initiated by nonpainful stimuli.

While the threshold for perception of pain is the lowest intensity of stimulus which may be recognized and is approximately the same in all normal individuals, the threshold at which patients react to pain varies considerably. Emotionally disturbed patients and those who already have some degree of pain generally show a lower threshold of reaction than do normal individuals. A person's reaction to pain depends considerably upon the association that the individual makes in the higher brain centers between painful stimuli and the interpretation of pain. Inasmuch as the reaction to pain includes not only voluntary reactions, but also those mediated through the autonomic nervous system, it may readily be appreciated that pain has a large emotional, as well as a purely physical, component. This dual aspect of pain makes it somewhat difficult for the examiner to differentiate completely the pain sensation from the reaction of the patient to pain.

Pain is subjective in character, and the examiner must depend upon what the patient relates to him in terms of quality, time of occurrence, location, intensity, and reaction to the pain. It is essential that he attempt to get the patient to be objective in his description of his discomfort to the end that his reactions to the pain will be completely divorced from his description of actual pain sensations. When this is accomplished, the examiner will be able to more fully evaluate the precise nature and location of the pain. Thus the patient who is able to tell the examiner that he has pain associated with the lower first molar when he bites on that tooth rather than describing all of his reaction to the pain makes it much easier for the examiner to arrive at a diagnosis. In evaluating symptoms of a painful nature, it is essential that the examiner assist the patient in discriminating between pain itself and his reaction to pain.

The diagnosis of the sensations of pain must be based on anatomic, physiologic, and psychologic considerations. Pain impulses set up by noxious stimuli are received by specific receptors known as free nerve endings which are scattered throughout the skin, mucous membranes, subcutaneous structures, and viscera. The impulses are carried through groups of myelinated and unmyelinated nerve fibers of various sizes at various speeds either directly to the posterior root ganglia in somatic nerves or indirectly in sympathetic trunks and through sympathetic ganglia to the posterior root ganglia via the white rami communicantes. The cell bodies of the sensory nerves, including those passing through the sympathetic chain, are located in the posterior root ganglia. From this area the dendrites or neurons enter the cord and penetrate to the region of the posterior horn. Here the impulses are shunted to a second neuron whose cell body is in the posterior horn. Pain impulses then cross to the opposite side of the cord and ascend to the lateral spinothalamic tract to the thalamus. These impulses then travel along additional neurons which extend to the postcentral area of the cerebral cortex.

Of special interest to the dentist is the transmission of sensory impulses by the peripheral branches of the trigeminal nerve. Pain impulses arising from pain-sensitive structures served by the peripheral branches of the trigeminal nerve are carried to the gasserian ganglion into the pons. In the pons the central fibers from the gasserian ganglion divide into short ascending and long descending branches. The long descending branches form the spinal tract of the trigeminal nerve and mediate all pain and temperature sensations. These branches terminate in the nucleus of the spinal tract in the medulla. Pain impulses are relayed from here to the thalamus and then to the sensory facial area from the postcentral gyrus of the cerebral cortex. The localization of perceived pain is most highly developed in the cerebral cortex, whereas the hypothalamus dictates the autonomic response and attitude of the patient to the noxious stimulant. Thus in the simplest conduction of the pain impulse, the spinal ganglionic, spinothalamic, and thalamocortical neurons take part. The cerebral cortex is necessary for the localization and evaluation of the intensity of the impulses, and the thalamus is important in the integration of pain.

Although all pain fibers enter the spinal cord through the dorsal root ganglion, the two varieties of pain known as superficial pain and deep pain have different routes of conduction by sensory fibers. Pain impulses from the surface of the body are generally carried in the somatic nerves and enter the spinal cord through the dorsal routes. This pathway is much more simple than that of the deep pain impulses, which are conducted to the cerebral nervous system by a variety of routes. Since deep-seated pain impulses may be carried by fibers attached to the blood vessels which join the autonomic nervous system, deep-seated pain may travel in association with autonomic nerves or with somatic nerves.

The quality of painful sensation depends to a large extent upon the origin of the stimulus. Several different clinically distinguishable qualities of pain have been found to exist: a bright pricking pain, a burning pain, and a deeper-felt aching pain. The bright pricking and burning pains have been associated with noxious stimulation of body surfaces. The bright pricking pain is thought to be carried in thick, rapidly conducting myelinated fibers, whereas burning pain is thought to be carried by slower conducting fibers of a smaller size. Pricking of the gingiva with a sharp explorer usually gives rise to an initial sharp pain of abrupt onset with a pricking quality and is then followed by a pain of slower onset which has a burning quality. Not only may the quality of pain vary, but also its intensity. The quality of pain from the deeper tissues differs from that of cutaneous or superficial areas in that it is more diffuse and long lasting and may tend to radiate. It is also more likely to be associated with nausea, slowing of the pulse, and a fall in blood pressue. Whereas superficial pain is fairly well localized, deep pain with its duller aching nature is more diffuse in character and is less accurately perceived. Localization of superficial pain varies according to the region, the number of sense organs present, and the frequency with which the organs are stimulated. Localization is highly developed in the hands, the lips, and tongue because of the abundance of sense organs and the amount of cortical training which has resulted from the identification of many objects. Localization of pain is poor in those areas in which there are but few sense organs and in which the cortical training necessary for the identification of objects is not well developed.

The localization of deep pain is likely to be poor and, in many instances, may be referred to a surface area of the body. Thus, pain from the teeth, jaws, tempo-romandibular joints, and other deep structures may be falsely localized and referred to the surface of the face. The exact mechanism of how this referral occurs is not well understood. The skin and mucous membranes may become abnormally sensitive to noxious stimuli because of a lowering of the pain thres-hold or because of an alteration of the excitability of central pain pathways so that various stimuli evoke a more intense sensation. Hyperalgesia of the skin and mucous membranes associated with a lowering of the pain threshold may be seen with inflammation. Hyperalgesia associated with alterations of the excitability of the central pain pathways supplying the skin and mucous mem-branes is sometimes seen in association with referred pain.

The diagnosis of superficial pain is based upon its quality, cause, intensity, localization, site, distribution, and duration. Two types of superficial pain may be recognized: a rapidly conducted pricking sensation which is bright and sharply localized and a slowly conducted burning sensation which is less sharp but fairly well localized. Deep pain is characterized by its quality, poor localiza-tion, and spread, and by associated phenomena such as hyperalgesia, hyper-esthesia, and tenderness. Deep pains are dull and aching in quality and are usually poorly localized. They have a tendency to spread to areas other than those which are stimulated. This spread may involve deep or superficial pathways or both and may give rise to "referred pain."

Two other types of pain which should be mentioned are central pain and psychogenic pain. "Central pain" arises in patients suffering from lesions of the thalamus or spinothalamic tracts. This type of pain is constant or recurrent in nature and is usually not well localized, and dysesthesia is readily elicited. Oc-casionally a patient will complain of pain for which no organic cause can be found. It must be remembered, however, that pain may be facilitated since perceptive centers in the brain may become hypersensitive after repeated stimulation. The patient who has had a pulpitis and still has the typical pain after the tooth has been removed presents an occasional problem to the dentist. The cortical threshold may be lower generally, as well as locally, and the effects of this may be seen in such individuals as neurasthenics who may be hypersensitive to any type of painful stimulus. It must also be remembered that psychoneurotic patients usually have a lower threshold of reaction to pain than do normal individuals.

Pain may arise from any of the pain-sensitive structures of the mouth and adjacent structures. Whether or not pain is produced is dependent upon the type of noxious stimulus and the pain sensitivity of the structures involved. A stimulus which may cause pain in the mucous membranes or skin may not produce pain in the muscles. The pain produced by a needle puncture of muscles is generally slight; however, it is severe in the presence of vascular disease or when the noxious stimulus is due to injection of a hypertonic solution. Pain is produced in muscles when in spasm, such as trismus, or in muscular cramps such as might be produced by tetany. Subcutaneous fat gives little pain when pierced by a needle or when it is cut, but if cutaneous nerves passing through the fat are injured, considerable pain may be perceived. Needle puncture of deep fascia is always painful. Tendons and the periosteum are sensitive to needle pricks or hypertonic solutions, and pain is a prominent feature of periostitis. Compact bone may be cut without pain, but pain may be produced when cancellous bone is cut. Joints are insensitive to a needle prick, knife cut, or cautery, but the synovial membrane is sensitive to inflammation, hypertonic solutions, and needle pricks. The arteries and veins may react painfully to needle puncture.

No pain sensations can be elicited from the enamel, but the dentin is somewhat sensitive, and the pulp is extremely sensitive to noxious stimuli. Free nerve endings are the only nerve receptors found in the pulp, and for this reason the pulp registers only pain regardless of the stimulus. Other complex receptors that register touch, cold, heat, pressure, and position sense are found throughout the oral mucosa, periodontal membrane, muscles, and adjacent structures. Pain associated with pulpitis is difficult to localize and may be referred to almost any area on the same side of the face supplied by the trigeminal nerve. Where pulpitis has involved the apical area of the tooth, localization of the area of involvement will be possible because of the stimulation of the other complex receptors in the periodontal membrane. Even in these instances the ability to localize pain varies considerably from one individual to another. Unfortunately, the lack of localization of a diseased pulp has led to the extraction of many healthy teeth. Inasmuch as pain may be referred from other regions to the teeth, jaws, and temporomandibular joints, patients may come to the dentist or be referred to the dentist under the misconception that the teeth must be at fault. Thus it is not uncommon for a patient to insist upon the extraction of a particular tooth upon which a fixation has been made when in reality the pain is referred from disease of the maxillary sinus or from the region of the neck.

It is obvious that the diagnosis of obscure pain even in the presence of dental disease should not be made without a complete evaluation of the character of the pain and the possibility of its arising from some source other than dental. It should also be remembered that pain may be referred from the teeth, jaws, and temporomandibular joints to other regions. It is not uncommon for pain in the ear and the temporomandibular joint region to arise from pulpitis of a lower molar. Pain arising from pulpitis of a lower molar may radiate to the eye, jaw, or ear, to other teeth in the same side of the face, or to the back of the head and neck. Similar referrals of pulpal pain may occur as a result of occlusal trauma; this pain should not be confused with pain of temporomandibular joint arthritis related to occlusal trauma.

The classifications of the symptoms of pain are generally made on an etiologic basis. Many terms have been used to designate a type of involvement of the peripheral nerve which gives rise to the symptom of pain. Two descriptive terms which are used loosely by clinicians to denote pain in the distribution of a nerve are neuritis and neuralgia.

The term neuritis has been used loosely to apply to diseases of the peripheral nerves which show evidence of inflammation or degeneration. More strictly, this term should be reserved for those changes which are inflammatory in nature. However, since it it is difficult many times to distinguish whether or not the condition is inflammatory or degenerative in character, the term neuritis can probably be best utilized to designate painful sensations which are more or less continuous, which are due to known causes, and which demonstrably alter the tissue. Thus the term neuritis may be considered as a diagnosis. The term neuralgia does not represent a disease entity but implies only a subjective symptom. Generally, however, this term is used to designate clinical syndromes such as trigeminal neuralgia, which is characterized by paroxysmal lancinating pain for which no etiologic basis or morphologic changes can be found.

The classification of neuralgia is based upon the character of the pain, the presence or absence of an etiologic basis, and a manner by which it can be relieved. In typical neuralgia the pain may be orientated along the distribution of the cranial or upper cervical nerves or their branches. In atypical neuralgia the pain may be diffuse and does not conform to the distribution of a nerve but rather to that of certain blood vessels. Typical and atypical neuralgias are further divided into major and minor types. Major neuralgias have the following similar characteristics: (1) unknown etiology; (2) periodic, lancinating, and very brief pain; and (3) can be relieved by interruption of the pain pathways. The minor neuralgias have the following similar characteristics: (1) a clinically apparent etiologic basis; (2) usually constant pain; and (3) can be relieved either by removal of the cause or by interruption of the pathways. Major neuralgias include trigeminal, facial, and glossopharyngeal neuralgia. Minor neuralgias include idiopathic pain involving the teeth, periodontal tissues, jaws, sinuses, temporomandibular joints, muscles, vessels, and nerves. Neuralgias of psychogenic origin are called psychalgias and are sometimes difficult to differentiate from trigeminal neuralgia. As with a typical facial neuralgia, the diagnosis of psychalgia must be made by exclusion and by psychiatric evaluation. Furthermore, the pain associated with psychalagia does not correspond to dermatomal peripheral nerve distribution or to the distribution of blood vessels. Neuralgia may be the precursor to organic disease and may be the only symptom which can be found. It may also be the symptom of inflammation of the nerves or the symptom of other disturbances. The evaluation of any neuralgia must be considered from a psychologic, somatic, and symptomatic standpoint.

Neuritis implies an inflammatory or degenerative change in the peripheral nerves and may be seen in relation to various forms of pulpitis, osteitis, periostitis, and other forms of specific disease which involve the nerves. In neuritis the inflammatory or degenerative changes may involve one or more nerves or the roots of the spinal nerves. The symptomatology associated with neuritis depends upon the location of the involvement and the character of the pain.

Headache

Headache is a term used to describe an ache or pain experienced in the region of the cranial vault. It is a subjective symptom and may be described in terms of quality, location, and intensity and its relation to other events. The cranium, the covering of the skull, any structure in the cranial cavity, and the adjacent structures which are pain sensitive may give rise to headaches. Headaches are characterized by the diffuse aching discomfort which is typical of the pain that is produced by visceral, vascular, or deep somatic disorders. Head pain which is sharp and localizable is more often due to neuralgias or lesions of the face. Headaches that arise from intracranial sources may result from traction, distention, or dilatation of many vessels in the cranial vault. Inflammation or other changes of the pain-sensitive structures of the head and direct pressure by tumors may also produce headaches. Headaches which arise from extracranial sources are due to sustained contraction of muscles of the head and neck and/or distention or inflammation of extracranial arteries. Headaches may also be migraine, histamine, or systemic in origin.

Of special interest to the dentist is the type of headache resulting from noxious stimulation of the teeth. This is not a common cause of headache, although it is clinically important. Pain in the head associated with a prolonged toothache is of two varieties: (1) that due to central spread of excitation and experienced in tissues supplied by the same and adjacent divisions of the fifth cranial nerve and (2) that due to sustained contraction of the muscles of the head and neck resulting secondarily from noxious stimuli arising in the teeth. Headache arising from a noxious stimulus may be eliminated by the use of a local anesthetic about the site of the noxious stimulus. Pain associated with contraction of the muscles of the head and neck will not be relieved by an injection of a local anesthetic. Even though a tooth may be seriously diseased, it cannot be considered to be the cause of a headache or neuralgia unless the pain can be eliminated by the use of a local anesthetic around the teeth.

Weakness

Weakness is a term used by patients to describe many subjective complaints that vary in their diagnostic significance. The complaint of weakness by a patient is generally so vague that it is almost meaningless unless the examiner evaluates this complaint in the light of more meaningful terms such as asthenia, lassitude, or faintness.

Persistent weakness characterized by lack of energy, lassitude, and undue fatigability may be associated with emotional disturbances or almost any type of serious disease. Malignant neoplasms, obscure chronic infections, anemia, metabolic and endocrine disorders, and nutritional deficiencies may produce lassitude. While early nutritional deficiency may be manifested only by lassitude, most diseases are accompanied by other signs and symptoms of disease. Asthenia is characterized by a generalized muscular weakness and feebleness which is common in senility, severe forms of common anemias, nutritional deficiencies, diseases of the thyroid glands, disorders of the locomotor system, and endocrine disorders such as Addison's disease. Many individuals complain of lassitude when they are suffering from any physical or emotional disorder; the evaluation of lassitude, then, must be approached from the standpoint of associated symptoms.

The patient may complain of frequent or occasional weak spells, fainting, and recurrent attacks of weakness. Since these attacks are usually of brief duration, the dentist is unlikely to see a patient during an episode of weakness; and the evaluation of this symptom will depend largely upon the history concerning the circumstances surrounding the recurrent weakness or syncope.

The most common causes of recurrent weakness and syncope are epilepsy, emotional disturbances, hypoglycemia, postural hypotension, and disturbances of cardiac rhythm. A history of recurrent attacks of loss of awareness or consciousness associated with abnormal movements or confusion is highly suggestive of epilepsy. In most instances the dental practitioner will find that the diagnosis of epilepsy has already been made by a physician. The knowledge that a patient has epilepsy and is taking Dilantin sodium is of special interest to the dentist in the prevention and treatment of gingival enlargement associated with the administration of this drug. Generally, patients have no idea of the relationship of epilepsy to gingival enlargement and do not tell the dentist they have the disease. It remains for the dental examiner to elicit this information by inquiry. A history of recurrent seizures and the presence of scars on the tongue and buccal mucosa from gnashing of the teeth should direct the examiner's attention to the possibility of the patient having epilepsy.

Dyspnea

Shortness of breath or dyspnea is a subjective sensation associated with a feeling of inadequate respiration. This symptom is of significance especially when it is related to muscle effort. Undue respiratory effort that is totally unrelated to the normal requirements for a particular activity is suggestive of abnormality. Dyspnea does not occur at rest in normal persons and only becomes apparent upon exertion when physical activity is strenuous or when the patient is obese, advanced in age, or out of "training." Shortness of breath that occurs with effort should be considered as pathologic only when it is out of proportion to that which normally occurs in an individual for that particular age, weight, and activity. Dyspnea associated with pathologic states may be seen in cardiac, pulmonary, and hematogenous diseases. Obstruction of the pulmonary tree, such as may be seen in patients with bronchial asthma and neoplasms, may also cause dyspnea.

The evaluation of a complaint of dyspnea in the absence of a complete physical examination can be made only on a relative basis. The dentist can only relate this complaint to other signs and symptoms which may be related to the dyspnea and can only evaluate the degree of dyspnea in terms of functional incapacitation (e.g., undue shortness of breath at rest or changes in the ability of a patient to carry out an activity which previously caused no dyspnea).

Other Cardiovascular Manifestations

Palpitation may be defined as an undue awareness of the beating of the heart. In itself it is usually of little significance except in certain cardiac arrhythmias. However, the suspicion of heart disease may be associated with this symptom in the minds of patients. Anxiety associated with palpitations, especially in those individuals who have been told that they have heart disease, is of considerable psychologic importance to the patient but may only serve to confuse the examiner. Palpitation is physiologic when associated with strenuous physical exercise. It is necessary that the examiner be aware of the patient's concept of what constitutes palpitation and what constitutes cardiac arrhythmia. Palpitation of the heart may be due to disorders of the mechanism of heartbeat, to the presence of organic or functional disorders outside of the heart or circulatory system (such as thyrotoxicosis, anemia, hypoglycemia), and to the use of tobacco, coffee, tea, and some drugs.

High blood pressure is usually not discovered by the dentist during clinical examination but is generally found by inquiry during the interview of the patient. When the dentist determines the blood pressure, he must be ready to evaluate his findings in terms of normal for that particular individual. When the patient offers the information that he has high blood pressure, the dentist must evaluate this information in terms of the signs and symptoms of high blood pressure. Hypertension is the symptomatic manifestation of an abnormal state of the circulation.

Hypertension may be renal, endocrine, or psychogenic in origin. Essential hypertension is a term used in various ways. It is used by some to indicate all hypertension except that due to pre-existing renal disease, by others to mean hypertension of unknown origin, and by still others to signify hypertension that is not malignant hypertension. The last term is generally used to indicate a persistent diastolic blood pressure of over 120 mm. Hg, vascular retinopathy, and early renal or cardiac insufficiency.

In this country an adult with a persistent blood pressure of 140/85 is considered to have a high blood pressure. In certain individuals, especially those predisposed to hypertension, a rise in both systolic and diastolic pressure may be caused by psychic factors such as anger, frustration, anxiety, and other emotional stimuli.

Although blood pressure may be recorded in the general practitioner's office with a mercury sphygmomanometer, the interpretation of the findings requires experience and knowledge usually outside the general practice of dentistry.

Even so, the history and examination, or the history alone, may present sufficient evidence to warrant referral of a patient to a physician for a more complete evaluation than could be accomplished by the dentist. Clinical symptoms that may accompany hypertension include headache, vertigo, and hemoptysis associated with respiratory tract bleeding from the rupture of a pulmonary arteriole due to vascular hypertension. Epistaxis is not unusual in hypertension.

Bleeding is a cardinal manifestation of disease which may arise from vascular dysfunction, blood vessel fragility, defects in blood coagulation mechanisms, and injury to vessels. In the oral cavity, bleeding is most commonly associated with gingival disease. Less common is hemorrhage due to defects in those factors concerned with blood coagulation. The latter is the most important as far as the life of the patient is concerned, but the former can be readily appreciated by the patient as a significantly important sign of gingival disease. It must be recognized that while gingival bleeding is usually the result of gingival disease, it may be the sign of systemic disease of great importance to the life of the patient.

Purpura is a manifestation of bleeding characterized by extravasations into the skin or mucous membranes. These may vary in size from small spots (petechiae) to large areas (ecchymoses). The most common purpuric areas in the oral cavity are petechiae associated with trauma. These may be readily seen on the soft palate as a result of coughing or as a result of physical trauma due to eating hard or sharp particles of food like toast or hot foods. Blood disorders such as leukemias, anemias, infections, subacute bacterial endocarditis, and splenic disorders may also produce purpuric areas in the mouth.

Frank bleeding associated with scaling procedures and extractions may be related to defects in those factors concerned with the coagulation of blood. This may be related to a quantitative deficiency in blood platelets, a qualitative deficiency of platelets, a deficiency of platelet thromboplastin, a lack of vitamin K, liver damage, drug intoxications, a decrease in fibrinogen, and an anticoagulant in the blood. The latter occurs frequently as the result of anticoagulant therapy in the treatment and prevention of coronary thrombosis. The patient's history is the most useful instrument in the prevention of hemorrhagic accidents from dental procedure. A past history of excessive bleeding should alert the examiner to an appraisal of a bleeding tendency. In the absence of a history of bleeding, the examiner must rely on the signs and symptoms of disorders which point to a hemorrhagic tendency. If these are found, an examination of the blood is indicated. Examination of the blood should show coagulation time, prothrombin time, bleeding time, platelet count, and clot retraction. The tourniquet test is also important. These tests may be carried out by qualified personnel in the dental office or by a physician to whom the patient is referred. In most instances the latter procedure will be the most expedient for a general practitioner.

Alteration of Weight

Excessive gain or loss of weight, especially of recent origin, is of more importance to the dentist than whether or not a patient meets the optimum for height, build, and age. Any deviation of the normal as expressed in terms of recent gain or loss of weight suggests the introduction of a new factor in the life of the patient. This may be the manifestation of disease or of physiologic adaptation to the individual's environment.

The most common cause of an increase in weight in childhood is that of normal growth and development. Pregnancy is another cause of physiologic increase in weight. Overeating is another factor in weight increase which must be considered in evaluating deviations of normal. Of considerable significance are those increases in weight due to metabolic and hormonal disturbances. Renal disturbances (nephrotic syndrome), congestive heart failure with water and salt retention, and glandular disturbances may bear an important relationship to increases in weight. Hormonal disturbances that may be responsible for excessive weight include hypothyroidism, hypogonadism, pituitary or adrenal disease, and adiposogenital dystrophy.

Recent weight loss may be digestive, hormonal, neoplastic, anorectic, pharmacologic, or psychogenic in origin. Digestive causes include vitamin deficiencies, diarrhea, vomiting, disturbances in mastication and deglutition, and dietary fads. Neoplastic disease of the digestive tract or of other areas may affect digestion with a resultant loss of weight. Hormonal disturbances include hyperthyroidism, diabetes mellitus, Addison's disease, and Simmonds' disease. Loss of appetite may accompany anxiety, pain, anorexigenic drugs, and excessive smoking and alcoholism. Loss of weight may also result from drug therapy.

Lesions

Objective signs of disease include those morphologic alterations of the soft tissues that are characteristic enough to be classified as specific lesions. Most lesions may be grouped into certain categories because of their rather consistent similar morphology, pattern of distribution, time of occurrence, duration, and presence of associated symptoms. The alteration in morphology of the tissue is so characteristic in many lesions that they may be classified as basic or *primary* types of lesions. Primary lesions may not retain their initial appearance and may be altered by trauma, mastication, maceration, movement of the tissues, and time itself. Those lesions which appear consecutively to the primary lesions are known as *secondary* lesions.

The diagnosis of many oral diseases is based upon the recognition of primary lesions. Because of the character of the oral mucosa, the primary lesions are not always as clear cut as those appearing on the skin. In many instances, however, the oral lesions will be a part of the over-all skin picture, and a referral to the skin will assist in making a more reliable evaluation of the oral lesions. Because of the rapid changes which occur to the initial primary lesions, secondary lesions are the most common lesions observed in the mouth. In an evaluation of any lesion in the mouth, the examiner must keep in mind those factors which might produce alteration in the primary lesions. An adequate history of the lesions may serve to indicate to the examiner what the initial lesion might have been.

Primary Lesions.—There are at least eight types of primary lesions which may occur in the mouth and on the skin in disease: macules, papules, nodules, vesicles, bullae, tumors, keratoses, and wheals.

Macules are flat, circumscribed alterations of tissue which may vary in size, color, and shape. The size varies from that of a pinhead to several centimeters. The color may vary from red and brown to white. Those of vascular origin are red to brown-red in color and may be called erythematous macules. Macules resulting from blood pigment (petechiae and ecchymoses) give rise to varying colors of red to brown in the oral mucosa. The erythematous macule represents simple erythema and is due to a localized congestion in the vascular bed; the color will fade on pressure. Petechiae and ecchymoses result from hemorrhage into the tissues; their color will not disappear on pressure. Pigmentary macules are brown to black in color and may be physiologic or pathologic in character. Examples of physiologic pigmentation are ephelides (freckles) and melanosis (melanoplakia); pathologic pigmentation may be seen in Addison's disease and in intestinal polyposis (Peutz-Jeghers syndrome). Macules may be transitory or permanent in character and vary in shape from circular, polygonal, and linear to polymorphous forms. (Fig. 1.)

A   B

C   D

Fig. 1. *Macules.* **A**, Ecchymosis associated with constant coughing. **B**, Hyperpigmentation of buccal mucosa in Addison's disease. **C**, Hyperpigmentation associated with chronic trauma. **D**, Physiologic pigmentation of the gingiva (melanosis gingivae).

Papules are circumscribed superficial elevated areas varying in size from a pinhead to about 5 mm. in area. They may be flat, conical, circular, and pointed to umbilicated. They vary in color from red, yellow, and white to bluish-red. The shape of the base may vary from round to more or less polygonal. The most common papule found in the mouth is that of lichen planus. Both the papule and the macule may provoke itching, burning sensations, or pain, or they may produce no symptoms at all either on the skin or on the mucous membrane. The surface may be eroded or overlaid with moist epithelial desquamations. (Fig. 2.)

Nodules are enlarged papules which are usually deep seated and involve the submucosa or lower dermis in the skin. They may also be slightly elevated

A   B

Fig. 2. *Papules*. **A,** Small raised lesion on the tongue due to accidental biting. **B,** Traumatic hyperplasia of a fungiform papilla.

A   B

Fig. 3. *Nodules*. **A,** Resolving granuloma pyogenicum; other similar lesions of varying sizes include reactive lesions such as fibroid epulis, traumatic fibroma, and fibroepithelial papilloma. **B,** Parulis or so-called gumboil associated with pulpitis of the maxillary first molar.

above the surrounding mucosa. They may be traumatic in origin or may be associated with rheumatoid arthritis, leprosy, and syphilis. (Fig. 3.)

Vesicles are circumscribed single or grouped elevations of epithelium of the skin or mucous membrane beneath or within which are collections of serum, plasma, or blood. The surface may be flat, globoid, or umbilicated and may be tense or flaccid in character. Where vesicles have not ruptured spontaneously or as the result of trauma, they may be seen characteristically in primary herpetic stomatitis, herpes simplex, herpes zoster, and varicella. (Fig. 4.)

Pustules are vesicles containing pus predominantly (e.g., impetigo).

Bullae or blebs are similar to vesicles except that bullae are larger and more deep seated and the roof of the cavity is more resistant to rupture than the

A   B

Fig. 4. *Vesicles*. **A,** Note the large vesicle located on the gingiva adjacent to the mandibular right cuspid. Its rupture will leave an ulcer like that seen in Fig. 11, *D;* its size approaches that of a bulla, and it is filled with a somewhat cloudy fluid. **B,** Small vesicle located on the upper lip characteristic of those seen in the early stages of primary herpetic stomatitis.

A   B

Fig. 5. *Bullae*. **A,** Bulla on the lower lip resulting from thermal injury; the character of the lesion differentiates it from a mucous retention cyst. **B,** Like most vesicles or bullae seen in the oral cavity, the one shown here has the collapsed roof; because of the deep involvement, the roof of a bulla tends to remain intact.

vesicle. (Fig. 5.) For this reason they are seen somewhat more frequently as primary lesions than vesicles. Bullae may be seen in pemphigus, Behçet's syndrome, and Stevens-Johnson syndrome or as the sequelae of trauma. The oral mucosa is commonly the first site to be involved in certain types of pemphigus even though the skin may be completely normal. Consequently it may be the alert dentist who may make the original diagnosis. The bullae of pemphigus, unlike the bullae of other disorders such as erythema multiforme, usually do not have an erythematous areola at the border of the lesion. Rubbing a nonvesiculated area may result in the formation of a vesicle or denudation of the mucosa or epidermis (Nikolsky's sign).

Tumor, cyst, epulis, exostosis, torus, papilloma, and polyp are terms which are used to describe variously sized and shaped growths that have the common clinical characteristics of tumescence. (Fig. 6.) These lesions may be reactive or neoplastic in character. Etymologically the term tumor merely means swelling. However, its present-day widespread usage to mean neoplasm or inflammatory

A   B

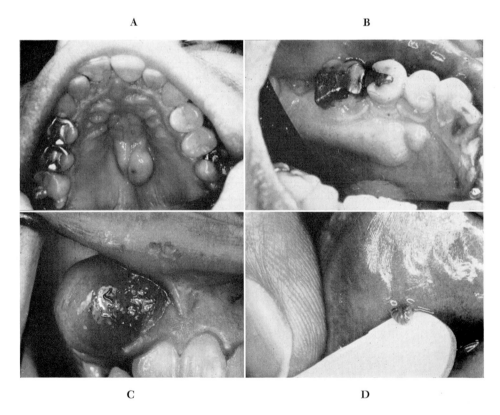

C   D

Fig. 6. *Tumors.* **A,** The lesion on the hard palate is a torus palatinus a blastomatoid lesion. **B,** The same type of bony tumescence on the mandible is called a torus mandibularis. **C,** A large soft tissue mass involving the alveolar mucosa and attached gingiva. The true nature of this type of lesion can only be determined by biopsy; its size clearly denotes its designation as a tumor. **D,** A small fibroepithelial papilloma.

enlargements has led to some confusion. More often than not the term is used to mean neoplastic disease. In view of the many blastomatoid, reactive, or non-neoplastic inflammatory enlargements which are present in the mouth, the use of the term tumor to describe these lesions does not appear to be justified. While many lesions that are generally non-neoplastic in character are characterized by tumescence, their clinical classification as tumors should be reserved until microscopic examination reveals their true identity. The examination of lesions which are characterized by tumescence should be directed toward the history of the lesion and its clinical features.

Thus one may speak of a lesion clinically in terms of tumescence, shape, size, base, surface texture, and the form which it may resemble. Tumefaction or tumidity refers to a swelling or the state of being swollen or edematous. The base of the lesion may be sessile, pedunculated, or stalked: sessile means attached by a broad base; predunculated means that the lesion is provided with a peduncle, pedicle, or a stem; polypoid merely means that the morbid enlargement resembles a polypus which is a broad descriptive term for a smooth and pedunculated epithelial tumor arising from a mucous surface.

The term papilloma refers to a small nipple-shaped epithelial tumor in which the cells cover fingerlike processes of stroma. Papillomatous refers to a morbid enlargement resembling a papilloma. While the terms polyp and papilloma have rather specific microscopic connotations and usually imply tumor in a neoplastic sense, the terms polypoid and papillomatous are somewhat less specific and may be used for clinical description of lesions regardless of their true nature. In general, a polypoid mass is attached by a more or less narrow peduncle and is rather spherical in shape; the attachment of a papillomatous mass is of the same dimensions as the mass itself, which is usually longer than it is wide. The clinical use of polypoid or papillomatoid (papillomatous) should in no way suggest the microscopic diagnosis of polyp or papilloma. The use of the term papillomatous or papillomatoid eliminates the necessity for referring to those non-neoplastic inflammatory enlargements as papillomas which imply a neoplastic character.

The surface of a lesion may be warty (verruciform or verrucous), papillate (filiform or fungiform), keratotic, ulcerated, fissured, or desquamated or flat, pointed, or horny, and the base of a lesion may be sessile or pedunculated.

Keratosis refers to an abnormal thickening of the outer layers of the epithelium of the mucous membrane or the skin. Keratinization of the mucous membranes usually takes place only on the gingiva in the mouth and never reaches the proportion that may be seen on the skin except in pathologic conditions. (Fig. 7.) Keratotic lesions of the mouth may vary in color from grayish-white to white or brown, depending upon the amount of extrinsic pigmentation present. Hyperkeratinization of the mucous membrane may be localized, circumscribed, focal, or diffuse in character. Common keratotic lesions of the mouth include focal hyperkeratosis, nicotine stomatitis, lichen planus, and leukoplakia. Chronic cheek biting, focal hyperkeratosis, and nicotine stomatitis are probably the most common forms of hyperkeratotic lesions in the mouth. Keratosis may be primary in origin, as in lichen planus, or secondary to trauma, as in nicotine sto-

A   B

C   D

Fig. 7. *Keratoses.* **A,** Lichen planus of the gingiva; there is a mild degree of hyper-keratinization present. **B,** Lichen planus of the buccal mucosa; the lacelike network is rather characteristic; only slight hyperkeratinization is present. **C,** Diffuse hyperkeratosis on lingual aspects of the mandible with raised and somewhat smooth surface; this is characteristic of early leukoplakia. **D,** Focal hyperkeratotic lesion presenting a verrucous surface. The malignant possibilities of this type of lesion are obvious; this type of lesion should be biopsied (excisional).

matitis. The latter type of keratinization may be considered as a secondary lesion. (Fig. 8.)

Secondary Lesions.—These lesions are the most common found in the oral cavity and include erosions (excoriations), ulcers, fissures, cicatrices, and desquamations.

Erosions are a kind of ulceration or loss of substance such as that produced on the skin or mucous membrane by trauma or as a sequel to primary lesions. They are usually superficial in nature and may be circumscribed, punctate, linear, or irregular in form. These lesions involve a loss of the outer layers of the mucosa and leave no scar on healing. Erosions in the mouth are usually moist in character and represent the necrosis and loss of the outer layers of the mucous membrane. Thus, moist erosions may be seen secondary to the collapse of vesicles and blebs or following the necrosis of the outer layers of the mucous membrane

A   B

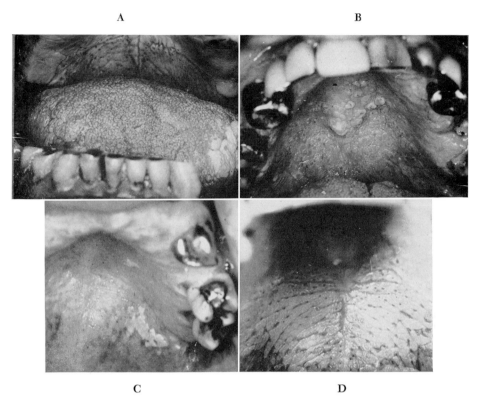

C   D

Fig. 8. *Hyperkeratinization.* **A-D,** Hyperkeratinization associated with nicotine-stomatitis. **B** shows the raised, punctate orifices of the mucous glands.

as in erosive lichen planus, desquamative gingivitis, or following traumatic wounds. (Fig. 9.)

Fissures are any clefts or grooves in the tissue that are normal or pathologically present. They may be superficial or deep, linear, radiating, longitudinal, or transverse. It is not unusual for these cracks or fissures to become inflamed. They occur frequently at the mucocutaneous junction of the mouth where extensibility of the tissue is essential to accomplish the necessary movements of the tissue. (Fig. 10.) Fissuring of the surface of the tongue is seen frequently and is not accompanied with inflammatory change unless the grooves are quite deep and accumulations of debris and bacteria occur. Scrotal tongue, angular cheilitis, and syphilitic rhagades show fissuring.

Ulcers are defects of the skin or mucous membrane which are deeper than erosions or excoriations in that they extend to the tissue beneath the epithelium. Ulcers should be examined for their size, depth, contour, base, edge, floor, secretion, duration, pain, evolution, and involution. The edges of an ulcer may be ragged, punched out in appearance, undermined, or everted. The base may be soft or indurated and its floor smooth, granular, glazed, pus covered, or hemorrhagic. Ulcers may be acute or chronic in nature and may be shallow or deep

Fig. 9. *Erosions.* **A,** Solar cheilitis with linear-shaped erosion. **B,** Retromolar erosion due to cheek chewing. **C,** Ulceration secondary to erythema multiforme bullosum. **D,** Erosion secondary to drug reaction (codeine).

Fig. 10. *Fissure.* Angular cheilitis due to mechanical trauma from a rubber dam.

in character. The outline of the ulcer may be circular, serpiginous, ovoid, crescentic, or irregular. Ulcers may result from physical agents such as heat or cold, chemical agents such as acids or alkalies, traumatic agents such as sharp teeth, dry toast, toothbrush bristles, or foreign objects in the mouth. They may appear secondarily to primary lesions or as a result of disease, either local or systemic in origin. Ulcers may be painless or indolent, or they may be extremely sensitive. Ulcers in the mouth are seen most commonly in association with acute necrotizing ulcerative gingivitis, herpetic gingivostomatitis, and herpes simplex and as a result of traumatic agents. (Figs. 11-13.)

Pseudomembranes may form on the mucosal surfaces as a result of pseudomembranous inflammation. The formation of a false membrane is a response of the mucous surfaces to a necrotizing agent. Because of the loss of surface epithelium, plasma exudes from the vessels and spreads on the eroded surface where it coagulates, enclosing necrotic epithelium in its fibrinous network. This occurs in acute necrotizing ulcerative gingivostomatitis; it may also be seen in diphtheria (Fig. 12, *C* and *D*).

Eschars are masses of dead tissue or sloughs produced by burning or chemi-

A   B

C   D

Fig. 11. *Ulcers.* **A,** Traumatic ulcer from biting the tongue—healing stage. **B,** Persistent traumatic ulcer with superimposed pyogenic infection. **C** and **D,** Recurrent herpetic ulcers.

A   B

C   D

Fig. 12. *Ulcers.* **A,** Periadenitis mucosae necrotica recurrens—early healing phase. **B,** Periadenitis—late healing phase. **C,** Acute necrotizing ulcerative gingivostomatitis. **D,** Acute necrotizing ulcerative gingivostomatitis—palatal lesion.

cal corrosives. Phenol and cresol may cause a firm, thick, dull-gray to brown eschar. "Aspirin burn" and phenol eschar appear white initially. Loss of the necrotic tissue leads to an ulcer. The laying down of fibrin on the injured surfaces may lead to a pseudomembrane. Phenol and "aspirin" eschars are the most common type seen in the mouth (Fig. 13, *A* and *B*).

Desquamation is a shedding of epithelial elements in scales or sheets which vary in size and shape and which may or may not cover an erosion. In general, scales occur as a result of inflammation. In the mouth, scales do not tend to accumulate as on the skin but are lost because of the continual wetting by the saliva. However, certain lesions such as leukoplakia and focal hyperkeratosis accumulate thick shiny masses of scales which give the lesion a grayish-white color. (Fig. 14.)

Crusts are the dry products of exudates from lesions occurring on the skin and lips. They do not usually appear in the mouth because of the maceration by saliva; however, they may be associated with scales and are termed moist desquamations. Crusts of the skin and lips are composed of pus, blood, dried serum, epithelial debris, and extraneous matter. The color varies according to the composition of the crust and may be yellowish to brown, depending upon the amount of pus or blood present. Crusts on the skin may be deep seated or superficial, while those of the lips tend to be superficial in character. Crusting appears most often on the lips of individuals exposed to the weather. Constant drying leads to crusting of lesions present on the lips. Such crusts tend to crack, fissure, and bleed because of the constant trauma associated with speaking and mastication. Crusts are seen commonly at the mucocutaneous junction of the lips in angular cheilitis, vesicular and bullous lesions, traumatic ulcers, and carcinomas. (Fig. 15.)

Crusts form only if conditions permit drying of coagulated blood, tissue fluids, and debris. Crusting does not occur on the moist surfaces of the mucous membranes; however, if the blood, serum, and debris become coagulated and entrapped in a fibrinous meshwork, a moist membranelike mass may cover an eroded surface. This may generally be scraped away to leave a bleeding surface. The surfaces of vesicles and bullae may collapse and cover the underlying tissue; they may be adherent or slough off in a short period of time. When the

A   B

C

Fig. 13. *Eschars.* A, Coagulation of buccal gingiva by phenol. B, Aspirin-induced mucosal necrosis; note two areas of contact, one on gingiva and one on buccal mucosa. C, Herpetic ulcer with secondary slough produced by silver nitrate.

A   B

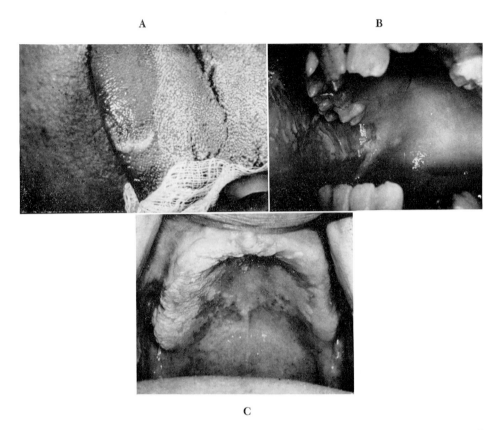

C

Fig. 14. *Desquamation.* **A,** Geographic tongue. **B,** Desquamative parakeratosis associated with cheek chewing. **C,** Desquamative hyperkeratosis associated with heavy smoking.

A   B

Fig. 15. *Crusts.* **A,** Syphilitic chancre; note deformity of the lip and serosanguinous crust. **B,** Crusted herpes labialis; note the conglomerate character of the lesion.

membranelike covering is lost, bleeding occurs, and a new pseudomembrane is formed (Fig. 13, *C*).

In addition to having an abstract descriptive knowledge of primary and secondary lesions, an examiner should also be able to detect and describe any lesion present in the mouth. Before a lesion can be related to one of the primary or secondary types of lesions, a systematic examination of the lesion must be made. First, it must be determined whether the present appearance of the lesion represents a lesion in its pure form (natural history), or if it is the result of involution or additional complications such as scratching, treatment, or injury, and whether multiple lesions are generalized or local in character. In addition, the color, shape, size, arrangement, base, and consistency of lesions should be noted carefully. When the objective symptoms are described, it is then possible to identify a lesion as a primary or secondary type of lesion. When the student becomes aware of basic differences in lesions of the oral cavity and is able to describe those lesions which are present, he will be able to utilize effectively the subjective information collected from the history and those facts collected in the clinical examination so that little difficulty will be experienced in arriving at a diagnosis. A knowledge of the type of presenting lesion does not unequivocally designate a specific disease. However, it does serve to orient the examiner to a particular field of inquiry that may in itself be narrow enough to permit a relatively easy differential diagnosis. For example, when an examiner identifies the presence of a predominating vesicular or bullous eruption, he knows in a broad sense that he may be dealing with a virus infection. Many diseases of viral origin can be named, but it is not our purpose here to do so since these can be found in almost any text of oral medicine or internal medicine; rather it is suggested that the examiner should at this time analyze his subjective and objective findings. Thus it might have been said that examples of virus infections are chickenpox, smallpox, herpes zoster, herpes labialis, and other distributions of herpetic eruptions. However, it must be remembered that physical agents such as poison ivy, poison, metals, or other irritative allergenic agents may also produce vesicles. Further, local parasites, infections such as impetigo, vesicular eczema, and scabies may also produce vesicular lesions. It is not expected that the student of oral diagnosis will be familiar with all possible diseases which may have vesicular eruptions, nor is it necessary to expect it since effective and efficient use of reference material allows a diagnosis to be made and at the same time enhances the training of the examiner.

REFERENCES

Adson, A. W.: Neuralgias of the Face; Diagnosis and Treatment, J. Internat. Coll. Surgeons 11:1-8, 1948.

Agnew, R. G., and others: Pain Problems in the Practice of Dentistry: A Symposium, J.A.D.A. 53:528-542, 1956.

Barison, H. L., and Wang, S. C.: Physiology and Pharmacology of Vomiting, Pharmacol. Rev. 5:193, 1953.

Bondy, Philip K.: Gain and Loss of Weight. In Harrison, T. R. (editor), Principles of Internal Medicine, New York, 1954, The Blakiston Co., Chap. 24.

Bonica, John J.: Management of Pain, Philadelphia, 1953, Lea & Febiger.

Christie, R. V.: Dyspnea: A Review, Quart. J. Med. **7**:421, 1938.

Cushing, H.: The Major Trigeminal Neuralgias: The Varieties of Facial Neuralgia, Am. J. M. Sc. **160**:157, 1920.

DuBois, E. F.: Fever and Regulation of Body Temperature, Springfield, Ill., 1948, Charles C Thomas, Publisher.

Engel, G. L.: Fainting, J. Mt. Sinai Hosp. **12**:170, 1945.

Friedman, Meyer: Functional Cardiovascular Disease, Baltimore, 1947, Williams & Wilkins Co.

Harrison, T. R. (editor): Principles of Internal Medicine; Part II, Cardinal Manifestations of Disease, New York, 1954, The Blakiston Co.

Lozner, E. L.: Differential Diagnosis, Pathogenesis, and Treatment of Thrombocytopenic Purpuras, Am. J. Med. **14**:459, 1953.

McAuliff, G. W., Goodell, H., and Wolff, H. G.: Experimental Studies on Headache; Pain From the Nasal and Paranasal Structures, Proc. A. Res. Nerv. & Ment. Dis. **23**:185, 1943.

Robertson, S., Goodell, H., and Wolff, H. G.: Headache: The Teeth as a Source of Headache and Other Pain, Arch. Neurol. & Psychiat. **57**:277, 1947.

Stead, E. A.: Fainting, Am. J. Med. **13**:387, 1952.

Ungerleider, H. E., and Gubner, R.: Extrasystoles and the Mechanism of Palpitation, Tr. Am. Therap. Soc. **41**:1, 1941.

Wolff, H. G.: Headache and Other Head Pain, New York, 1948, Oxford University Press.

Wolff, H. G., and Wolf, S.: Pain, Springfield, Ill., 1948, Charles C Thomas, Publisher.

Case history

Taking a history is probably one of the most important parts of the examination of a patient, yet it is generally the least understood and most undervalued prerequisite to the process of formulating a diagnosis that exists today in the practice and teaching of clinical dentistry. The case history constitutes the foundation not only for an intelligent approach to diagnosis, but also for the establishment of a successful patient-dentist relationship. Only from an accurately taken and carefully interpreted history can diverse symptoms of disease be grouped into a meaningful pattern. All too often a diagnosis or the chance to prevent gross pathologic alterations by disease is missed because the examiner fails to uncover the earliest and detectable clues to disease. This may be largely avoided if the subjective sensations of the patient are brought out in a history. To attempt to make a diagnosis without systematically utilizing the patient's knowledge of the disease is not unlike the proverbial stories about a ship without a rudder.

There are occasions when it appears that a diagnosis is plainly evident by inspection alone; however, three important considerations are likely to be overlooked without at least a brief history: (1) coexistent disease may be present that will go undetected unless the patient is allowed to express his complaints; (2) the attitude of the patient, which is so important to the establishment of rapport, is often disregarded; and (3) all too often a diagnosis may appear to be obvious, yet it may be masking a serious and extensive disease.

A case history need not be extensive; it may consist of only a few questions if adequate coverage is thereby provided. However, it must be pointed out that the art of taking a history entails a knowledge of how extensive a history should be for any given occasion. This ability requires practice, and the diagnostic acumen of a clinician is generally directly related to his ability as a historian. There are at least two instances when a case history should be extensive, detailed, and arranged not only to cover the patient's immediate complaint, but also to include all historical facts relating to the patient's oral and systemic health: (1) all case histories which are being taken by a student for training in oral diagnosis should be as complete as possible until such time as he demonstrates his ability to reduce the length and coverage, yet still have an adequate history, and (2) a case history which is to be the basis for periodic follow-up health examinations should initially be as thorough and complete as possible irrespective of no apparent relationship to the patient's complaint.

The approach to the patient is as important to the case history as the interpretation of the findings, since the information obtained is dependent upon the proper rapport between the patient and the clinician.

Obtaining a case history is a procedure which requires the utilization of all the knowledge and experience a dentist has accumulated from his basic science and clinical training. The history is often called the subjective examination of the patient since it contains information which the patient tells the historian. Each case history presents the dentist with circumstances which are unlike any of his other cases, yet similarity between cases is often the basis for sound judgment and diagnosis. Obtaining a history provides the dentist with an opportunity to hear the patient's complaints and symptoms and also to determine his general health and well-being. It provides clues to diagnosis, focuses attention to specific areas in need of comprehensive evaluation, and alerts the dentist to the need of special precautions he must use in carrying out treatment procedures.

A case history should be brief and concise, yet it should contain all of the information required by a given situation. Unfortunately, no short cut is available for the inexperienced historian to assure brevity and accuracy; however, a uniform procedure will ensure the inclusion of all the necessary details. The historian must direct the patient toward the subject at hand at all times, condensing and sorting the pertinent information from the irrelevant. A history that is lengthy and poorly organized is a time-wasting procedure and usually discourages further efforts.

The procedure is primarily a diagnostic effort; however, most patients will be favorably impressed with the interest shown in their health by the dentist. The confidence of the patient is often won during the first meeting with the patient, and, since the history is usually taken on the patient's first visit to the dentist, it provides the dentist with an adequate opportunity to develop proper rapport with his patient. While primarily a diagnostic procedure, a thorough, well-written case history often serves as evidence of professional competence in medicolegal cases. Errors of treatment by the dentist vary from those which cause minor inconvenience to the patient to those of a very serious nature, and most of the errors may be predicted from information in the case history.

There should be no necessity for justifying history taking. As a diagnostic procedure it is invaluable, as a legal aid it is important, and as a factor in the improvement of patient relations it is most satisfying.

A clear understanding of the objectives of a case history will guide and improve the efforts of any practitioner: (1) to arrive at a tentative diagnosis of the patient's chief complaint, (2) to determine any systemic factor which might affect the formulation of a diagnosis, and (3) to determine any systemic condition requiring special precaution prior to or during dental procedures to protect the health and life of the patient. Advantages of obtaining a case history include establishment of a written record which will serve as a diagnostic instrument; protection of the dentist from possible disease contact; establishment of a basis for future reference; and provision of a document which will serve as legal evidence of professional competence.

The basic method for history taking is that of the direct interview with the patient. In the direct interview the historian questions the patient in an orderly fashion, following a basic pattern of questions. He makes notes during the interview and afterward compiles the important information he has obtained. Other methods have been devised which are intended to decrease the time needed for the interview. Two such timesaving methods are the use of a printed questionnaire and the use of a printed check list of information. Whatever the method used, it must serve the purpose of obtaining important information.

APPROACH TO THE PATIENT

The technic of history taking involves the dentist's initial behavior with the patient and the development of rapport with the patient. The interview should be more than the mere recording of answers to a set of questions; it must establish confidence and induce the patient to reveal eventually all the details relative to his or her illness. The attitude of the examiner must impart to his patient that he is not hurried and that he is completely interested in the patient's welfare. In order to establish confidence, the examiner must be patient and sympathetic and explain all the factors relative to any question he is asking; he must never express surprise or shock at anything the patient may reveal, and he must be able to talk in terms that the patient will understand and feel at ease with. If the patient appears to be embarrassed, shows evidence of emotion, or hesitates to answer a question, it is obvious that the question touches strongly on the patient's emotional life and probably will have to be delayed until a later time. The examiner should sympathetically endeavor to have the patient express his complaints in simple language unadorned by a self-diagnosis derived from past experiences of friends.

In order to examine children it is necessary to gain their confidence. Initially, too much attention should not be given to the child, and it helps to place children at ease in the dental office if the dentist appears busy. Questions of a general nature may be asked first to establish the interest of the child, and then later, when this has been accomplished, questions relating to the history may be asked more effectively. Questions regarding the chief complaint and the present illness are better answered by the child, whereas questions regarding past history, family history, and social history are best answered in cooperation with a parent.

PLAN OF HISTORY TAKING

The taking of a history should be systematic and should follow a definite outline. Following a definite order either mentally or with a written outline tends to prevent the omission of pertinent information that might otherwise be forgotten. By placing the patient's complaint first, the patient is permitted to recount the complaint and symptoms that brought him to the examiner. The following outline is one which is commonly used in taking a history:

Chief Complaint
Usually the answer to the question, "What prompted you to seek dental treatment?"; should be limited to a word, phrase, or sentence

Present Illness
Chronologic account of the patient's chief complaint and related symptoms; should include all relevant material since the time of onset of the complaint

Past History
All material of a nature to reveal the patient's dental and general health prior to the onset of the present illness; should include constitutional diseases, serious illnesses, manifestations of allergic states, and accidents or operations

Family History
General health of family, history of mental disease, cause of death of parents if deceased, history of chronic infectious diseases in the family, history of dental problems in the family, etc.

Personal and Social History
Marital status: Duration, health of partners, pregnancies, number of children, etc.
Habits: Use of drugs and medicines, tobacco, biting habits, and other oral habits
Occupation: Exposure to occupation hazards, working schedule as related to dental appointments, type of work, etc.
Personality: Moody, inclined to worry, complaining, meticulous, sociable, easygoing, etc.
Weight: Recent loss or gain of weight with possible causes

Systems Review
Head:
>   Headache
>   Eyes: Vision, diplopia, inflammatory disease
>   Ears: Hearing, tinnitus, vertigo
>   Nose: Obstruction, epistaxis, frequent "colds"
>   Throat: Hoarseness, tonsillitis, sore throat

Cardiorespiratory: Chest pain, dyspnea, orthopnea, angina, palpitations, murmurs, hemoptysis, cough, night sweats, rheumatic fever

Gastrointestinal: Digestion, mastication, sore tongue, sore gums, saliva, occlusion, toothaches, devitalization of teeth, extractions, appliances, pyorrhea, nausea, vomiting, diarrhea, and abdominal pain

Genitourinary: Dysuria, nocturia, hematuria, oliguria, polyuria, edema

Catamenia: Menopause, menorrhagia, metrorrhagia, dysmenorrhea, menarche

Neuromuscular: Paresthesia, anesthesia, paralysis, convulsions, neuralgias, arthritis, joint pains, limitation of motion, tremors, luxation and subluxation of mandible, centric relation, centric occlusion, closure pattern

The case history should follow this or a similar outline so that the examiner covers a certain minimum field of information which in itself may call attention to the patient's symptoms and significant items of past history as well as facilitate the oral interview and establish rapport with the patient. The following elaboration of the outline has for its objective the presentation of all the facts that may have influenced the patient's health up to the time of the interview.

Chief Complaint(s), Symptom(s)

The chief complaint (C. C.) is a symptom or symptoms described by the patient in his own words relating to the presence of an abnormal condition. It is not necessarily answered by the question, "Why did you come to the dental clinic?" because the patient's answer may be, "I need a checkup," "I want a bridge," or "My dentist told me to come." These should not be used as chief complaints because they are not symptoms. There is usually a reason *why* a patient believes he needs a checkup, a filling, or a bridge, or a reason *why* he has been referred by a dentist or physician. The chief complaint(s) is subjective in nature and is related to an uncomfortable or abnormal sensation. It is necessary that the chief complaint be a symptom because complaints expressed as symptoms leave no room for doubt regarding the patient's problem. Using expressions of desire or discontent for the chief complaint allows the patient to assume that the examiner knows why he wants a filling or a new plate, and also allows the patient to establish his own diagnosis and treatment plan. If the examiner attempts to use the statement, "I came for a checkup," he is faced with the enigma of analyzing his chief complaint in terms of date of onset, type of onset, location, character, and related symptoms. A chief complaint is the patient's expression of disease, and that disease is what is to be treated—not the patient's diagnosis or desire.

It is quite possible that the patient has no chief complaint. This is a significant finding and should be recorded. However, a complaint may not be easily elicited or easily described, or it may not be of such magnitude that it can be localized by the patient, since people vary in their ability to accommodate for abnormal conditions. Such conditions as bleeding gums, bad taste, rough teeth, or vague pain which may have been troublesome to the patient at first may later become unapparent as he becomes accustomed to the symptoms. Symptoms of toothache and periodontal abscesses may be foremost in the patient's complaint, yet mask the symptoms of a more generalized disease. It is possible to overlook a chief complaint because the patient is not familiar with diagnosis or treatment procedures and is under the misconception that the examiner is aware of the condition causing his trouble.

Shaping the Complaint.—Since the patient does not express his discomfort or distress in terms of scientific symptomatology, many times it takes insight and ability on the part of the examiner to analyze the complaint, and he may be called on to use all his skill in order to arrive at the exact nature of the symptom. When a complaint lacks the scientific details of formal symptom terminology, it has to be interpreted scientifically and accurately by the dentist if he is to find a rational basis for a diagnosis. The interpretation of the complaint and its conversion into more precise usable information are salient features of making a diagnosis.

The complaint which a patient makes to the dentist may be invested with special meanings and associations above and beyond the meaning given to more scientific definitions. It may be shaped by past experiences and by cultural and circumstantial forces. If a patient has had past experience with a symptom occurring in a particular disease, similar symptoms will cause the patient's complaint to be unconsciously molded by the comparative situation.

In order for a patient to have a complaint, he must be aware of some abnormal disturbance. This awareness varies from one individual to another. At what intensity of distress the patient will make his complaint known to the dentist depends upon the individual and upon many other factors such as age, stress, preoccupation, health, fatigue, social custom, perception, and past experience. A complaint may be couched in terms of location, dysfunction, or the extent of incapacitation that results from the disturbance. Either consciously or unconsciously many patients will try to fool not only themselves, but also their dentists regarding complaints for fear that some disturbance will be found which is greater than they are prepared to accept. It must be remembered that patients' complaints are usually not objective; they are almost always colored by biased opinions.

The reaction of a patient to a particular symptom may vary with his mental attitude or preoccupation. For example, a toothache during a student's examination period may cause considerable distraction, whereas the same toothache may produce very little distraction at a time when he is enjoying himself, or he may be able to tolerate the pain well during the examination period but become quite distraught when required to wait a short time for treatment. The perception of a symptom may be acute for one patient, yet a symptom of the same intensity may be of no importance to another.

Another factor which may shape the complaint is the inability of the patient to communicate his abnormal experience to the examiner. This may be due to the patient's lack of ability to express himself or to the fact that he has never experienced such symptoms previously and lacks terminology for an adequate description of his symptoms or complaint. While it is true that the lay and dental vocabulary are different, the dentist may give considerable help to the patient by assisting in the proper use of comparisons. However, the tendency to lead a patient to an incorrect history must be guarded against. Many times patients will complain of poorly defined sensations, e.g., a vague sensation in the back part of the mouth, pressure on the chest, a feeling that one side of the mouth is higher than the other, and the like. In these instances the dentist should help the patient by suggesting the proper descriptive terms. Gestures, facial expressions, bodily attitudes, and physical demonstrations by the patient represent his inability to express himself, but they are actually a part of his means of communication.

It should be remembered that the complaint is also shaped by the memory of the patient. Many times he forgets the symptom itself and recalls only his reaction to it. This is probably because the psychic component of distress is often so much more upsetting than any physiologic manifestation of disease. The complaint may be complicated by the fact that some individuals feel that to complain about anything even in the most diminutive fashion will brand them as a coward or as a malingerer. Many patients feel that a visit to the dentist for anything except the most dire toothache is to be avoided; as far as they are concerned, a visit to the dentist is only a step toward a full denture.

The age of the patient apparently influences the quality of the complaint. Young children are usually more concerned about what is going to happen to them than they are about any particular discomfort they may have. Other patients, while they may be concerned about their discomfort, are probably more concerned with the significance of the symptoms. It would appear that adolescents are more concerned with their activities, such as examinations, classes, dates, and ball games, than with describing any discomfort unless it is of an acute nature. Even in acute problems they are usually more concerned with what is going to be done than with relating what their problem is. While it is usually true that younger patients have keener symptom perception than older people, they are less able to describe their symptoms. On the other hand, while elderly patients may be dulled in their mental processes, they are much better able to tell the dentist about their troubles because of experience in expressing themselves and past experience with symptoms.

The prestige of the dentist and his demeanor may also shape the quality of the complaint. It is not uncommon for patients to assume that the dentist is well aware of their complaint and will need but a minimum of information from them. Many times older patients are reluctant to give a young examiner anything but a cursory review of their disturbance, especially in a system review if they do not understand its intent. On the other hand, many patients feel that a young examiner does not have much experience and needs all the assistance they can give him. Some persons feel that gray hair and age are expressions of experience and ability and that no help from them is needed by a sage to make a diagnosis of their ailments.

The examiner must be quick to assess the feelings of the patient regarding his approach to them and must be ready to adjust to that type of patient-dentist relationship and examination which will establish the greatest harmonious relation. The dentist who rigidly approaches all patients in the same way will be successful only with those who appreciate his particular personality and methods.

The complaint may be shaped in one direction if the patient finds that his examiner is sympathetic, but it may be shaped in an entirely different way if he finds there is no expression of sympathy. However, an over sympathetic examiner may have to listen to much irrelevant material. Some patients do not resent a matter-of-fact approach to their initial complaint, while others deeply resist this approach and seek to channel their complaints to a more receptive mood on the part of the examiner. Many patients seek confirmation of their complaints and an authoritative acquiescence from the examiner and, when these are not forthcoming, choose another complaint in the hope that the new complaint will be confirmed.

When a patient knows a disease exists and has had some experience with it in the past, he is likely to interpret all his symptoms in terms of this known disease. Thus a patient who has a knowledge of an impacted asymptomatic molar may attribute any symptom relative to his teeth or jaws to the impaction and shape his complaint in terms of this abnormality. The patient who has been told at some time that he has heart disease is likely to be especially reactive to palpitations and to describe them in terms all out of proportion to their significance and severity.

The publicity given to certain diseases for the purpose of educating the public in the early recognition of the disease may also affect the complaint. It is not infrequent for patients to become aware of an innocuous lesion of the mouth such as lichen planus and to attribute imaginary changes in the lesion to cancer simply because they are afraid of cancer. Since such diseases as pyorrhea, syphilis, gonorrhea, and tuberculosis are not considered to be socially acceptable, many patients are reluctant to couch their complaint in terms that might draw attention to these diseases; instead, they let the examiner find out for himself a history or symptoms of these diseases. Also, many patients steer clear of all symptoms which might suggest a serious or hopeless significance. It may be only after a great interval of time or until the distress has become acute that the patient is willing to make known his complaints. In many instances in which a particular diagnosis is feared, a patient may attempt to hide or disguise the salient symptoms (e.g., symptoms such as dysphagia associated with cancer phobia) or present them in such a way as to keep the examiner from making the feared diagnosis. Some patients apparently nurture symptoms which are more attractive to them, and at the same time they tend to minimize in their mind symptoms less acceptable to them even though they know them to be more significant. For example, there are patients who believe that the esthetic result of a particular appliance is not in keeping with their own views, yet, in the opinion of the experienced prosthodontist, the results obtained are the best possible for that patient. Such patients may complain severely of malfitting dentures with the hope that their continued distress and complaint will force the prosthodontist to remake an appliance with the esthetic result they think is more suitable to them. Not infrequently, older patients with full dentures think they should have "white pearly teeth" like those of young movie stars.

The duration of the complaint is of considerable significance. The time it takes for a disease process to develop affects the complaint expressed to the examiner at the time of the examination. The patient has difficulty in remembering early symptoms and is concerned with more recent symptoms which may be of a more severe nature. His inability to locate the symptoms is also significant. Those symptoms which are well localized usually tend to be well defined by the patient. On the other hand, those which are diffuse, radiating, and seem to travel are difficult for him to define clearly. It must be remembered that poorly defined symptoms may be organic or psychogenic in origin. A patient may complain of an uncomfortable feeling in his teeth and about gnashing of the teeth (bruxism) and yet be completely unaware of other symptoms of psychogenic origin.

Educated complaints are difficult to assess. Those patients who have a knowledge of the symptoms of a particular disease may shape their complaint to correspond with the symptoms of that disease. This occurs frequently with self-diagnosis and when a friend has had the same symptoms. The frequency, duration, and magnitude of symptoms appreciably affect the complaint given to the examiner. For example, an occasional mild pain of short duration in a tooth is often considered inconsequential, whereas continuous pain of the same intensity that interferes with working, sleeping, or pleasure is considered consequential.

It is necessary to determine the patient's chief complaint because it is his immediate and chief concern. It is also the basis for determining the remainder of the history and the treatment plan. The chief complaint is not necessarily the patient's latest complaint and is never a diagnosis. An analysis of one or more chief complaints and their mode, time of onset, course of development, character, and related symptoms constitute that part of the history termed present illness.

Present Illness

The present illness (P. I.) is a chronologic account of the chief complaint and associated symptoms from the time of onset to the time the history is taken. New complaints in the order of their appearance and relation to the chief complaint should be recorded. When possible, quantitative statements should be made, e.g., "pain of toothache severe enough to keep patient from sleeping, from eating, from working;" "dyspnea after climbing one flight of stairs though previous climbing brought no onset of symptoms;" "pain sharp and lancinating in character, constant, and associated with chewing food."

The first statement should be a brief account of the date of onset of the chief complaint, type of onset, character, location, relation to other activities such as movement, eating, sleeping, cold, heat, reading, etc., and association with the complications.

Each symptom should be expanded by detailed inquiry concerning development and relation to other symptoms in the same system in which the complaint lies; e.g., if sore tongue is a symptom, an attempt should be made to determine whether or not any symptoms associated with this disorder are present that may be suggestive of systemic disease such as pernicious anemia. One may suspect congenital syphilis when the patient complains of the poor esthetic quality of a notched incisor, but the presence of other associated signs and symptoms such as mulberry molars, interstitial keratitis, deafness, mouth rhagades, saddle nose, and family history should be investigated before suggesting a diagnosis of syphilis.

Negative as well as positive symptoms should be listed in order to more fully establish the identity and severity of disease. For example, a tooth that has previously reacted painfully to cold and then to "hot" and then reacts neither to "hot" nor cold suggests pulp necrosis. If diabetes mellitus is considered an associated factor, other positive signs and symptoms such as polyphagia, polydipsia, polyuria, predisposition to pyogenic infections, periodontal abscesses, and decreased salivation should be investigated. The present illness record should include the patient's personal reaction to a disease. When the life of the patient is not at stake, he may not view the disease with any great concern. The treatment of such persons sometimes presents a problem because of the lack of cooperation. The treatment plan and prognosis may have to be modified to meet the existing conditions. The present illness record should also include constitutional symptoms such as recent loss or gain of weight, fatigue, fever, night sweats, and a statement from the patient as to the probable cause.

Previous diagnoses, medications, and treatment related to the chief complaint should be described as to form, intended purpose when known, and apparent effect. Just as the existence of a previous diagnosis and treatment of tuberculosis of the lung have a bearing on chest surgery, the previous diagnosis and treatment of Vincent's infection will have a bearing on the diagnosis and treatment of existing periodontal disease. The patient's adjustment to his environment and the effect of his disease on personal relationships should be mentioned briefly in the present illness and expanded in the social history. It is important to know why the patient came to you, why he was referred, what he had been told to expect, and what he believes to be the cause of his chief complaint.

A comprehensive and valuable write-up of the present illness necessitates a good basic knowledge of diseases of the oral cavity so that the interviewer is able to trace out leads given him by the patient during the interview. In many cases the historian will have considered some possibilities of the diagnosis during the interview which will direct his questioning. The possibilities considered must be both from the standpoint of elimination as a diagnosis and from the standpoint of requiring further investigation. Since the present illness deals with the details of the chief complaint, adequate time and careful questioning at this point in obtaining the history may save time and disappointment.

Past History

For the purpose of simplicity it is well for the dentist to consider the past history in two parts: the past dental history and the past medical history.

Dental History.—The past dental history, or a patient's past history of dental treatment, often provides the dentist with valuable prognostic, as well as diagnostic, information. In obtaining such a history, the historian must always be aware of how the patient is presenting the story. Patients who have been dissatisfied with dental treatment in the past often distort a history and lead the historian to believe that they have been victims of a series of incompetent dentists when in reality they have been indifferent and neglectful toward their dental health. In most cases patients will be willing and cooperative at this point in the interview, since it is their opportunity to tell of their dental experiences. It is also an excellent opportunity for the dentist to determine the reactions of patients to dentistry in general and more specifically to the procedures which they have experienced in the past.

The following is a list of details which should be investigated in the past dental history.

OUTLINE OF PAST DENTAL HISTORY

1. Frequency of visits to a dentist
2. Frequency of dental prophylaxis
3. Past experience during and following local anesthesia
4. Past experience during and following extractions
5. Past periodontal therapy, the condition which required the therapy, and the type

of treatment which was given (scaling, occlusal adjustment, subgingival curettage, gingivectomy, and drug application)

6. Past orthodontic treatment: a positive history should include the condition which was treated, the length of time of active treatment, the nature of the appliances used in treatment, and whether a retainer is still required
7. Dental appliance history: length of time appliance worn, whether or not modified such as rebase or addition of teeth, personal care of appliance
8. Fixed bridges: length of service, comfort, modifications
9. Fixed canal fillings: length of time present, apicoectomy
10. Surgical procedures in and about the mouth other than extractions, nature of the tissue removed, manner in which it was removed, recurrences

The frequency with which a patient is accustomed to visiting a dentist provides the historian with information regarding the interest of the patient in his dental health. The frequency of dental prophylaxis may be a valuable guide in evaluating periodontal conditions which are present and provides the dentist with prognostic information. A knowledge of a patient's past experience during and following the administration of a local anesthetic may alert the dentist to the necessity for investigation into possible allergy to the anesthetic agent, or such information may allow him to anticipate possible syncope during the administration of local anesthetics in future appointments.

Patients who have had extractions must always be questioned regarding the healing process and whether or not they experienced any excessive hemorrhage following the extraction. Of particular interest are those individuals who have experienced prolonged bleeding and infections following extractions. In such patients it may be necessary to obtain further systemic evaluation before proceeding with additional extractions.

A patient who gives a history of periodontal therapy should be questioned regarding the type of treatment and the time in the past it was received. The particulars of the type of treatment should be obtained so that the present status of the periodontal structures can be adequately evaluated. The patient should be questioned specifically about whether or not the treatment included complete scaling, occlusal adjustment, or surgery. In many cases it will be found that treatment consisted only of drug applications; insofar as possible, the type of drug used should be determined. The planning of future periodontal treatment for a patient who gives a history of previous treatment may depend largely upon the type of treatment the patient states he has received previously and the present clinical status of his periodontal tissues.

A patient giving a history of orthodontic treatment may present clinical findings which will be explained on the basis of the past treatment. An example of such a clinical situation would be the finding of root resorption on the dental radiographs of a patient who has had orthodontic treatment. If a retainer is still required, the patient should be questioned closely as to whether or not he follows instructions in the use of the retainer.

In obtaining a history from a patient who wears a removable dental appliance, such as a partial denture or a removable bridge, it is important to get a detailed account of the length of service of the appliance, whether or not the original appliance is being worn, and whether modifications have been required as the result of neglect on the part of the patient. It is just as important to determine from the partially edentulous patient who does not present with an appliance in his mouth whether or not he has ever worn a removable appliance. Many such patients are unable to tolerate the appliance either because of discomfort or because of a defective appliance. Patients who wear complete dentures offer a special problem in history taking. They should be questioned about the cause of the loss of their natural teeth and as to whether the original complete denture was placed immediately or whether the edentulous ridges were allowed to heal for a period of six weeks to a month before the dentures were inserted. In patients in whom the original complete denture was inserted immediately, it is important to determine whether the denture has been rebased since it was originally placed.

While questioning the patient about his past dental history, the dentist is afforded the opportunity of gaining insight into the patient's interest and attitude toward dental health. The patient 50 years of age or older whose oral reconstruction is a choice between complete dentures and partial dentures may be a better candidate for complete dentures if his past dental history shows that he has taken little interest in the care of his mouth at any time in his life. The past dental history of a patient may, in many cases, provide information which is the deciding factor as to the type of treatment that is to be rendered that patient. When existing conditions are dependent upon past treatment, the diagnostic value of the past dental history cannot be overestimated.

Medical History.—The past medical history is that part of a patient's health history which is related to past systemic diseases, injuries, and operations; it may be related directly or indirectly to dental treatment. If the dentist is ever to perform a lifesaving act in his practice of dentistry, his best opportunity will present itself when he takes a careful past medical history. Many of the procedures carried out in dental practice and many drugs prescribed in dental practice are potentially fatal to certain patients. It is the moral, ethical, and legal responsibility of the dentist to determine who these patients are so that he may take the necessary precautions during dental procedures or avoid the use of certain drugs which may have a harmful effect on the patient.

In general the past medical history contains information relative to childhood diseases and their sequelae, serious illness, injuries and operations, irradiation, and allergy.

Childhood Diseases.—A history of rheumatic fever may be listed under childhood diseases although the disease is known to occur in adulthood. The importance of a history of rheumatic fever cannot be overemphasized. It is important for the dentist to have a good fundamental knowledge of the clinical manifestations of rheumatic fever so that he may question his patients intelligently when a history of the disease is suspected. Rheumatic fever has varying degrees of severity; however, the degree of severity of the initial disease cannot be directly related to the residual damage left by the disease. The residual effect of rheumatic fever which is of primary interest to the dentist is endocardial damage. Such damage is usually located at the mitral valve so that in many cases stenosis of the mitral valve becomes a cardinal sign of the sequelae of the disease. The fact that the mitral valve (and at times the aortic valve) is often involved makes it possible for the physician to hear a murmur when auscultating the heart. These murmurs are usually quite characteristic and indicative of damage produced by rheumatic fever. However, it is conceivable that the damage produced by rheumatic fever could be mild enough so as not to produce changes in the endocardium which would result in a heart murmur. This presents somewhat of a dilemma to the dentist in trying to determine whether or not to carry out prophylactic measures which are indicated because of a history of rheumatic fever. In such cases the conservative procedure is to carry out the prescribed prophylactic measures.

It has been known for many years that dental extraction and prophylaxis are quite frequently related to subacute bacterial endocarditis (Horder). Subacute bacterial endocarditis (S.B.E.) almost always occurs in individuals who have a history of rheumatic fever or congenital heart disease. Prior to the advent of penicillin and the other antibiotics employed in its treatment, subacute bacterial endocarditis was considered to be a fatal disease within a period of one year. At the present time, while the number of fatalities has been decreased as a result of the use of antibiotics, the disease is still taking the lives of approximately 18 per cent of those who develop it. Various studies indicate that the disease is precipitated by a number of causes, all of which permit the entrance of microorganisms into the blood stream. Included among the various modes of entry into the blood are dental extraction, prophylaxis, vigorous manipulation of infected root canals, upper respiratory infections, tonsillitis, septic abortion, and traumatic manipulation of the lower genitourinary tract. Of all these precipitating causes, dental procedures have been incriminated in from 13 to 22 per cent of the cases (Seabury, Millard).

Subacute bacterial endocarditis is a disease which carries with it a tremendous morbidity rate in spite of the ever-decreasing mortality rate. Seldom is a patient successfully treated for this disease in less than a period of four weeks. The treatment itself consists of massive daily doses of penicillin over a period of from four to six weeks. This in itself implies a long period of inactivity as well as a great expense involved in medication, hospital bills, and physician's fees. Unfortunately, the emphasis on the decreasing death rate in subacute bacterial endocarditis is made while little attention is given to the actual morbidity rate associated with the disease. Even so there is no excuse for a dentist carrying out procedures which may possibly allow entrance of bacteria into the blood stream of individuals who give a history of either rheumatic fever or congenital heart disease without first giving the patient maximum protection with an appropriate antibiotic.

Unfortunately, subacute bacterial endocarditis may occur at any age, and it may be difficult for a dentist to appreciate the importance of a history of rheumatic fever or congenital heart disease in an elderly individual who has already undergone several extractions without premedication and has escaped subacute bacterial endocarditis. Such circumstances must be attributed to good fortune since the next extraction or dental prophylaxis may be the one to precipitate subacute bacterial endocarditis. Another important factor to be considered in prophylaxis against subacute bacterial endocarditis during dental procedures is the fact that in many cases the disease is precipitated by an upper respiratory infection. In patients who give a history of rheumatic fever or congenital heart disease it is wise to delay any dental treatment which will cause bleeding during the period when the patient has an upper respiratory infection. In addition, the patient should be urged to receive adequate medical attention from his physician during the course of such an infection.

It is the responsibility of every dentist to know the procedure for prophylaxis against subacute bacterial endocarditis while procedures which cause bleeding are carried out in the mouth. Information on subacute bacterial endocarditis prophylaxis is readily available to the dental profession.°

A positive or negative past history of childhood diseases may be of importance to the dentist, particularly when oral manifestations of childhood diseases are found in young patients. It is not unusual for a child to present for dental treatment because of a tender swelling in the parotid region. In such a case, a negative history of mumps and a lack of any dental infection which might cause such a swelling suggest the possibility that the patient has mumps. Certain soft tissue findings in the oral cavity of a young patient may suggest the presence of measles, scarlet fever, or chickenpox.

A history of primary herpetic gingivostomatitis may also be of importance in the young patient who presents with a sore throat and mouth, since the differential diagnosis of secondary herpes and other vesicular diseases is at times dependent upon a history of the primary attack of herpes. Occasionally, necrotizing gingivitis is mistaken for primary herpes. The natural history of herpes and necrotizing gingivitis precludes the latter in young children.

Serious Illness.—A history of serious illness is obtained in the past medical history and should include such diseases as tuberculosis, coronary thrombosis, strokes, venereal diseases, jaundice, congestive heart failure, hypertension, and diabetes.

A person who has had tuberculosis requires continued care throughout his lifetime. With modern treatment many cases of tuberculosis are arrested and the patients live normal lives following the initial bout with the disease. However, these persons should be examined at regular intervals by their physician for possible recurrence. It is of interest to the dentist to see that such patients receive their regular checkups for the protection of both the patient and the dentist.

Coronary thrombosis is a common finding in middle-aged men today, and at present the use of anticoagulants is in vogue in the treatment and prevention of this disease. Anticoagulants are also used for the treatment of thrombophlebitis to prevent pulmonary embolism as well as for the treatment of vascular problems involving the eye. Anticoagulant therapy has become more popular in recent years and in some areas has found popular use in the diseases

---

°The American Heart Association has published a pamphlet entitled *How the Dentist Can Protect His Patients from Bacterial Endocarditis.* Dentists can obtain copies of this pamphlet from the American Heart Association office or from their local Heart Association.

just mentioned. Obviously, if a patient is receiving anticoagulants, such procedures as dental extraction, gingivectomy, deep scaling, and other dental procedures likely to cause extensive hemorrhage are contraindicated until the normal coagulation mechanism of the blood has been restored. It may be necessary to seek the cooperation of the physician when emergency situations arise. By using the proper drugs, a physician can restore the normal clotting mechanism within a period of twenty-four hours. When this can be done without undue hazard to the patient, it may be desirable to do so in order to allow the emergency procedure to be performed.

Strokes or vascular accidents often involve areas of the brain which result in mental, as well as motor nerve, changes. Since they are frequently associated with hypertension, it may be necessary for the dentist to employ proper precautions prior to treatment in order to avoid undue apprehension on the part of the patient. Because victims of stroke who have motor nerve damage often find it difficult to care for the mouth properly, this must be taken into consideration in the treatment of periodontal disease and in extensive reconstruction of the mouth.

A past history of syphilis should prompt the dentist to carry out certain precautions in the examination of the patient with the consideration of possible reinfection in mind. In addition, he should be aware of certain well-known oral changes that occur during the tertiary stage of syphilis. The date and type of treatment given for syphilis may provide important information.

Gonococcal temporomandibular joint arthritis is known to occur in some patients following the infection of the lower genitourinary tract. The possibility of combined infection with both the gonococcus and the syphilis spirochete should not be overlooked.

A history of jaundice should alert the dentist to the necessity for autoclaving needles used for administering local anesthetics because of the possible transmission of infectious hepatitis or serum jaundice through the use of contaminated needles. Further, a history of jaundice may suggest residual liver damage and the possibility of decreased prothrombin level in the blood. Jaundice may be the result of chronic alcoholism as well as metastasis of neoplastic cells to the liver. It may suggest a hemolytic anemia or obstruction of the bile ducts. The effects of liver disease on the prothrombin level of the blood should always be kept in mind when the possibility of liver disease exists and when the dentist is considering a dental procedure which will cause bleeding.

The patient in whom congestive heart failure is well controlled presents no problem to the dentist in carrying out normal dental procedures. However, when a patient is known to have congestive heart failure that is being controlled by a physician, consultation with the physician is indicated in the event that he may desire that certain precautions be taken. A patient who gives a history of congestive heart failure should be questioned carefully as to the proper control of his cardiac problem. If he has not returned to his physician since the initial treatment, he should be advised to do so since the possibility of recurrent heart failure exists.

Hypertension may be either benign or malignant and has long been a consideration by dentists relative to the use of vasoconstrictors in local anesthetics. It is known that moderate amounts of epinephrine, as used in routine administration of dental anesthetics, produce no appreciable rise in blood pressure. The patient's apprehension prior to dental appointments should receive more attention as a possible source of increasing blood pressure than the use of epinephrine in dental anesthetics. When a patient who is known to be hypertensive shows apprehension prior to dental appointment, premedication with a suitable barbiturate is indicated.

Diabetes mellitus is a disease which should be understood rather well by the dentist in order that he may recognize its clinical manifestations and the potential problems that it presents in dental treatment. Diabetes which occurs early in life tends to be less well controlled than that which occurs during middle age. In general, diabetic persons show a greater susceptibility to infection than normal individuals, and this must always be considered in dental extraction and treatment of periodontal disease. The possibility of a patient suffering from insulin shock in the dental office is not too remote, and, if the history of diabetes is known prior to the dental treatment, proper precautions can be taken in order to prevent serious complications. Oral infections should be treated vigorously and promptly. This is particularly true in the patient with so-called "brittle" or juvenile diabetes. Any infection in the body, whether in the foot or in the oral cavity, upsets the insulin requirements of the diabetic patient. When an oral infection exists, it must be treated promptly and the patient must be advised to see his physician regarding readjustment of insulin requirements. The increased susceptibility to infection, combined with the effects of infection on insulin requirements, requires that the diabetic patient maintain good oral health at all times.

Injuries.—Injuries to the face often involve the maxillary and mandibular bones, the teeth, and the temporomandibular joints. If a history of injury exists, it is necessary to determine its extent, the area involved, and the time it was received. A history of injury may seem insignificant to a patient, but not infrequently an acute temporomandibular arthritis may develop any time from days to months after the injury. Initially an injury might not be severe enough to produce symptoms of acute temporomandibular joint arthritis; however, subsequent chronic minor trauma from occlusal irregularities may be sufficient to precipitate an acute traumatic temporomandibular joint arthritis.

When teeth are present in an area which has been injured, radiographic examination and vitality tests of the teeth in the associated area are indicated. The vitality of teeth should be determined in the arch involved in the injury, in the opposing arch, and in areas beyond the area of injury. Occasionally radiographic radiolucencies may be explained on the basis of previous injury to an area of bone. In questioning a patient relative to injuries he may have received, such things as auto accidents, accidental falls, and contact sports should be considered as possible sources of injury to the face.

Operations.—Any surgical procedure which has been performed on a patient may be potentially important to the dentist. The date of operation and the results reported to the patient by the surgeon should be determined. In the case of operation for neoplastic disease, the type of neoplasm and the area from which it was removed should be indicated in the history. Special consideration should be given to those neoplasms which have a tendency to metastasize to bone, especially the jaws. Although metastatic neoplasms are not commonly seen in the jaws, they nevertheless do occur. Operations involving the head, neck, and facial regions should receive particular attention from the historian since it may become the duty of the dentist to provide follow-up examinations for patients who have received surgical treatment for a variety of conditions involving the mouth and jaws.

Irradiation.—Radiation therapy is being used effectively and extensively in the modern treatment of cancer, and certain immediate long-range effects of this type of therapy are of concern to the dentist. The immediate effects are primarily related to an extremely sore mouth; this reaction to irradiation subsides in a period of from four to six weeks. The long-range effects are of more significance to the dentist in that they dictate certain precautionary measures for him to observe. When neoplasms in the mouth are irradiated, frequently the bone of the jaws is also subject to the radiation. This may result in a change in the vascularity of bone to such a degree that recovery from even minor trauma may be inhibited. Thus, in many instances, a past history of irradiation of the bone around the teeth contraindicates the extraction of the teeth in this area for the lifetime of the patient. In addition to the bones being irradiated, the salivary glands are frequently in the path of ionizing radiation. This may result in a loss of function of salivary gland tissue with a complete cessation or marked decrease in salivary flow. Without the normal detergent action of adequate salivary flow, patients frequently develop rampant dental caries and progressive periodontal disease.

All forms of ionizing radiation have a similar effect on bone and salivary gland tissue whether the irradiation be from x-rays, radium, or radon. Whenever a patient gives a history of irradiation, it is wise to consult with the radiologist who rendered the treatment and discuss with him the extent of dental treatment that may be carried out without risking the possibility of osteoradionecrosis.

Allergy.—A history of allergy, drug intolerance, and drug reaction is important to the dentist because of the relationship of the manifestations of these conditions to oral diagnosis and treatment. It is well known that dental procedures and dental drugs may elicit allergic or allergic-like manifestations. It is also true that patients present themselves for diagnosis of oral lesions which are manifestations of a reaction to a drug. Thus it is imperative that the dentist be aware (1) of the possibilities that a particular oral manifestation may have an allergic basis; (2) that a past history of an unfavorable reaction to a drug which is to be used in dental treatment may require careful consideration before it is used again, if at all; and (3) that while satisfactory evidence is still lacking that those patients with the so-called atopic diseases (hay fever, asthma, eczema, or hives) actually develop allergic reactions to drugs more often than those without them, nevertheless, clinical experience clearly shows that when allergic reactions do occur in this group, they tend to be more severe than in the nonallergic group.

Every dentist should be well acquainted with the basic concepts of allergy and hypersensitivity and with the various manifestations of allergy. Since it is not unusual for a patient who is allergic to one allergen to be allergic to several, a history of any type of allergy may be of the utmost importance. Since a wide range of allergens may produce allergic changes in the oral cavity, the dentist must know a variety of allergens and must be able to recognize allergic reactions in the mouth. At times when an allergic reaction in the mouth is suspected, it may be necessary for the dentist to carry out a detailed account of the patient's history of allergies and, in some cases, to request the patient to keep a diary of daily activities in order to determine the allergen.

Another important phase of the history of allergy is related to the administration of drugs in the dental office. With the wide variety of drugs available, there is an accompanying wide variety of allergic responses to these drugs. It is possible for the dentist to avoid producing an uncomfortable and perhaps incapacitating or even fatal allergic reaction to the drug he prescribes by obtaining a careful history regarding allergy to various drugs prior to their administration. Indiscriminate use of valuable drugs, particularly antibiotics, should be avoided in order to lessen the possibility of sensitizing the patient unnecessarily. The dentist should avoid dispensing drugs without first determining whether or not the patient is allergic to the contents of those drugs. This is particularly true of the patient who is given "pain pills" by the dentist and assumes that they are some potent analgesic and not aspirin. Patients who are allergic to aspirin show a particularly severe asthmatic type of reaction to the drug and may die in an acute asthmatic attack following its ingestion (Walton). An increasing number of untoward reactions to penicillin are being seen, and, although few in number, they are most generally severe and occasionally fatal. The serum sickness type of reaction to penicillin which occurs from a week to ten days after the drug is given often incapacitates a patient for a period of ten days and requires vigorous care for relief.

Clinical reactions to drugs may appear as true allergic responses to proteins, as a dermatitis, or as reactions not characteristic of allergy to proteins (Carr). Those reactions to drugs which are seen in allergy to proteins include systemic anaphylaxis, asthma, allergic conjunctivitis, rhinitis, urticaria, angioedema, serum sickness syndrome, and polyarteritis nodosa. Those reactions to drugs not characteristic of allergy to proteins include deleterious effects to the blood and drug fever.

Anaphylactic shock is a term used primarily to designate a reaction in experimental animals, but a group of clinical signs and symptoms resembling anaphylaxis may be seen in human beings. The manifestations of anaphylaxis have been seen following the administration of penicillin. Systemic anaphylaxis is characterized by sudden onset, asthmatic dyspnea, urticaria, angioedema, weakness, nausea, vomiting, fall in blood pressure, syncope, respiratory failure, and death. These reactions may result rapidly in death or may not occur at all. It does not necessarily follow that all of the foregoing reactions will occur. Of special significance are the multiple reactions, including anaphylactic shock, which may accompany iodism. More cases of iodism have been attributed to contrast media than to any other cause (Alexander). Thus the use of a contrast media for outlining cysts and periodontal pockets or for other uses such as in disclosing solution, should always be preceded by questions regarding possible allergy to iodine. Reactions to iodine include direct chemical burns, generalized dermatitis related to external use on small areas, and urticaria, purpura, and dermititis.

Bronchial asthma is an expression of drug hypersensitivity. It may occur alone or in association with urticaria, rhinitis, or hay fever. It differs from the alveolar congestion and bronchospasm of anaphylactic shock. While aspirin is one of the most common causes of bronchial asthma, many other drugs may induce it.

Conjunctivitis may be seen following topical or systemic administration of drugs. It is often a prominent feature of the Stevens-Johnson syndrome. Conjunctival suffusion may be seen in conjunction with hay fever and with vasomotor rhinitis.

Urticaria refers to the phenomenon of whealing and is one of the most common reactions to drugs. It may occur as angioedema of the lips in penicillin hypersensitivity, as angioedema and bullous eruptions in iodine reactions, and in reactions to tannic acid, streptomycin, sulfonamides, and vitamin B_{12} concentrate.

Urticaria, sneezing, rhinitis, migraine, hay fever, and gastrointestinal upsets should also be considered. Positive statements should be included as to the patient's reaction to dust, pollen, food, sunlight, and drugs like aspirin, penicillin, local anesthesia, oil of cloves, mercury, sulfonamides, and iodine. Occupational diseases, metal intolerances, herpes simplex, hives, etc. should be considered in the past history and included in the record of the present illness where applicable.

Urticarial manifestations appearing after administration of antibiotics such as penicillin, chlortetracycline (Aureomycin), oxytetracycline (Terramycin), and chloramphenicol (Chloromycetin) may be present in patients who present an immediate type of allergic sensivity. Penicillin or the involved antibiotic acts as a hapten and conjugates with a body protein to yield the complete antigen. Another reaction to the antibiotics may be an erythema of the ninth-day type which is characterized by a generalized macular, maculopapular, morbilliform, rubelliform, or scarlatiniform eruption usually accompanied by mild or almost absent constitutional symptoms and appearing from seven to ten days after administration of the antibiotic. Still another type of reaction to the antibiotics, more especially penicillin and chlortetracycline, is the "id" type of reaction characterized by eczematoid, erythematovesicular, and desquamating eruptions affecting more generally the feet, hands, and groin. Associated symptoms are not usually constitutional in nature. The onset is early in the couse of treatment, usually within twenty-four hours. Urticaria due to penicillin may subside while the drug is being used, may fail to recur when the drug is readministered, or may reappear periodically for many weeks after its use has been stopped.

Many drugs may produce systemic reactions similar to those described for the allergic reaction to therapeutic antiserum. As in serum sickness, symptoms appear between the first and second week after administration of the drug. The syndrome of fever, urticaria, arthralgia, and lymphadenopathy is known as the serum sickness pattern or syndrome. Peripheral neuritis and renal manifestations may also be a part of the drug reaction.

Periarteritis nodosa may be induced in susceptible individuals by iodides, hydantoins, sulfonamides, and serums.

Dermatologic manifestations of drug hypersensitivity must be differentiated from physical trauma and irritation. Sensitization of the skin does not necessarily imply that the mucous membranes are sensitized (Rostenberg). The most common dermatologic manifestations of drug hypersensitivity are allergic contact-type dermatitis, urticaria, and the exanthematous eruptions. Denture-sore mouth, polypoid hyperplasia of the palate, and black hairy tongue associated with overgrowth of yeast or fungus organisms should not be considered generally as allergic phenomena. Denture-sore mouth, characterized by erythema and at time hyperplasia, is more often than not the result of trauma rather than true sensitivity to the acrylic resins (Nyquist). It is possible, though rare, that poorly or inadequately processed acrylics will contain sufficient monomer to produce an untoward reaction of the mucosa. Erythema multiforme refers to a multiplicity of lesions (macules, papules, vesicles, and bullae) which may occur as the result of drug hypersensitivity. The salicylates and sulfonamides are the most frequent offenders; however, these lesions may occur with serum sickness and penicillin, barbiturates, and other medication.

"Fixed" drug reactions may occur with the use of the antibiotics as well as with the usual drugs causing this type of reaction, e.g., phenolphthalein and sulfanilamide. Clinically the eruptions consist of circumscribed areas of erythema, edema, and scaling which slowly subside when the antibiotic is withdrawn. Such lesions usually leave a residual pigmentation. Readministration of the drug brings about a recrudescence of the lesions in the same area.

Local anesthetics are not infrequently the cause of contact dermatitis. They may also cause death but probably not through true allergy or immune mechanisms. Local anesthetics may be divided into two groups: those which are chemically related to one another and whose basic structure permits cross-reaction and those which are not chemically related and do not cross-react (Alexander). Thus, when an unfavorable reaction to one of the local anesthetics in the first group occurs, an anesthetic should be selected from the second group whose members are not chemically related. A complete listing of the members of each group may be found elsewhere (Alexander). Briefly, the first group includes those local anesthetics containing procaine hydrochloride and the second group includes lidocaine (Xylocaine) and others.

Local anesthetics may produce contact dermatitis, serum sickness syndrome, and asthma. Gilman classified the reactions to local anesthetics as follows: (1) manifestations due to toxic influences such as excitement, delirium, convulsions, and respiratory failure; (2) an immediate type of reaction arising from a disturbance of the circulatory system, consisting of pallor, increased pulse rate, fall in blood pressure, and syncope; and (3) an allergic reaction manifested by asthma.

Diagnosis of allergy to drugs is generally based on the information obtained from a history. Patch testing for contact dermatitis should be done by one experienced in their application and interpretation since they may occasionally cause severe and distressing local reactions. Skin tests are of no value in the diagnosis of other allergies, and it is possible to elicit a true positive response with the development of a severe systemic reaction.

Blood dyscrasias may be produced by drugs through destruction of circulating blood elements or depression of the bone marrow. Such disorders may be produced by mechanisms other than hypersensitivity. Blood changes produced by drugs include granulocytopenia, thrombocytopenic purpura, and aplastic anemia.

Antihistaminic drugs may also frequently give rise to drug reactions. The more common side reactions are drowsiness, sleepiness, dizziness, headache, insomnia, nervousness, nausea, vomiting, constipation, diarrhea, and dryness of the mouth. Severe and rather bizarre reactions include delirium, narcolepsy, shock-like states, labyrinthitis, cardiospasm, urinary retention, fever, syncope, and dermatitis. These reactions have been thought to occur more commonly in allergic persons. Allergic reactions such as asthma and contact eczema, as well as arthralgia and urticaria, have also resulted from the use of antihistamines.

Potentiation of analgesic agents has been reported for many of the ataractic drugs. A history of the use of these tranquilizing agents should alert the dentist to the possibility of potentiation of narcotic analgesics which he may be prescribing. Since the tranquilizers do not have an analgesic property, the effect of potentiation is a true one and not one of summation. Adverse reactions, side effects, and toxicity, as well as habituation and addiction to the ataractic drugs have been reported in the literature (Hughes).

The importance of an adequate history concerning the use of drugs to be used for a patient in the treatment of disease by a dentist cannot be overemphasized. Since an allergy to a drug generally does not occur spontaneously, a previous single exposure to a drug does not assure the dentist that an untoward reaction will not result from his administration of a drug. However, an adequate history of a previous reaction to a drug may well prevent the occurrence of an unfavorable reaction. To further emphasize the need for a history, one only has to consider the widespread use of aspirin, the most common drug in use, which causes severe allergic reaction; yet the knowledge of this fact is not widespread among the members of the dental profession or the laity. While the number of cases of aspirin sensitivity is small in relation to its very extensive use, the untoward effects are often striking and dangerous to the patient and therefore should not be treated lightly. The dermatologic manifestations of an allergy to aspirin include urticaria and extensive angioneurotic edema involving the face, tongue, and palate. Systemic manifestations include bronchial asthma and constitutional or anaphylactic shock. Since in many instances there is a record of antecedent allergy, asthmatic patients should always be asked about previous use of aspirin and whether or not any untoward reaction occurred from its ingestion. While sensitivity to aspirin may be mild and go undetected, such a sensitivity may become more severe with subsequent administration.

Family History

The family history (F. H.) should include the most important conditions that have tendencies to be inherited as well as an indication of the possibility of infective contact as in tuberculosis. Diabetes mellitus, cancer, allergy, and nervous and mental disorders are important. The record of an illness with unusual hereditary tendencies, such as hemophilia, should contain information concerning relatives more distant than the immediate family. Information regarding ages of living parents or ages at time of death and also cause of death is useful in determining familial patterns. Hereditary and familial patterns are important in primary erythroblastic anemia, osteogenesis imperfecta, hemorrhagic telangiectasia, hereditary opalescent dentine, hereditary craniofacial dysostosis, supernumerary teeth, missing teeth, malocclusion, and other disturbances.

Personal and Social History

The personal and social history should include a brief summary of the patient's marital status, occupation, financial status, type of personality, habits, and religion. The excessive use of alcohol is an important consideration in general anesthesia and is important in the nutritional status of the patient. Cirrhosis of the liver and vitamin B complex deficiency states may arise from alcoholism. Excessive use of alcohol may at times result in poor patient cooperation. Tobacco is important because of its relationship to leukoplakia and verrucous carcinoma of the oral mucosa, oral hygiene, and nicotine stomatitis. Habits such as nail biting, tongue thrusting, pipestem chewing, pencil chewing, thread biting, tooth tapping and jiggling, and improper use of toothpicks should also be recorded if they have important relationships to abnormality in the mouth.

Problems imposed by illness, treatment schedules, financial arrangements, care of children, unemployment, time off from work, distance from the office, and the likelihood of the patient having to move to another area before completion of the treatment should be considered.

Personal hygiene may sometimes indicate what to expect in the way of home care. Education and intelligence are factors that must be considered when determining treatment to be carried on at home. The methods of toothbrushing and the home care the patient has been using, as well as the number of times daily he may carry out these procedures, are important. The manner in which the patient takes care of his toothbrush should also be indicated.

Systems Review

The systems review permits organization of some of the apparently unrelated symptoms. It also decreases the possibility of overlooking important symptoms by including other areas of the body and giving the examiner logical sequence for a complete review of the patient's history. Negative statements should never be used as the answers to questions concerning the various systems. Positive statements leave no doubt as to their meaning and indicate that the subject has been covered with the patient. The rote one-breath question, "Have you had a cough, hemoptysis, edema, night sweats, cardiac trouble, loose teeth, pyorrhea, measles, mumps, or rheumatic fever?" is to be avoided. Questions in the system review should be directed toward the signs and symptoms that have not been brought out in the record of the present illness and should give the examiner a better idea of the patient's health.

Head.—Although the structures of the head are a part of the respiratory, gastrointestinal, nervous and other systems and could be made a part of those respective systems under the *Systems Review*, the functional and anatomic integration of the eye, ear, nose, and throat suggest their grouping and review together.

Headache.—The presence or absence of headaches or past head injuries should be recorded. Headaches fall into two major categories according to their origin: those that arise mainly as the result of stimulation of intercranial structures and those that occur on stimulation of tissues outside of and adjacent to the skull. The headaches of major concern to the dentist are migraine, hypertension, temporal arteritis, eye, sinus, and those associated with teeth, temporomandibular joint, or muscles of the head and neck. Diffuse headaches associated with disease of the teeth or pain in the teeth if prolonged may also be increased by severe sustained contraction of the muscles of the head and neck. The most commonly encountered headaches are migraine and those of sustained muscle contraction associated with anxiety and emotional tension. The teeth do not remain obscure as a cause of neuralgia or other facial pain. Dental pulpitis and pain associated with exposed dentin may be the cause of local pain or referred pain, but it is doubtful from clinical experience that such conditions are the source of headaches. Thus impulses arising from the teeth and associated with headache, although clinically important, are not a common cause of headache.

Usually a headache associated with a diseased tooth or teeth may be evaluated by the use of a local anesthetic about the tooth in question, since anesthetizing the diseased tooth will eliminate headache and other pain. However, generally in such instances tenderness and ache in the muscles of the neck and back of the head are still present. Headaches with intervals of complete freedom from pain do not have their origin in diseased teeth. The extraction of diseased teeth for the relief of such headaches is not justified. The rationale for treatment should be directed toward the alleviation of the disease of the teeth; if, in the course of treatment and restitution of the tooth, the neuralgia, headache, or other facial pain is eliminated, then the tooth can be considered responsible for the headache. However, teeth should never be extracted solely for the purpose of determining by exclusion the cause of the headache.

As previously stated, when noxious stimuli arise from the teeth, the infiltration of a local anesthetic about the source of noxious stimuli will eliminate the headache. However, pain and tenderness associated with noxious stimuli arising in the muscles of the head and neck usually remain for several hours. In the case of noxious stimuli arising from the teeth, the sustained muscle contraction is found in the masseter and temporalis muscles, in addition to the muscles of the occiput and neck. Therefore, headaches from sustained contractions of the muscles of the face, head, and neck are secondary to noxious impulses arising from the teeth. Some instances of extreme headache and toothache may result from traumatic occlusion. In addition to the headache, there may be associated pain of the face or temporomandibular joint. The patient may be indirectly aware of this association and may attempt to hold the jaw in a particular manner, thus inducing sustained contractions of the muscles of mastication and of the face, head, and neck. In these instances, probably the headache is due primarily to sustained contractions of these muscles.

Eyes.—The patient should be questioned concerning inflammation and pain in the eyes. A certain amount of information may be gained by asking questions relating to spectacles. Pertinent conditions associated with defective vision, yet showing little or no evidence of ocular affection, include squinting eyes, nystagmus, toxic states due to renal disease, alcohol, tobacco, lead, and quinine, migraine, diseases of the visual cortex, severe hemorrhage, etc. At times photophobia is associated with any headache experienced chiefly in the front or on the top of the head. It is commonly noted in patients with migraine headaches, nasal and paranasal disease, and muscular spasm headaches. (Any reaction to light by the eye must be interpreted in relation to the intensity of the light used. No one can be expected to stand the dental unit light shining directly into the eyes, and this should not be used as a criterion of photophobia.)

Occasionally following extractions of teeth and other dental operations, there may be lacrimation and slight reddening of the conjunctiva on the side of involvement. There also may be erythema on that particular side. The skin over the painful area may be hyperalgesic and accompanied by extensive motor reactions. Afferent impulses from injured periodontal tissues of an extraction site may produce a diffuse headache caused by noxious impulses arising from these injured tissues. These impulses give rise to excitatory processes in the brain stem which spread to exert their effects on many trigeminal structures.

Ears.—The presence or absence of deafness, tinnitus, vertigo, or discharge should be noted. Many children's diseases may affect the auditory nerve, producing various degrees of deafness. Mumps occasionally produce a profound type of deafness without middle ear involvment. Many drugs, especially quinine, salicylates, arsenic, nicotine, mercury, and alcohol, can produce a nerve type of deafness in susceptible people. Interference with the blood supply to the labyrinth as may occur in patients with the various anemias or arteriosclerosis can affect hearing. Eighth cranial nerve deafness in a few cases may be due to syphilis, especially in the late form. The duration of the deafness, history of onset, and related symtpoms are important factors to be recorded, especially if they relate to the chief complaint and/or correlated symptoms. Vertigo in patients with Meniere's syndrome should not be associated with symptoms of temporomandibular joint dysfunction. Deafness and vertigo have been suggested as symptoms of Costen's syndrome, but these are not acceptable with present concepts. The relationship of Meniere's disease with periodontal disease or abscessed teeth has not been established. Vertigo and dizziness may be associated with the eighth cranial nerve, brain disease, epilepsy, migraine, severe anemia, or drug reactions.

Nose.—Colds must be distinguished from allergic symptoms. Frequent colds give some indication of the resistance of the patient. In children sinusitis may give rise to symptoms that are thought to be due to frequent colds. Postnasal drip may be due to an allergic rhinitis, foreign objects, sinusitis, or lesions. Epistaxis may be associated with rheumatic fever, and a history of frequent nosebleeds should lead to questions regarding other symptoms of this disease. Nasal hemorrhage is frequently present in patients with hypertension and various blood dyscrasias, or it may be the result of various chemical irritants such as mercurial and phosphorus poisoning or local conditions such as trauma in the anterior septum where Hassalbach's venous plexus is located. In addition to the function of smell, the nose prepares the air for use by the lungs. It cleans, moistens, and warms inspired air. Breathing through the mouth instead of the nose has an injurious effect on the tissues of the respiratory tract and the oral cavity and is also a factor in maldevelopment of the facial skeleton and malocclusion of the teeth because of the displacement of the normal growth forces. Most individuals have a strong tendency for nasal respiration; however, if the nasal passageways are blocked, the individual will, of necessity, breathe through the mouth.

At this time in the system review some information relative to the problem of respiration through the mouth instead of the nose should be obtained. During the clinical examination, the effects of mouth breathing as well as whether or not habitual mouth breathing is occurring can be determined. However, at this time subjective information relative to the altered function is of importance in later direction of the clinical examination and many times determines the necessity for referral to the rhinologist. Habitual mouth breathing may be due to anatomic malformation such as nasal obstruction, enlarged tonsils, engorged nasal mucosa, and a deviated nasal septum. Probably the size of the airway, plus additional factors such as nasal and/or pharyngeal obstruction, is the predisposing factor in the mouth breather. Thus a narrow airway coupled with engorgement of the vascular bed or enlargement of the lymphoid masses in the pharyngeal airway may very well result in varying degrees of mouth breathing. Mouth breathing due to the physiologic hyperplasia of the pharyngeal lymphoid tissue usually occurs between the fourth and twelfth years. Since the lymphoid mass begins to atrophy after the twelfth year, the mouth breathing becomes less frequent because of the decrease in the obstruction to breathing through the nose. However, in many instances mouth breathing is a residual habit even after the nasal obstruction is removed.

While few patients will admit that they are chronic mouth breathers, a review of some of the factors which predispose to mouth breathing, as well as a review of the precipitating factors, may well bring out the need for examination in this particular area. Allergy, chronic rhinitis, sinusitis, nasal polyps, and a deviated septum are factors which may be important in the etiology. Nasal obstruction is quite common during sleeping hours and is especially prone to occur when the patient is lying on his back. Some children have an open-mouth habit but do not necessarily breathe through their mouths. However, this habit itself may lead to mouth breathing because when the mouth is open it is easier to breathe through it than to breathe nasally. In mouth breathers or in persons with the open-mouth habit, hyperplastic gingivitis, especially of the anterior portion of the mouth, is likely to occur.

Mouth breathing is a common habit and presents important clinical problems. To treat gingivitis associated with mouth breathing or to intercept certain types of malocclusion associated with mouth breathing, it is necessary to determine the type and character of the mouth breathing. This information will greatly influence the treatment planning. In many instances mouth breathing will be treated by the rhinologist and also by the dentist. Certainly the dentist is in the position to correct habitual mouth breathing after the obstruction, if there is one present, has been treated by the rhinologist or in patients in whom no organic obstruction is noted. In many instances, however, the elimination of a possible organic obstruction should be determined by the rhinologist. Whether or not there is a necessity for detailed clinical examination for mouth breathing many times is determined during a system review. Testing for nasal and oral breathing that can be done by the dentist and the determination of a rationale for referral to a rhinologist will be discussed briefly in Chapter 8 under clinical examination of the patient and indications for referral of patients to specialists. A history of nasal obstruction, allergic rhinitis and sinusitis, atrophic rhinitis, nasal polyps, or deviated nasal septums coupled with a complaint of difficulty in breathing through the nose, should direct the examiner's attention to a thorough examination of the structures which may be affected by mouth breathing and to a more complete examination of this area than might ordinarily be given. Careful observation of the patient during the history taking offers many clues to the direction one must take for a more thorough evaluation either by a more detailed review of this area or by a more detailed clinical examination. (See references for additional details of the etiology and diagnosis of mouth breathing.)

Throat.—A few exploratory questions concerning the throat should be asked even though a patient's complaints are not directed to the throat. The review should cover hoarseness, tonsillitis, and sore throat. Persistent hoarseness should be considered as due to a neoplasm until proved otherwise. Frequent episodes of sore throat and tonsillitis are significant factors in thumb sucking, tongue thrusting, and mouth breathing and are important historically in the evaluation of rheumatic fever. The differential diagnosis of herpetic stomatitis and acute necrotizing gingivitis is facilitated by a positive history of sore throat and dysphagia prior to the onset of oral lesions. Complaints about the throat should direct the examiner to specific areas of consideration during the clinical examination.

Gastrointestinal System.—A review of the gastrointestinal system serves to systematically recall to the patient's attention any symptoms of disease in this tract, including the mouth, that may have a bearing on his present illness and treatment. The information obtained may be of value because (1) disease that is manifest in the mouth may be the hallmark of more extensive systemic disease; (2) it is helpful in calling to the examiner's attention the patient's basic desire in seeking dental service, especially if the disturbances of the gastrointestinal tract are considered by the patient to be due to oral conditions such as poor chewing ability, ill-fitting dentures, or periodontal disease; and (3) the diagnosis of many conditions in the mouth is dependent upon the proper evaluation of the condition of the remainder of the system; viz., the nutrition, especially an older debilitated patient, is in many instances dependent upon the proper and comfortable mastication of a proper diet.

More patients have complaints involving the gastrointestinal system than any other system. A complete review of this system should include questions regarding nausea, vomiting, regurgitation, indigestion, anorexia, dysphagia, constipation, diarrhea, hematemesis and melena, jaundice, loss of teeth, toothache, flatulence, excessive thirst, abdominal pain, hemoptysis, bad taste, food impactions between the teeth, salivary changes, difficulty in mastication, pyorrhea, bleeding gums, canker sores, bad breath, loose teeth, pain, pain or sensitivity to heat, cold, or foods, vague feelings of discomfort of the teeth and gums, gumboils, and sharp edges on the teeth.

While patients frequently tend to underestimate the significance of complaints relative to this system and habitually attribute their discomfort to "something I ate," it is well known that the hallmark of many diseases may be manifest by symptoms in the gastrointestinal system. Such diseases as anemia, allergy, syphilis, vitamin deficiency, leukemia, and acute infections frequently present their chief symptoms in the gastrointestinal tract. A consideration of the symptoms common to the gastrointestinal tract lends itself to their artificial division into three main groups: (1) anorexia, dsyphagia, nausea, and vomiting; (2) constipation, diarrhea, and dysentery; and (3) symptoms referable to the oral cavity.

Other than oral complaints, nausea and vomiting are among the most frequent symptoms referable to the gastrointestinal tract. While the symptoms themselves may appear to point toward a stomach disorder, reflexes which cause nausea and vomiting may rise virtually in any part of the body or nervous system. They may be induced by pain and other sensations and intoxications, by unusual strains and efforts, by emotions and psychic disturbances such as fear, and by other conscious or unconscious mechanisms. Vomiting may be associated with almost any disturbance; unless it is qualified by some other symptom, the act itself may be of little diagnostic importance. The physiologic basis for the symptoms of nausea and vomiting appear to be a diminution in the functional activities of the stomach and alterations in the motility of the duodenum. There are apparently two ways of stimulating the organism to vomit: those which are central in origin and those which are peripheral in origin. Both vomiting stimuli act upon the vomiting center. Nausea and vomiting may be encountered in patients with acute infectious diseases, acute abdominal emergencies, chronic indigestion, diseases of the heart such as chronic heart failure, metabolic disorders such as the crises of thyrotoxicosis, Addison's disease, and disorders of the nervous system. In other instances the effects of drugs and poisons, laryngeal irritation, and psychogenic causes may produce vomiting.

Vomiting may be differentiated from regurgitating. Regurgitation implies an expulsion from the esophagus of undigested food retained because of some obstruction such as occurs with cardiospasm, esophageal varices, or a diverticulum, or an expulsion of gastric contents without preceding nausea. Regurgitation is of dental significance because of the acidity accompanying this type of activity and the decalcification of the teeth. In many diseases such as carcinoma of the stomach in the early stage and chronic indigestion due to lesions of the stomach, the cause of nausea and vomiting may not be readily apparent.

Indigestion is a term with no specific meaning that is generally used to mean those symptoms following eating such as heartburn, nausea, epigastric fullness, flatulent pains in various combinations, and belching of gas. Nausea and vomiting may also accompany severe cases of so-called indigestion.

Anorexia is a symptom which means lack of appetite and hunger. Clinically, it occurs in so many conditions of ill health, both psychogenic and organic in origin, that its diagnostic significance has little value. However, it may be present in patients with poor oral hygiene, ill-fitting dentures, painful teeth, and periodontal disease. Decreased weight should be associated with this symptom if it occurs in an individual who has just recently had dentures or some other type of dental treatment or in middle-aged or older persons whose appetite previously has been good. In a system review, vomiting should be related to the time, volume, contents, relation to food intake, and means of relief. If the volume is small, especially in the morning and after meals, it is often functional; if copious and occurring at night or late in the day, this suggests obstruction. When food content from the day before is seen, obstruction should be suspected. Bile stain indicates an obstruction below the pylorus. Coffee-ground color indicates blood decomposed by acid.

Complaints of persistent indigestion related to a lack of dentures or to new dentures should not be taken lightly. While the indigestion may be psychogenic in origin due to the new dentures, it is also likely that such persistent distress may well be due to more serious conditions in the gastrointestinal tract. As previously mentioned, the complaint is the patient's communication in his own terms about his symptoms, but the interpretation of the complaint is the responsibility of the dentist. In many instances the patient already had a complaint of indigestion prior to the time the dentist was consulted. Not knowing the true significance of his complaint, the patient may well have considered that his difficulty was due to ill-fitting dentures and that new ones would take care of his complaint of indigestion.

There are symptoms so universally associated with unimportant illnesses that scant attention is given to them, with the result that serious disease is sometimes neglected. For example, a hoarse voice due to carcinoma of the larynx may be permitted to go untreated for a considerable length of time under the misapprehension that it is due to laryngitis. In the same manner a patient may seek out a dentist for treatment of ill-fitting dentures under the mistaken idea that his indigestion is due to the ill-fitting dentures.

Dysphagia, which means difficulty in swallowing, is a symptom which is usually of special significance to the dentist because of its relation to his field of interest. It may be due to mechanical obstruction in the esophagus, to lesions of the mouth, pharynx, or larynx, or to disturbances of the neuromuscular components used in swallowing. The most common cause of dysphagia is mechanical obstruction of the esophagus, and by far the most common obstruction of the esophagus is due to carcinoma. Thus the first and most important symptom of carcinoma of the esophagus is difficulty in swallowing. Dysphagia from carcinoma usually has a gradual onset but may suddenly become progressively increased until even liquids are unable to pass through the esophagus. Regurgitation and pain are usually inconspicuous or absent. It can be readily understood that the dentist is in a prime position to evaluate changes in the swallowing ability of his patients. Dysphagia may also be due to disturbance in neuromuscular mechanisms. The Plummer-Vinson syndrome is generally considered in this category since the difficulty of swallowing in this condition resembles that due to a neuromuscular disorder; the actual cause of dysphagia is not clear. Patients with this syndrome are usually middle-aged women who present the characteristics of a chronic idiopathic microcytic anemia in conjunction with signs of vitamin B complex deficiency. Thus dysphagia, anemia, and atrophy of the mucosa of the upper gastrointestinal tract are symptoms of this syndrome. These patients also usually have relative degrees of acrodynia and sore mouths. Spoon-shaped fingernails are not uncommon findings. In some instances hyperkeratotic white plaques may be found on the buccal mucosa and throughout the mouth. These lesions apparently have a tendency to regress to carcinoma. Symptoms of dysphagia considered in the system review should include a reference to the time of onset and its relationship to hoarseness, coughing, and eating.

Constipation is an undue delay in the evacuation of feces. Diarrhea is the elimination of watery feces with excessive speed. Constipation is the most common of all symptoms referable to the gastrointestinal tract. While some investigators do not consider constipation, per se, to be physiologic, much attention has been placed on changes of bowel movements in an attempt to increase the awareness of the public to the possibility of cancer of the gastrointestinal tract. While it is popularly thought that at least one satisfactory bowel movement a day is sufficient and that less than this constitutes constipation, such factors are quite variable and some healthy persons will form a stool of normal consistency which is passed only every two or three days. These individuals are not constipated, for the stool has not been excessively dehydrated in its passage through the distal colon and has not been unduly delayed in evacuation. Constipation and diarrhea may be central, reflex, or mechanical in origin. The emphasis placed on constipation as a symptom is probably unwarranted. However, when constipation is recent and progressive, a serious psychogenic or organic cause must be suspected. The onset of constipation after middle life should raise a suspicion of organic disease of the bowels, especially if the disorder is progressive.

Diarrhea is as difficult to define as constipation. There are disturbances which by any standard can be called diarrhea. These are more likely to be termed dysentery than diarrhea. The concept of diarrhea varies with the training, education, culture, and habits of the patient. Recurrent or chronic diarrhea may follow acute infectious dysentery. There are diarrheas caused by neoplasms, protozoa, bacterial molds, drugs, worms, allergies, radiation, vitamin deficiencies, and other specific agents. Diarrhea of brief duration is commonly due to dietary indiscretion, food intolerance, or infections by organisms of the salmonella group. Prolonged diarrhea suggest some type of infection, and it may be due to bacillary dysentery, tuberculosis, enteritis, dietary deficiency, or such intractable disorders as idiopathic ulcerative colitis or regional enteritis. The latter are usually severe enough to force a patient to see a physician, and the dentist is only indirectly concerned with these diseases.

A positive history of hematemesis (vomiting of gross blood) and melena (passing of tarrish stools) are, with rare exceptions, manifestations of hemorrhage in the upper digestive tract. Peptic ulcers are the most common cause of hematemesis. Carcinoma of the stomach and portal hypertension are less frequent causes. While hematemesis and melena may be due to a large number of disorders, it must be kept in mind that about 90 per cent of all cases are due to primary intragastric diseases.

Jaundice is a term which refers to a discoloration of the skin with bile pigments. The scleras, skin, and to some extent the mucous membranes assume a greenish-yellow hue; however, the intensity of the jaundice color varies greatly. The bile pigments causing the discoloration are derived from the red corpuscles. The term yellow jaundice often means more to the patient than to the dentist. However, the dentist should always check misinterpretation of the sallow complexion of general ill health by asking the patient about the urine and stool color and the doctor's statement at the time of the discoloration. Jaundice may be separated clinically into primary obstructvie, hemolytic, and hepatocellular types. *Obstructive jaundice* may be due to lesions within the lumens of the bile ducts, lesions in the wall of the bile ducts, or lesions causing compression of the bile ducts. *Hemolytic jaundice* is caused by excessive breakdown of erythrocytes and a rapid production of bilirubin. The causes include pernicious anemia, sickle cell anemia, malaria, certain drug sensitivities (e.g., sulfanilamides, chemical agents such as acetanilid, lead, and bile salts), erythroblastosis fetalis, and Cooley's anemia. *Toxic* or *infective jaundice* is associated with portal cirrhosis, allergy (such as arsphenamine, sulfanilamide, mercury, etc.), hepatitis, amebiasis, leptospirosis, and yellow fever. Thus jaundice is a *symptom* of an underlying disturbance located in the liver, bile ducts, gall bladder, or a combination thereof.

It is important to know historically when teeth have been lost, reasons for loss, sequence of eruption, presence or absence of disease in formative periods, presence or absence of toothaches, location, and presence of drainage in the mouth. In periodontal therapy it is significant to determine whether or not teeth were lost because of dental caries and/or because of periodontal disease. It is important to know how long the presence of disease has existed and if the loss of teeth is associated in any way with an acute disease process in the past. The presence of many periodontal abscesses with sudden loss of tissue tone suggests the possibility of uncontrolled diabetes mellitus.

A statement that a toothache is without apparent cause is usually due to the observer's inability to make a diagnosis. Such conditions as sinusitis, anemia, cardiac failure, very slight trauma, pregnancy, menses, angina pectoris, mumps, neuroses, changes in altitude, and trigeminal neuralgia may many times produce toothaches without the presence of obvious disease in the tooth.

In some instances there is a direct time correlation between the occurrence of gastrointestinal disturbances and the insertion of a new partial or complete denture or the extraction of several teeth. Gastrointestinal disturbances associated with the insertion of dentures may be psychogenic in origin due to increased salivation or may be coincidental with more serious disorders not attributable to oral changes. Sensitivity reactions to denture material are not common and are exceedingly difficult to demonstrate due to the common occurrence of denture-sore mouth from ill-fitting dentures. Poor patient preparation without attention to what the patient expects from new dentures might well be the basis for some of the so-called "poor-denture" patients and untoward reactions.

Cacogeusia (bad taste in the mouth) may be due to blood, pus, stagnant food, debris, or metals. The presence of a metallic taste should lead to investigation of metal intoxication with a consideration of occupational hazards. Pus from periodontal pockets and periodontal abscesses gives a particularly disagreeable taste, although many degrees of appreciation of these factors are present from one individual to the next. The establishment of an appreciation of what a clean mouth feels like is one phase of dental education and home care. Food impaction is a common cause of the feeling of bad taste. A history of food sticking between the teeth is suggestive of functional inadequacy in the area of impaction. Since the olfactory sense accounts for much of a person's ability to taste, the history of bad taste should lead to questions concerning conditions of the nasal passage. An associated productive cough may well mean that there is some pulmonary disease such as bronchiectasis or tuberculosis. Malfunction of the cardia with the regurgitation of food particles is not a too frequent cause of bad taste. In making an evaluation of bad taste in the mouth, it is necessary to determine the duration and association of other factors such as coughing, vomiting, gastric disturbances, sinusitis, colds, etc. The quality of the taste (sweet, sour, salty, or metallic) should be determined and evaluated.

Increased flow of saliva may be associated with metal intoxication, mercurial therapy, wearing of dentures, Vincent's infection, herpetic stomatitis, and other functional disorders. Decreased salivation (xerostomia or dry mouth) is seen following irradiation, in old age, and with functional disorders. Decreased salivation and dry mouth may, in some degree, be caused by obstruction of the salivary gland ducts by inspissated material or calcareous deposits. Dry mouth and drooling are terms used by patients to describe the symptoms of a change in the quantity of the flow of saliva. A history of endemic parotitis may at times aid in making a differential diagnosis, since it is unlikely that a patient who has had bilateral mumps is suffering from this disease when presenting with an enlargement of the parotid glands.

When a patient has previously been fitted with a prosthetic appliance but now keeps it in a drawer and never uses it or just uses it on special occasions, questions should be asked regarding the complaints associated with the appliance. A review of the conditions in the past allows a better understanding of the problems to be encountered by the practitioner as well as a chance for patient education. The same is true of patients who, when told of periodontal diseases, are troubled because previous treatment was supposed to have cured the condition. An adequate history of previous diseases of the oral structures in relation to further treatment is necessary not only to bring out objective dissatisfaction, but also to learn of personality problems that have to be considered for successful treatment of the patient.

A patient who expresses difficulty in masticating food may do so because of painful teeth, malocclusion, periodontal disease, insufficient occlusal surfaces, temporomandibular joint disease, oral lesions, muscular dysfunction, or lack of training after long disuse. The most frequent cause of such difficulty is loss of posterior teeth without replacement. In some instances, tipping and extrusion of posterior teeth, especially third molars, may lead to trauma of the temporo-mandibular joint through occlusal disharmony. Very frequently the patient may trace his difficulty to the loss of teeth, placement of restorations, or eruption of third molars.

A history of orthodontic treatment should include the reason for the treatment and the apparent results in terms of the patient's satisfaction.

Genitourinary System.—The principal historic manifestations of disorders in the urinary system are dysuria, polyuria, hematuria, and edema. In a review of this system, positive statements regarding a history of these manifestations of disease, as well as venereal disease, should be made. A history or the presence of disorders is of importance to the dentist because of the relationship between oral health and the general health of the patient. The value of the information obtained may be found in the following relationships: (1) Manifestations of serious metabolic disorders such as diabetes mellitus are frequently suspected because of disorders of urinary function, viz., polyuria. While this symptom may be transient, it may also be of primary consideration in directing the examiner's attention to other contributory symptoms of diabetes mellitus. (2) Edema which is generalized or limited to areas particularly susceptible to accumulations of a transudate because of dependency or laxness of the skin is of dental significance because of the frequent association with cardiac insufficiency. This factor, as well as other diseases of renal and nutritional disorders, is of primary concern to the oral surgeon contemplating surgical procedures. (3) A history or presence of venereal disease is of importance because of its possible relation to disease of the mouth, such as syphilitic glossitis, Hutchinson's incisors, and mulberry molars, and because of possible contraction of the disease by the dentist. Rarely gonor-rhea may lead to acute pyogenic arthritis of the temporomandibular joint.

Questions regarding venereal disease require tactful inquiry by name and symptom: e.g., gonorrhea, "clap," penile discharge in the male; vaginal discharge with low abdominal pain and dysmenorrhea or a disease diagnosed as "inflam-mation of the tubes" in the female; and syphilis, "bad blood," "haircut," chancre, or prolonged "needle treatments for bad blood." Tests of food handlers and premarital tests usually suffice to obtain valuable information concerning serology; patients should be questioned about previous tests when veneral disease is sus-pected.

Catamenia.—The menstrual history is of importance as an index to a woman's health and as a means of detecting an early sign of genitourinary cancer and a bleeding tendency. Odontalgia, mucosal ulceration, salivary gland swelling, and gingival hemorrhage are associated with menstruation in some women. Preg-nancy complicates dental care in several aspects; increased carbohydrate intake in patients with so-called morning sickness may contribute to an increase in the rate of dental caries. Dental appointments may necessarily be avoided in the morning when "morning sickness" is a factor.

So-called pregnancy gingivitis, gingival "tumors," and the tendency for an increase in the severity of an existing gingivitis may be seen in pregnant women. The apparent increase in gingivitis may be due to several factors, including less inclination on the part of women to maintain good oral hygiene because of an "ill feeling" and because of hormonal imbalance and vascular changes during this period.

The climacteric should be evaluated in the female patient because of the changes occurring in the mucous membranes and because of the psychic factors involved. The main symptom of the menopause is the so-called hot flush which is often accompanied or followed by sweats. Such flushes may occur for no apparent reason or may occur in association with a temporary psychic unrest— dental procedures involving discomfort, etc. They usually affect only the upper portion of the body and produce a sensation of warmth over the chest, head, and neck. The skin may flush and turn red, and there may be a sensation of choking and suffocation. Flushes are likely to appear during the night as well as during the day. Other symptoms, such as tinnitus, palpitations of the heart, loss of appetite, bitter taste in the mouth, flatulence, nausea, vomiting, abdominal cramps, diarrhea, or constipation (or both) may be produced. The patient may have headaches ranging from an occasional dull ache to an intense ache that lasts for days and weeks. The hot flushes may cause the hands and the whole body to tremble. Vague pains such as backaches, numbness, and tingling sensations may also be present. Induced menopause may result in the same symptoms. The development of symptoms of anxiety, depression, tension, or hysteria in the premenstrual period is a well-recognized and accepted feature of the menstrual cycle in the female.

In the menopause there is a decrease in ovarian function and sufficient hormonal imbalance in some patients to produce marked symptoms. Along with the shift in hormonal balance, in many patients there appears to be a marked shift in stability of the autonomous nervous system. As a result there are frequent discharges of sympathetic activity which result in the symptom called hot flushes and in nervousness, etc. The other symptoms which appear during and after the onset of the menopause are due to the gradual decrease of estrogen. This decrease makes itself manifest by a gradual decrease in the thickness of skin and mucous membrane and in the size and tone of muscles, the appearance of atrophy of the vagina, the endometrium, and the breasts, and a relative decrease in the formation of bone matrix. This latter condition results in senile osteoporosis because of the relative failure of osteoblastic activity to provide an abundant organic matrix for the deposition of calcium. This is more marked in some patients than in others. Such senile osteoporosis is evident by radiographic examination in many patients, especially in the mandible. In some instances these areas of radiolucency have been mistakenly described as pathologic conditions.

While men may suffer from symptoms of the climacteric, this is very uncommon and should not be emphasized since it is probably of no clinical significance. In women, osteoarthritis may first become symptomatic at the time of menopause. When complaints of osteoarthritis are already present, symptoms may be sharply accentuated with the onset of the menopause. It must be remembered that age, wear and tear, trauma, abnormal occupational stresses, congenital and developmental defects, infection, and neuromuscular disease are all considered to be causes of osteoarthritis, and thus it may be difficult to assess the importance of the menopause in the etiology of osteoarthritis of the temporomandibular joint. Clinically, osteoarthritis of the temporomandibular joint is asymptomatic even in the presence of extensive articular damage.

Premenstrual tension and dysmenorrhea are often accompanied by menstrual irregularity and premenstrual stain. Premature occurrence of amenorrhea after less than the average span or normal menstrual cycles is called early menopause. The onset of female climacteric before the age of 45 years is definitely abnormal and is probably related to an early depletion of primordial follicles. Thus it is possible for an individual in the early menopause to show the characteristic menopausal symptoms, including osteoporosis of the mandible and atrophic gingival changes.

Between the ages of 45 and 50 years there is progressive irregularity in frequency, duration, and amount of menstrual flow until an only occasional period or spotting occurs; complete amenorrhea then occurs. A recurrence of bleeding after a period of amenorrhea in patients over the age of 45 years must be considered to be due to ovarian or uterine neoplasms until proved otherwise. Hyperhidrosis, rapid gain in weight, atrophic arthritis, and osteoporosis are not uncommon findings following the menopause.

It is obvious how the symptoms of the climacteric may present problems in diagnosis and treatment of dental conditions. In patients with gynecologic disorders following menopause it is not uncommon to find sore and tender mouths and certain forms of gingivitis. Patients in the menopause commonly complain of dryness or a burning sensation in the mouth. Lesions of the buccal mucosa consisting of irregular grayish-white areas which are expressions of atrophic changes are not infrequently mistaken for leukoplakia or lichen planus.

The dentist should not overlook the psychic factor in his evaluation of any dental problem in the patient in the menopause, since the "human equation" may be of considerably more importance than technical perfection. For example, dentures may be technically perfect, yet some patients, because of emotional imbalance during the menopause, may not be able to adjust and train themselves in their use.

Neuromuscular System.—A complete review of the neuromuscular system should contain at least sufficient questions to assure an adequate coverage of any history of syncope, convulsions, anesthesias, paresthesias, paralysis, mental confusion, memory loss, sudden changes in temperament, bruxism, neuralgias, neuroses, trismus, and myositis. The extent of the review will depend in part upon the type of information to be obtained and in part upon the emphasis that may be directed toward this system, especially from the *chief complaint* and *present illness.* Of primary interest to the dentist are the relation of syncope to dental procedures, paresthesias and anesthesias related to dental extractions or traumatic injury, major and minor neuralgias of the mouth and face, bruxism associated with occlusal dysfunction, and oral, systemic, and psychic changes associated with convulsions, mental confusion, and cerebral damage.

Syncope or fainting may result from psychic stimuli, emotional upsets, hypodermic injections, pressure on the carotid sinus, postural hypotension, myocardial infarction, hyperventilation, hypoglycemia, hysteria, and occasionally from heart disease. When there is a positive history of frequent syncope, the patient should be questioned regarding the time of onset, position of patient at onset, duration of a syncope, and any alleviating circumstances. Orthostatic syncope associated with rigid attention and lack of muscle movements is of much less significance than recumbent syncope. A past history of syncope is very likely to be related to emotional upsets or apprehension; however, a complete history should cover the possibility of other factors that may have been responsible.

Syncope should not be confused with the transient blackouts of petit mal (epilepsy) because posture and activities may be little affected during the blackouts. Unconsciousness, arising from circulatory disorders that cause cerebral ischemia, varies from momentary fainting (postural syncope) to prolonged unconsciousness, e.g., apoplexy. A history of convulsions should be described as to the presence or absence of self-injury from falling, tongue biting, and cheek biting since these factors rarely accompany hysteria.

Anesthesias and paresthesias should be described as to location, duration, mode of onset, and associated symptoms. Transient perioral numbness or paresthesia of both hands is a common symptom of hyperventilation. It is not uncommon for a patient to complain of anesthesia and paresthesia of the side of the face and lips following extraction of a difficult third molar. These symptoms usually subside, but occasionally they may persist. Not infrequently, when damage to the mandibular nerve is great, traumatic neurofibromas may develop and the patient may be troubled with varying degrees of discomfort.

Inquiry into a history of paralysis of the mouth and face should include questions concerning transient or developing muscular weakness and the development of speech defects not related to dentures. In tertiary syphilis (paresis) the gait is often shuffling, and the patient may not be able to keep his eyes off his feet while walking. An ataxic gait, while somewhat characteristic in itself, may occur in many conditions and diseases besides tertiary syphilis. In general, an individual who has been seriously debilitated will initially have difficulty in walking in addition to other manifestations of weakness. Cerebrovascular accidents (CVA) may cause a patient to be paralyzed in any portion of the body. It is not uncommon for a patient who has experienced a cerebrovascular accident to have a complete or partial paralysis of the muscles of facial expression and mastication on one side of the face. Such a patient has difficult problems in oral hygiene as well as problems in restorative dentistry. Those with severe paralysis affecting an arm may find it difficult to place or to remove partial dentures.

A history of bruxism may be difficult to obtain at the first interview since many patients are unaware of this condition. It may be necessary to ask the patient to determine its presence for himself. He may be completely unaware of any clenching or grinding habits even though there may be clinical signs of their presence. Other members of the family may be aware of this condition, especially when the bruxism occurs when the patient is asleep. Bruxism is of extreme importance in the etiology of traumatic occlusion and its basis must be determined, whether it be psychogenic and/or occlusal in origin.

A complaint and history of odontalgias and referred pain require careful questioning about the time of onset, duration, type of pain, extent, spread, and factors such as heat, cold, and eating that may be the precipitating agent.

Bones and Joints.—A review of the bones and joints may contain questions directed toward previous trauma, pain, swelling, heat, limitation of motion, duration of symtoms, mode of onset, mode of relief, association of complaint with the use of the bone or joint, previous history of infantile scurvy, rickets, fractures, osteomyelitis, poliomyelitis, cerebral palsy, muscular atrophy, and hemophilia. When a chief complaint and related symptoms are located within this system, a detailed account much more extensive than that just indicated may be necessary before an adequate coverage of the system can be considered to have been accomplished. While the primary concern to the dentist is the review of the bones and joints of the masticatory system, diseases of the bones and joints outside this area may be of significant importance to the formulation and treatment of oral disease.

Certainly no dentist would consider the evaluation of the temporomandibular joints complete without a consideration of the other joints of the body, since the same disease may also be present in the other joints. In some instances the diagnosis of temporomandibular joint disease may be dependent upon the presence or history of disease elsewhere in the body. The question of whether or not the historian should cover the bone and joint system more extensively will depend upon the type of examination and the presence of disease in the bones and joints of the masticatory system.

When a history of joint disturbances is suspected, questions should be asked relating to trauma, muscular imbalance, degenerative diseases, neuropathic joint disease, specific infectious arthritis, acute rheumatic fever, rheumatoid arthritis, and the effects of movement. When the attention of the examiner is directed toward the temporomandibular joint, a more complete review of the symptoms of disease of this joint must be carried out.

It must be remembered that the temporomandibular joint is only a part of the masticatory system and that, as a functional part of this system, diseases and other components may reflect to the temporomandibular joint. Thus the symptoms of temporomandibular joint abnormality may be associated with injuries to the jaw, occlusal disharmony, oral habits, faulty dental therapy, lack of replacement of lost teeth, and bruxism. It is not uncommon for a patient with arthritis of the joint to complain of painful sensations in the ear or around the temporomandibular joint which have no organic origin within the temporomandibular joint or ear. In these instances the patient may consult a otolaryngologist first and be told that he has no ear disease. With such a history the examiner should make a detailed inquiry for symptoms of dysfunction not only of the temporomandibular joint, but also of other components of the masticatory system.

The most important symptoms of disturbances of temporomandibular joint are related to various degrees of trauma. Complaints associated with acute symptoms can usually be related to a known traumatic injury. Following the injury there is a painful restriction of mandibular movements and in some instances pain of a continuous nature. Chronic trauma related to chronic subluxation of the temporomandibular joint and occlusal disharmony are the most frequent causes of disturbances of the joint. These symptoms include clicking or snapping noises upon moving the mandible, unilateral mastication with restriction of mandibular movements, and referred pain to the ear, occipital and temporal regions, and in some instances the neck, tongue, jaws, or sinuses. The patient will often have remissions of the symptoms but occasionally will have acute exacerbations.

Symptoms involving the temporomandibular joint may also arise from disease of the joint itself. Rheumatoid arthritis, degenerative joint disease, infective arthritis, rheumatic fever, bursitis, and nonarticular rheumatism may produce symptoms of pain and limits the jaw movements. Systemic symptoms may be present with infective arthritis, viz., fever, chills, sweats, malaise, and anorexia.

Atypical facial neuralgias, Meniere's disease, headaches, and psychogenic complaints may be difficult for the examiner to evaluate in a differential diagnosis of temporomandibular joint disturbances. Thus, when a complaint involves the temporomandibular joint, it is important that the examiner be aware of the other factors which may produce complaints referable to the joint. A diagnosis of temporomandibular joint dysfunction should be based on the examination of the joint and on obtaining and evaluating a history of the patient's complaints. Though the physical examination of the joint is a necessary procedure, initially it is probably not as important as proper collection of the facts concerning the patient's complaint. Because of the common relation of occlusal dysfunction to temporomandibular joint dysfunction, examination of the occlusion is of primary importance. However, a careful analysis of the complaint and associated symptoms should be made to rule out other causative agents.

There may not be a characteristic or prodromal illness prior to the onset of inflammation of the joints in rheumatoid arthritis; on rare occasions it may involve the temporomandibular joint first. The nature and intermittent character of complaints with remissions and exacerbations associated with swelling and stiffness of joints suggests rheumatoid arthritis. The proximal interphalangeal joints almost always are involved ultimately. Almost all disorders of joint function are characterized by the association of two or more related symptoms. An investigation of these symptoms would generally lead to an understanding of the related complaints and of the underlying basic disturbance. For example, in a complaint of chronic joint pain it is significant to know that recently a third molar was extracted and that prior to this there was frequent subluxation of the mandible. While it is possible for the extraction itself to be responsible for the complaint, the prior chronic subluxation must be evaluated before treatment can be instituted. While a patient is primarily interested in alleviation of the pain in the temporomandibular joint, treatment of symptoms, such as injections of cortisone or hyaluronidase into the joint space or immobilization of the jaws, will probably not give permanent relief. However, a complete review of the masticatory system will serve to direct the examiner in his examination to the underlying basis for the disturbed function of the joint and provide a rational basis for therapy. It is to be expected in the example given that the examiner will find evidence of disturbed occlusal harmony and that a permanent therapy must include an occlusal adjustment. The third molar may well be responsible for the occlusal disharmony, but in view of the persistent complaint the clinical examination will probably show additional occlusal disharmony. Thus the chronology of the complaints and a clinical examination of the occlusion are both necessary before adequate therapy can be undertaken. Moreover, an adequate history and examination will serve to rule out other possible causative agents.

In some instances an examiner may elicit the symptoms of temporomandibular joint disturbance and also occlusal disharmony but fail to discover significant symptoms of emotional disturbances. This often results in poor treatment planning and ineffective therapy since no therapy for the adjustment of the occlusion and palliation of the temporomandibular joint symptoms can be adequate in the presence of perpetuating emotional disturbance. Thus the examiner must be adept in collecting the facts, have a basic knowledge of the disease processes responsible for the symptoms collected, and be able to synthesize these two components in the formulation of a diagnosis.

REFERENCES

Alexander, H. L.: Reactions With Drug Therapy, Philadelphia, 1955, W. B. Saunders Co.

Carr, E. A.: Drug Allergy, Pharmacol. Rev. **6:**365-424, 1954.

Comroe, B. I., Collins, L. H., and Crane, M. P.: Internal Medicine in Dental Practice, ed. 3, Philadelphia, 1949, Lea & Febiger.

Dingman, R. O., and Hayward, J. R.: The Value of Writing Case Histories, J. Oral Surg. **5:**123, 1947.

Emslie, R. D., Massler, M., and Zwemer, J. D.: Mouth Breathing, J.A.D.A. **44:**506-521, 1952.

Fulton, M., and Levine, S. A.: Subacute Bacterial Endocarditis With Special Reference to Valvular Lesions and Previous History, Am. J. M. Sc. **183:**60-77, 1932.

Gilman, S.: The Treatment of Dangerous Reactions to Novocain, New England J. Med. **219:**841, 1938.

Herrmann, G. R.: Clinical Case Taking, St. Louis, 1945, The C. V. Mosby Co.

Horder, T. J.: Infective Endocarditis, Quart. J. Med. **2:**289-329, 1909.

Hughes, F. W.: New Psychotherapeutic Drugs, J. Indiana M. A. **50:**293, 1957.

Landa, J. S.: The Dynamics of Psychosomatic Dentistry, Brooklyn, 1953, Dental Items of Interest Publishing Co., Inc.

Massler, M., and Zwemer, J. D.: Mouth Breathing; Diagnosis and Treatment, J.A.D.A. **46:**658-671, 1953.

Meakins, J. C.: Symptoms in Diagnosis, ed. 2, Boston, 1949, Little, Brown & Co.

Millard, H. D., and Tupper, C. J.: Subacute Bacterial Endocarditis: A Clinical Study, J. Oral Surg., Anes. & Hosp. D. Serv. **18:**224-229, 1960.

Modell, Walter: The Relief of Symptoms, Philadelphia, 1955, W. B. Saunders Co.

Nyquist, G.: A Study of Denture Sore Mouth, Acta odont. scandinav. (supp. 9) **10:**1-154, 1952.

Rostenberg, A., Jr.: Eczematous Sensitization, Arch. Dermat. & Syph. **56:**222-232, 1947.

Seabury, J. H.: Subacute Bacterial Endocarditis, Arch. Int. Med. **79:**1-21, 1947.

Walton, C. H., and Bottomley, H. W.: Allergy to Aspirin, Canad. M.A.J. **64:**187-190, 1951.

Clinical examination–general

The clinical examination of a patient should be based on a discipline that will enable an examiner to identify the cause of disease for which a patient seeks help and to detect disease which is unknown to an apparently well patient. The principles should be the same for the complete, screening, or emergency type of examination. The clinical examination, regardless of its purpose, is not a diagnosis but a step toward diagnosis, and the discipline by which it is carried out is the same irrespective of the omission of some of the elements of the complete type of examination. Therefore the fundamentals necessary to carry out a complete and thorough examination should be the basis of knowledge for all practitioners who seek to satisfy the principles of an adequate clinical examination. The practitioner who is well grounded in the methods of a thorough and complete examination is generally in a position to know what elements can be omitted without interfering with the formulations of a complete diagnosis even though it is necessary to utilize the screening or emergency type of examination.

The omission of some of the elements of a complete examination for the purpose of screening patients is justifiable only when the limitations of the omission are well understood. The justification for an incomplete or emergency type of examination is based upon the relative efficiency of such an examination in the recognition of obvious disease and the relief of symptoms. This use, even when its limitations are known, does not justify teaching it in a course of oral diagnosis to the exclusion of a complete discipline which is so necessary for the development of competence in oral diagnosis. Once all the elements of a complete examination are mastered, the type of examination or its contents may be easily modified to meet the circumstances. Therefore all the procedures necessary to carry out a complete examination will be given here.

PRINCIPLES

The clinical examination is based on the principles of inspection, palpation, percussion, and auscultation. In general, these technics are applicable to the examination of the entire mouth and adjacent structures. All too often the examiner uses only the procedure of inspection. This is a mistake since palpation, percussion, and auscultation may be of considerable value in the examination of many areas and conditions.

Inspection is the systematic visual assessment of the patient under examination. By inspection, assessment may be made of the color of the skin and mucosa; surface contours and proportions of the body and its parts; functional movement; and various bodily states which reflect in part the physiologic and psychologic constitution of the individual. Thus, the examiner uses inspection every moment he is looking at his patient, noting anatomic, physiologic, and psychologic landmarks. Surface contours are influenced by the state of development of the musculature and the amount of fat in the superficial tissues. The prominences produced by underlying structures and easily seen in a thin person may be obscured in a fat one. In a thin individual, muscles of mastication such as the temporalis and masseter may be easily seen either when they are at rest or during function, whereas in a fat person the form and size are usually obscured even during function. Tumescence from a pathologic state such as enlargement of any of the glands of the neck may be obscured in an obese individual, whereas in a thin one a surface contour may be markedly changed and easily seen. Despite the fundamental similarity of structure in all patients, individual variations do occur. Almost everyone is familar with the differences in musculature and other anatomic features of the various races. Thus certain peculiarities of external form are characteristic of certain people. A slight asymmetry affects both the proportions and the movements of the body and its parts.

Palpation is a procedure whereby the examiner feels or presses upon the structures or portions of the body. An examiner skilled in the palpation of the normal body structures and their variations will find this procedure of significant value in discovering conditions outside the range of normal. The method of palpation depends upon the area to be examined. In some areas, such as the floor of the mouth, bimanual palpation is the method of choice (Fig. 16, *A*). Bidigital palpation is the method of choice for the lips (Fig. 16, *B*). With these methods, the intervening tissue is pressed and gently rolled between the two hands or fingers. The use of two hands or fingers allows for greater depth of coverage and movement of the tissues than is possible with the use of only one hand or finger. Also, with two hands more support can be given to those tissues which are freely movable than is possible when only one hand is used against unsupported tissue. At other times two hands are used to inspect the same structures on each side of the body; this is bilateral palpation (Fig. 16, *C*). This method gives the examiner some basis of comparison provided both sides are not abnormal. In addition to the comparison of bilateral structures for abnormalities, the examiner must keep in mind what should be normal in the average individual. Adequate palpation does not require undue pressure on the tissues with resulting discomfort to the patient; the procedure should be such that it causes very little discomfort.

By palpation the competent examiner is able to tell much about the tissue he is evaluating. It is necessary that he have an adequate knowledge of the anatomic and physiologic states of the tissue he is to consider. Only by practice will he learn to differentiate muscle tissue, glandular tissue, tendinous tissue, and

Fig. 16. *Palpation.* **A,** Bimanual palpation. **B,** Bidigital palpation. **C,** Bilateral palpation. **D,** Palpation of the teeth for mobility. **E,** Direct palpation to determine movement of a tooth during function. **F,** Palpation by compression; note fingers are held together to determine texture of underlying tissue.

osseous tissue in their normal anatomic and functional relationship. In the palpation of a salivary gland, the examiner should determine its boundaries, the density, attachments, anatomy of the surface, and relationship to other structures. Where possible, palpation and expression of saliva is desirable to allow inspection of the saliva and its freedom of flow. The palpation of muscle should reveal its boundaries, attachments, consistency, size, changes during function, and the presence or absence of tenderness. Palpation of bones should be done to reveal normal bony landmarks such as fossa, joints, tubercles, and muscle attachments; normal bones should be nontender and nonyielding except in areas of contiguous cartilage. Bones should be tested also for continuity, at rest and during function. Bilateral palpation for alterations in size and form is a desirable procedures.

Where possible, the potential spaces should be examined for the presence of density changes; accumulations of pus may fill the spaces and give the area a hard boardlike density. Palpation of the surface of the mucous membrane and skin is also an especially desirable procedure; texture, density, and resilience are significant factors in the examination of these tissues. Palpation of the teeth should consist of manual movement of the teeth by the examiner (Fig. 16, *D*), feeling for excessive movement of the teeth during functional movements of the jaws while chewing, and feeling for excessive movements of the teeth when the teeth are in contact and various excursions of the mandible are being performed (Fig. 16, *E*). In palpation of the skin, its texture, resilience, density, and lubrication should be considered. Depending upon the location, as much of the surface of the hand or fingers as possible should be brought to bear on the part to be inspected. Thus, where circumstances permit, the fingers should be held together and the hand should remain flat (Fig. 16, *F*).

Percussion is the technic of striking the tissues with the fingers or an instrument so that the examiner may listen for the resulting sounds. The response of the patient to the procedure is also noted. Percussion is valuable for the evaluation and localization of inflammation of the periodontal membrane and secondary pulpitis. In many instances tenderness of the teeth may be localized to a single tooth because of the response of the patient to the technic of percussion. Changes in the character and density of the supporting tissues and the amount of alveolar bone surrounding a tooth may be evaluated to a certain extent by the sounds elicited by percussion. The difference in the sound produced may be easily appreciated by comparing percussion notes of the teeth on one side of the mouth with their counterparts on the opposite side. In general, a tooth with normal support will give rise to a rather high-pitched sound, whereas one with less support or less dense support will give rise to one of lower pitch. A difference in the percussion note of a given tooth and that of its counterpart on the opposite side of the arch does not necessarily indicate the presence of an abnormality of the supporting structures. In any case variations of the normal, as well as the presence or absence of other contributory signs and symptoms of disease, must be taken into consideration.

The composite sound of percussion which is produced by the patient tapping his teeth together in centric relation or in acquired centric occlusion is of value in making a general appraisal of the degree and localization of premature contacts. A light tapping of the teeth together from the rest position of the mandible may serve to elicit or to demonstrate hypertonicity and spasticity of the muscles of mastication. Tapping of the muscles themselves may also produce the same effect. Percussion of the teeth is best carried out with the handle of an explorer (Fig. 17, *A*). It should be directed at right angles to the incisal, occlusal, lingual,

A

B   C

Fig. 17. *Percussion.* **A,** Percussion of teeth with instrument handle. **B,** Direct percussion to elicit nerve response. **C,** Indirect percussion; note that pleximeter finger is percussed immediately over point of contact.

buccal, or labial surfaces. Very light tapping is all that is necessary, and it goes without saying that pounding is entirely unnecessary. A pain response or an abnormal percussion note may be elicited when the percussing instrument is directed in any or all directions.

The technic of percussion of muscle and bone consists of sharply tapping the area to be tested with the tips of two or three fingers. An area is tapped twice and the sound or response compared with that produced in its like area on the other side of the face. The fingers should be flexed to a right angle at the first interphalangeal joint (Fig. 17, *B*). This method of percussion is of value in observing muscle reflex mechanisms of the mandible, muscle tenderness, hypertonicity of the muscles of mastication as evidenced by localized contraction at the site, and a demonstration of Chvostek's sign (in latent tetany, tapping over the facial nerve in front of the ear causes twitching or spasm of the facial muscles).

Percussion applied by tapping bone with the finger-tips may be useful in locating tender areas in the mandible or maxilla. Percussion to determine the density of structures such as bone is best carried out by placing a finger of one hand on the area to be evaluated and striking it a blow with the tip of one of the fingers of the other hand (Fig. 17, *C*). The middle finger of one hand (pleximeter finger) is held firmly but not uncomfortably against the bony structure to be percussed. The middle finger of the other hand (plexor finger), flexed at a right angle at the first interphalangeal joint, is used to strike the pleximeter finger two quick sharp blows. The action is done entirely by the wrist, and the plexor finger is removed quickly from the pleximeter finger to prevent dampening of the sound. Differences in the density of the bone and underlying structures may be clearly differentiated where they exist. As in palpation and inspection, like areas on two sides of the face must always be compared.

Auscultation is the act of listening for sounds produced within the body. The development of a sense of hearing for the various sounds of interest to a dentist is one of the least appreciated facets of the clinical examination. Unless the examiner's attention is receptive to the sounds of abnormal breathing, clicking and snapping of the temporomandibular joints, vocal fremitus, and other abnormal sounds, it is quite likely that a complete appraisal and diagnosis of a patient's abnormality may be overlooked in many instances. While it seems unlikely that any dentist would undertake therapy in an asthmatic or dyspneic individual with abnormal breathing sounds without further systemic evaluation, it does happen, for it is not uncommon to completely overlook this phase of auscultation. This may be further emphasized by pointing out the failure of many clinicians to recognize snapping and clicking of the temporomandibular joint as a symptom of disturbance of this joint. Another use of auscultation which appears to be overlooked by many is the determination of the relationship of oral structures to the production of normal speech. The loss of teeth, placement of artificial teeth, cleft palate, and muscle paralysis can give rise to serious impairment of speech. Another abnormal sound of considerable significance to a patient wearing full dentures is constant clicking of the teeth during speaking and mastication.

Occasionally a patient will complain of a peculiar "squeak" that may be elicited by clenching of the teeth. The cause of such an abnormal sound may be difficult to locate and may necessitate special procedures. However, it is usually caused by the abnormal movement of teeth whose approximating surfaces have been restored with improperly finished amalgam. The sound is not unlike that of the "tinner's cry" of fresh amalgam being squeezed. The placement of flat wax dental floss between the contact areas of the suspected teeth may serve to localize the offending restorations.

CLINICAL EXAMINATION OF THE PATIENT—GENERAL

The clinical or physical examination of the patient should include the exposed parts of the body and the structures of the mouth. A logical and orderly scheme of examination should be practiced. While the physical examination may consist of only an examination of the affected part as determined by the chief complaint, only a thorough and complete examination as indicated in the following outline can be expected to produce a high yield of unsuspected disease or even the "obvious" disease. The examination procedures should follow that given in the accompanying outline.

OUTLINE OF GENERAL CLINICAL EXAMINATION

General Appraisal (including temperature, pulse rate, and blood pressure when indicated)

Head
Skull—facies, facial form, symmetry
Eyes—scleras, pupils, eyelids, conjunctival lesions
Nose—deformity, obstructions, mouth breathing

Skin
Pigmentation, hair, texture, scars, lesions
Fingernails—biting, disease

Neck
Lymph nodes, scars, lesions, swelling, tenderness, pulsations, deviation of the midline

Jaws
Symmetry, anteroposterior relationship, closure pattern, lateral and protrusive movements
Temporomandibular joints—clicking, snapping, swelling, tenderness

General Survey

The clinical examination should begin with a general appraisal or survey of the patient's well-being; it begins when the patient is first observed. This part of the examination will allow the dentist to make an over-all evaluation of gross alteration of body habitus, state of nutrition, body build, constitution, intellectual achievement, personality, speech, mental alertness, psyche, and general hygiene. When indicated, the examiner should record body temperature, pulse rate, blood pressure, weight, and respiration.

The examination of the exposed parts of the body is not to be considered a medical examination but rather a review of parts immediately related in health and disease to the mouth and to dental treatment; this review is within the scope of the responsibility of the dentist in rendering a health service. In the general survey an attempt should be made to evaluate the individual in relation to his disease, including his psychologic adjustment to his disorder. Observations should be included that relate to the natural course of the disease and alterations caused by therapy.

The general survey does not take the place of a routine systematic clinical examination; however, it does serve to facilitate the examination by directing the examiner's attention to certain areas or systems for a more detailed consideration than might be otherwise considered routinely. The general appearance of a patient may suggest such entities as pernicious anemia, thyrotoxicosis, tic douloureux, tabes dorsalis, or an endocrine disturbance, yet the true nature of the disease remains to be substantiated by further detailed examination. Therefore, early in the clinical examination, the findings from the general appraisal will serve as a guide for the rest of the examination.

Constitution and stature of an individual represent not only characteristics of inheritance, but also the influence of the endocrine system. Inasmuch as diseases of the endocrine system may affect the characteristics of stature and body build, variations from the range of normal may characterize a particular disturbance of the endocrine system.

Examination of a child should begin with a general appraisal of the status of general growth and development. The examiner may use anthropometric charts showing so-called norms of growth and development at various age levels, provided he keeps in mind that each child has his own pattern of growth and development. It is more significant to know that a child is consistently within the same percentiles for weight and height than it is to know whether or not he is tall or short, overweight or underweight. It must be kept in mind that there may be no sharp line of differentiation between the normal and abnormal child in respect to the features of body build or growth such as size or rate of growth. However, it is well to know how growth and development can be influenced by such factors as genetics, disease, malnutrition, and endocrine disturbances. This phase of the examination is of considerable importance in the interception of malocclusion, diagnosis of malocclusion, and the formulation of an orthodontic treatment plan.

It is not the purpose of this book to point out and describe all the findings in disease that may relate to abnormalities of body build, growth, and development. While great variations of body build do exist in the range of normal, and and the body habitus of all individuals may not be characteristic enough to fit into a clear-cut category, it is to be expected that the student and practitioner will have a sufficient knowledge of the range of normal to detect abnormal body proportions and qualitative abnormalities of secondary sexual characteristics. It is most important that they develop an appreciation for variations from the normal in growth and development of children and for variations of body build and stature in adults. Descriptions of the normal constitution and body habitus and the effects of disease upon growth and development can be found elsewhere. The primary consideration of the dentist in his clinical examination of the patient is to recognize that abnormalities of constitution and body habitus may play an important part in the diagnosis and treatment of oral disease.

It is not unusual for the experienced examiner to sum up the appraisal of the patient's weight and nutrition by the phrase "well developed and well nourished." This does not simply imply well-developed musculature or an abundance of avoirdupois. The phrase "well developed" should be used to mean normal body proportions consistent with the size, age, and sex of the individual. The phrase "well nourished" should be used to mean the absence of any evidence of disease due to malnourishment. Weight is only one feature in the nutritional state of an individual. Probably the most common disorder in this country is obesity. Thus the term "well nourished" means the absence of evidence of avitaminosis, hypoproteinemia, iron deficiency, mineral deficiency, and excessive variation in the person's ideal weight.

A partial survey of the neurologic and musculoskeletal systems can be made from an observation of an individual's gait. There is considerable variation in normal gait; however, systemic and local disease, especially of the feet and the hip joints, may markedly influence gait. Diseases involving pyramidal and extrapyramidal tracts, cerebellar disease, and other diseases involving posture columns may produce rather characteristic abnormalities of gait; e.g., ataxic patients may keep their eyes fixed on the floor while walking with a shuffling gait and a patient with hemiplegia associated with apoplexy (cerebral vascular accident) usually walks with a circumduction of the hip with plantar flexion and inversion of the foot and with the flexed arm of the afflicted side held rigid. Thus the presence of an abnormal gait may be somewhat diagnostic and also introduce the examiner to the possibility of paralysis in other areas, i.e., facial muscles and those of mastication. It goes without saying that the examiner must attempt to identify the areas which are involved since dental treatment many times will be dictated by the extent and location of the paralysis.

The patient's body temperature should be recorded if the presenting complaint involves constitutional symptoms that include fever. In taking oral temperatures, the thermometer should be left in place for at least three minutes. The bulb should be placed under the tongue and the mouth should be kept closed. The use of hot or cold fluid just prior to taking the temperature may lead to erroneous results. Fever is a reaction of the body to physical or somatic disturbances. The degree of elevation of body temperature depends on many factors, the two most important being the type and severity of the pathologic process and the individual reaction of the patient to the disease. Increased pulse rate, increased respiratory rate, and increased basal metabolic rate usually accompany fever. The most common cause of fever is the response to local or systemic infectious agents such as bacteria and viruses. Another cause is malignant neoplasms. This is especially true in the lymphomatous diseases, including the leukemias. Injuries may cause a rise in body temperature. Thus fever may be related to specific injury to the central nervous system or to dead or dying tissue. The most common causes of fever in patients seen by the dentist are abscessed teeth, acute necrotizing gingivitis, and herpetic gingivostomatitis. The severity, type, character of onset, and time relationship of the fever to tissue lesions are significant factors in the differential diagnosis of herpetic gingivostomatitis and acute necrotizing gingivitis.

When a patient's history is being taken, his speech should be evaluated because of its frequent importance as a diagnostic clue. Disorders of speech may be of no diagnostic importance or may be associated with neurologic lesions, inability to enunciate, disturbances of the larynx, harelip, cleft palate, nasal obstruction, or other serious diseases. For example, an anxious and tense individual is likely to speak rapidly and at a high pitch; however, these same speech mannerisms are likely to be present in the thyrotoxic patient. A chronic alcoholic or an individual with general paresis may have difficulty in speaking and in enunciating; such difficulties should alert the examiner to the possibility of the presence of disease. Though hoarseness may be associated with a cold or an upper respiratory tract infection and is usually of a transitory nature, persistent hoarseness may suggest the presence of a tumor or paralysis of the vocal cords. Of special interest to the dentist are lisping associated with tonguetie, inability to pronounce labials associated with harelip and/or cleft palate, and difficulties of enunciation related to loss of teeth, encroachment on the tongue space, ill-fitting dentures, and macroglossia.

Respiration should be noted for rate and rhythm if surgery is to be done and there is a past history of heart disease, lung disease, or asthma. In the patient with asthma, orthopnea may or may not be present and wheezing may be present on expiration and inspiration. With asthma, the accessory chest and neck muscles labor to push the air in and out of the lungs. In left ventricular failure, which the dentist is not likely to see except as an associated complaint, expiration takes little effort, and orthopnea is usually present. Observation of respiration is done only to recognize signs of respiratory embarrassment. The presence of respiratory embarrassment, however slight, should be evaluated. It is under these circumstances that precautionary measures should be taken and in some instances a medical referral made.

The pulse should be taken whenever heart disease is suspected or has appeared in the patient's history. While the stethoscope reveals more than the pulse rate, the average practicing dentist is not equipped or trained to auscultate sounds of the heart. However, it is possible for him to palpate one of the larger peripheral arteries rather easily and to discover the presence of cardiac disease. The radial artery is most often used. In addition to noting any thickening of the arterial wall (quite common with advancing age), the course of the artery, its compressibility and fullness, and its rate and rhythm should be evaluated. In general, tortuosity is indicative of arteriosclerosis; a palpable cordlike structure in both diastole and systole is seen in patients with hypertension; a full, or bounding pulse is found with increased cardiac output, after exercise, and in persons with hyperthyroidism and similar conditions; a rapid and "thready" pulse may occur when there is an insufficient quantity of blood and weakened ventricular systole; a pulse with a sharp rise and fall with a sharp summit and wide pulse pressure (Corrigan's or water-hammer pulse) is typically present in patients with aortic regurgitation and may be found to a certain degree in those with anemia and hyperthyroidism.

Tachycardia and bradycardia should be noted and correlated with the patient's history of cardiovascular disease. Without auscultation of the heart, it is impossible to actually evaluate either of these two signs. Tachycardia, bradycardia, and heart irregularities may be normal findings, but in the presence of a history of cardiac disease such findings give basis for medical referral.

Palpitations of the heart may be considered as an awareness of the pounding, rapidity, or irregularity of heart action. While some forms of palpitation may be extremely serious, the phenomenon usually causes distress beyond its significance. The dentist is usually confronted with immediate concern when a patient complains of an awareness of pounding of the heart. Occasionally the symptoms include tachycardia and paroxysmal arrhythmias. These symptoms may produce fright, weakness, vasomotor disturbances, or collapse. It is not uncommon for the disturbances in rhythm to cause this type of distress and yet cause no interference with cardiac efficiency. These symptoms may arise in any normal individual exposed to dental procedures, especially when treatment tends to cause anxiety. Occasionally the use of drugs or anesthetics will cause tachycardias or cardiac arrhythmias. Thus disturbances in rhythm of the heart occur not only in normal individuals under unusual circumstances but also in patients who have heart disease. A history of cardiac arrhythmias prior to dental operation or oral surgery may serve to direct the treatment of the patient by the dentist in case such conditions arise while he is treating the patient. If there is a history of heart disease, the onset of tachycardia may be a threat to the patient. If a patient is known to have auricular fibrillation and is using a drug to slow the ventricular rate, it is well to know that he has taken such medicine prior to dental procedures.

Other findings of significance in the evaluation of a patient with heart disease are malar flush, clubbing of the fingers, and distention of the neck veins. A malar flush may indicate hypertension, fever, or mitral stenosis. Cyanosis and clubbed fingers may be related to pulmonary disease or heart disease. Pronounced substernal pulse may be due to aortic insufficiency, hypertension, or an aneurysm. If a patient who is seated in a dental chair and breathing normally has significant distention of the neck veins, heart disease or mediastinal obstruction should be suspected.

When oral surgery is considered and symptoms suggest the presence of cardiac disease, a determination of blood pressure should be made. In most dental offices this procedure is not routine; its use is limited to emergency situations. In those instances where the other examination procedures indicate the presence of cardiovascular disease, the recording of the patient's blood pressure hardly seems necessary. However, in instances of transient or recurrent hypertension, it would appear wise to record the blood pressure prior to surgical procedures.

The brief evaluation of the patient's cardiac status should not be considered as exhaustive or final. Whatever precautions the dentist may take for the safety of his patient are taken for the purpose of referring the patient, when necessary, for more adequate evaluation. Thus the emphasis on the cardiac evaluation is not upon the discovery and diagnosis of cardiac disease itself but upon the discovery of signs of cardiac disease that might be of significance in dental treatment.

In most instances it might appear to the casual observer that a general appraisal of the patient is not warranted since the yield of information appears to be small. Fortunately most clinicians make a gross appraisal of a patient's health without being really aware of it. Actually it takes but little more concerted effort to broaden the scope of the practitioner's awareness of his patient's general appearance. It is the development of a systematic awareness that enables the good diagnostician to detect all the significant deviations from normal health. Obvious signs of disease may be entirely lacking in the oral region, yet the examiner's considered general appraisal of the patient may dictate to him the necessity for a medical referral for the patient's good. Even the simplest considerations of the patient's health and well-being are obvious signs to the patient of the dental practitioner's interest in him as a whole individual. All too often the criticism of "playing doctor" is leveled at the conscientious dental practitioner showing any interest in his patient other than to search for dental caries. This criticism cannot be justified except in rare instances where a dentist enters into those areas which are unrelated to his responsibility and for which he is not qualified by training.

Head

The examination of the head should include a brief review of the skull (including facies, facial form, symmetry) eyes, and nose. The objectives of this part of the examination are to evaluate briefly those abnormalities of the head which may be related to the patient's general well-being and to evaluate those abnormalities which may be directly or indirectly related to the diagnosis and treatment of disease within the province of the dentist. The primary consideration is the recognition of abnormalities. The next procedure is the interpretation and evaluation of the results of the examination. How the examiner handles the facts which he has collected will depend to a large extent upon his ability to determine which findings are contributory, which are related to predisposing and exciting causes, and which are related to the signs and symptoms of oral disease. Thus the prerequisites to formulation of a diagnosis are the collection of the facts and a descriptive knowledge of those diseases responsible for the observed abnormalities.

Once it is recognized that an abnormality exists, it is possible for the examiner to make an evaluation of it in terms of disease processes. The recognition of the abnormality will be considered here; the relationships of these abnormalities to disease will be found more aptly in those textbooks concerned with descriptions of disease. The primary purpose of the examination of the head is not to make a diagnosis of disease but to recognize the presence of an abnormality which can, with proper knowledge of the signs and symptoms of disease, be related to oral disease. Therefore, the examiner's attention should be initially concerned with the discovery of those features of the head which are outside the range of normal. To be concerned primarily with the diagnosis of an abnormality generally precludes the recognition of any disease other than that of which the examiner has a descriptive knowledge. This is especially true in the examination of the head since many clinicians are familiar with only the most important abnormalities of the head and are unaware of the relationship or importance of abnormalities of the skull, eyes, and nose to diseases of the oral structures.

Skull.—The external features of the cranium may give some clue as to congenital deformity, growth and development, asymmetry, general effects of disease, and endocrine disturbances. Deformities of the skull can be more readily determined by an examiner who has acquired an appreciation for the normal through systematic observation. The contour and size of the skull varies considerably within the normal limits, and even extreme deviations from normal may not indicate any disturbance. However, mild degrees of altered contour and size which may be difficult to detect may be due to a pathologic disturbance. This should not imply futility but rather the need for considered observation.

The presence of signs of disease, injury, and operations may play a signifi-

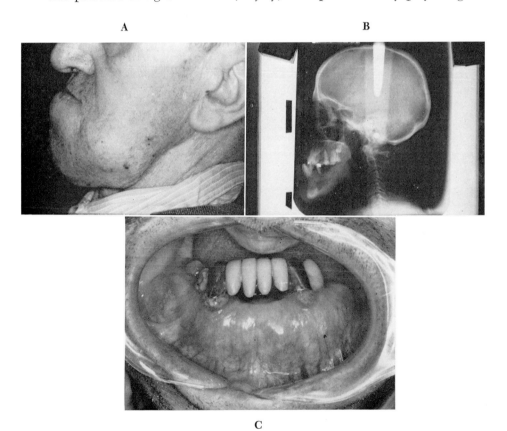

A   **B**

C

Fig. 18. *Paget's disease.* **A,** Marked enlargement of mandible with prognathism and lateral enlargement. **B,** Radiograph showing prognathic enlarged mandible of patient shown in **A. C,** Enlarged and expanded mandible of patient shown in **A.**

cant role in the evaluation and differential diagnosis of disease of the mouth and adjacent structures. Textbooks on pathology and oral medicine are usually replete with descriptions of abnormal findings of contour and size of the skull. Pictorial descriptions of an abnormally large head related to hydrocephalus, osteitis deformans (Fig. 18), leontiasis ossea, and acromegaly are well known. The "square head" which appears abnormally large (though actually it is not) is frequently attributed to prominent "bosses" of the frontal bones and may occur in the healing of the bone lesion of either rickets or congenital syphilis. Less well known is the importance of the signs of injuries and operations of the head. The scar of an operation for tic douloureux, intracranial tumor, or gunshot wound may be the basis for dysfunction of the oral structures.

The term facies refers to the appearance of the patient's face as a whole. The appearance may be suggestive or characteristic of certain disease conditions. Of special interest to the orthodontist is the adenoid facies seen in children. It is characterized by a thin face, pinched nose, high arched palate, mouth breathing, and, frequently, a languid expression. Other rather characteristic facies include those of acromegaly (Fig. 19), cherubism (Fig. 20), goiter (Fig. 40, A), mongolism (Fig. 21, A and B), cretinism (Fig. 21, C), achondroplasia, myxedema, and Cushing's disease (Fig. 22). The facial appearance may show evidence of dehydration, i.e., dry wrinkled skin with sunken cheeks and hollow eyes. The face may also show evidence of edema, i.e., pale and puffy; this may be especially prominent beneath the eyes. The facies of the chronically ill and the psychiatric patient may also be of diagnostic significance.

Examination of the profile facies may reveal much about the positions of the teeth and jaws. The "Andy Gump" type and the "Hapsburg" jaw are fairly characteristic signs of malocclusion, malfunction, and/or maldevelopment (Fig.

A   B

Fig. 19. *Acromegaly.* **A,** Marked enlargement of tongue. **B,** Thickening of skin has resulted in thick lips and lids, broad nose, coarse features, and enlargement of hands with thick blunt fingers and heavy palmar pads. (Courtesy Dr. Stefan Fajans.)

Fig. 20. *Cherubism or familial fibrous dysplasia.* **A,** Note fullness of lower face providing a round or square face. **B,** Bilateral involvement of angle and body of mandible with destructive lesions which produce bulging of buccal plate. **C,** More severe example of cherubism; note symmetrical enlargement of lower face. (**A** and **B,** Courtesy Dr. William G. Shafer; **C,** courtesy Dr. Carl Witkop.)

A   B

C

Fig. 21. *Characteristic facies in mongolism and cretinism.* **A,** Mongolism; note transverse grooves on tongue and characteristic mongoloid facies. **B,** Profile of typical mongoloid facies. **C,** Typical facies and habitat in cretinism. (**A** and **B,** Courtesy Dr. Joseph Hartsook; **C,** courtesy Dr. William Beierwaltes.)

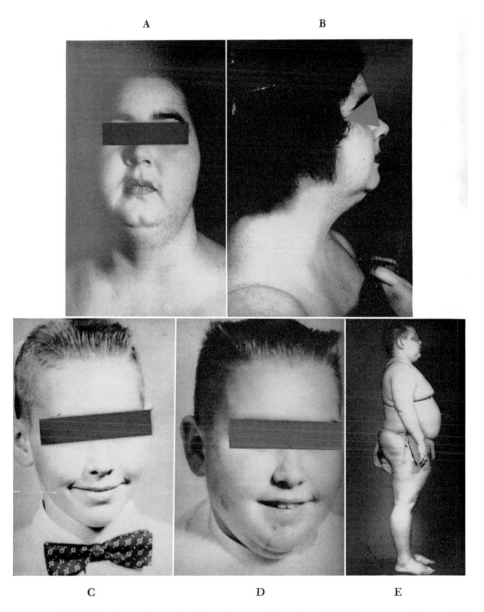

A   B

C   D   E

Fig. 22. *Cushing's syndrome.* **A,** Moon face and hirsutism. **B,** Enlargement of fat pad of upper back ("buffalo hump"). **C,** Early development, 9 years of age. **D,** Progress of disease with development of round facies, 14 years of age. **E,** Further progress of disease with greater change in face and development of typical habitus. (Courtesy Dr. Stefan Fajans.)

23). The facial profile should be evaluated not only in terms of osseous structures, but also in terms of the muscles supplied by the fifth and seventh cranial nerves. Extreme malpositions of the teeth are seldom seen without accompanying muscle strains and unilateral contractions of the facial muscles.

Symmetry must also be considered. Normally the skull and face are fairly symmetrical; however, perfect symmetry is not usually found, and the two halves

A   B

Fig. 23. *Facial profile.* **A,** Prognathism associated with Angle's Class III malocclusion. **B,** Retrognathic mandible.

A   B

Fig. 24. *Facial asymmetry.* **A,** Note droop of left angle of mouth and wide opening of left eye at rest. **B,** Note inability to retract left angle of mouth and to close left eye.

of the face and skull will invariably differ somewhat. A demonstration of this fact may be shown by producing two faces from a photograph whose negative is cut vertically in the center and using each half to make a complete print. It is necessary that the examiner develop an appreciation for asymmetry of the face in order to recognize skeletal defects that may have an important bearing on growth and development of the jaws, to properly evaluate past injury, and to recognize the presence of disease whose beginning may be manifest only in slight facial asymmetry. The most common asymmetries encountered by the dentist are seen in association with alveolar abscesses, abscesses of the soft tissues, paralysis of the facial nerve (Bell's palsy, Fig. 24), functional and organic malpositions of the jaws, tumors, diseases of the parotid glands, and post-traumatic swelling (Fig. 25).

A   B

C   D

Fig. 25. *Facial asymmetry.* **A,** Swelling due to extension of periapical infection. **B,** Nodular lateral swelling produced by actinomycosis. **C,** Lipoma producing facial asymmetry due to smooth, soft swelling over entire lower two-thirds of lateral face. **D,** Involvement of the space of the body of the mandible by infection.

The obvious signs of gross enlargement which give the face and jaws asymmetry are important; however, even more important are the slight degrees of asymmetry that herald the onset of disease. Thus the emphasis is upon the slight degree of asymmetry and its recognition rather than simply upon gross deformities. This does not mean that gross deformities are unimportant; it does suggest that most examiners will see the obvious signs of asymmetry but will fail to recognize equally significant signs of slight asymmetry. The cause of jaw and facial asymmetry may be skeletal, muscular, glandular, occlusal, or soft tissue in origin. Asymmetry may be manifested only when the mandible is opened (Fig. 26). Functional deviation of the mandible may be due to a disturbance of the temporomandibular joints, muscle disturbances, and disturbances of neurogenic origin. Deviation of the mandible when the teeth are occluded may be skeletal or occlusal in origin. Not infrequently disharmony between centric relation and acquired centric occlusion will result in a midline deviation of the mandible. This deviation may be grossly apparent or observed by comparison of the midline of the maxilla and mandible. Deviation of the midline may also be due to malposition of the teeth; therefore, the mandible must be placed in centric relation to determine whether the deviation is due to occlusal disharmony and premature contacts or to malposition of the teeth.

The analysis of facial form is of considerable importance in the evaluation and diagnosis of malocclusion. Its relation to the development of occlusion will be found in Chapter 5.

Eyes and Adnexa.—The eye is more commonly affected by constitutional disease than any other organ or system. The information gained from the history and from a brief clinical examination may indicate the true nature of oral disease and the necessity for additional investigation by an ophthalmologist. The dentist must limit his examination to subjective findings derived from the patient's statements and from a general inspection of the eye and adnexa for gross departures from the normal. While the ocular manifestations of systemic disease

A   B

Fig. 26. *Functional asymmetry due to temporomandibular joint ankylosis.* **A,** Closure. **B,** Opening; note shift of mandible to the right.

Fig. 27. *Exophthalmos.* Graves' disease with characteristic protrusion of the eyes. (Courtesy Dr. William Beierwaltes.)

not infrequently herald widespread or distant disorders, the dentist cannot recognize many of them because of their location in the eye beyond his examination. However, many diseases may be manifest in a location which he may observe by simple inspection. The objective signs of disease which may be seen by the dentist include Argyll Robertson pupil, exophthalmos, conjunctival petechiae, nystagmus, pigmented pingueculae, interstitial keratitis, corneal ulcerations, lid lag, widening of palpebral fissures, icterus, ptosis of the eyelid, miosis, and exudation.

Ptosis is dropping of an eyelid due to paralysis of the levator palpebrae superioris resulting from dysfunction of the third cranial nerve. The cause may be congenital in origin or may be due to any condition such as tabes dorsalis, multiple sclerosis, and neoplastic or inflammatory disease. In Bell's palsy, there is inability to close the lid, and the constant irritation causes excessive lacrimation (Fig. 24). Exophthalmos (Fig. 27) is a protrusion of the eyeball and is a characteristic finding in Graves' disease. Lid lag may be demonstrable in patients with thyroid disease. As the eye is rotated downward, the lid fails to follow synchronously. Corneal ulcerations, infrequent blinking, and widening of the palpebral fissures are also likely to be present in the patient with hyperthyroidism and exophthalmos.

The sclera is normally bluish-white, and variation in this color may be readily appreciated by simple inspection. Icterus may be seen in the sclera. Of dental significance is the relationship of blue scleras to osteogenesis imperfecta, and odontogenesis imperfecta. The conjunctiva may give valuable signs of vitamin A deficiency (Bitot's spots) and jaundice and may contain petechiae associated with subacute bacterial endocarditis and purpuras. Interstitial keratitis may give the cornea a grayish ground-glass appearance. This, as well as the other elements of Hutchinson's triad (notched incisors and middle ear deafness), is seen in congenital syphilis. Vitamin A deficiency may be manifest in the cornea by keratotic changes. Riboflavin deficiency may also produce changes, although these are difficult to see with the naked eye. The corneal reflex may be lost with sensory disturbances of the trigeminal nerve.

The change in the *pupil* most significant to the dentist is miosis associated with tabes dorsalis (Argyll Robertson pupil) and the pinpoint pupil of the narcotic addict. Pupils of unequal diameter may be of congenital origin or may be related to disease of the nervous system. Some ocular-oral syndromes of dental significance include Behçet's syndrome, consisting of a recurrent iritis, aphthae in the oral cavity, and ulcerations on the genitals; Stevens-Johnson's syndrome, consisting of a severe conjunctivitis in association with an eruptive fever and stomatitis (the lesions are of an erythema multiforme character); and Sjögren's syndrome, consisting of conjunctivitis due to dryness and stomatitis due to diminished secretions of the mouth and pharynx.

Nose.—An examination of the nose should include observations of gross deformity (saddle nose of syphilis [Fig. 28], achondroplasia, fracture, lesions), inflammation of the turbinates with possible relation to toothaches not otherwise placed as to origin, the presence of discharge and its relation to postnasal drip, allergy, lesions, epistaxis, and nasal obstruction, and the ability of the patient to breathe through his nose. Obstruction of the nasal cavity may be due to polyps, foreign objects, large turbinates, tissue hypertrophy, and habit. The relationship

A   B

Fig. 28. *Saddle nose.* **A** and **B**, Congenital syphilis; note disproportionate development of maxilla and mandible in patient shown in **A**.

A   B

Fig. 29. *Mouth breather.* **A**, Note short upper lip and exposure of gingiva. **B**, Note outline of gingival hyperplasia.

of nasal breathing to mouth breathing is of primary consideration to periodontal and orthodontic therapy. (Fig. 29.)

Chronic mouth breathing may result from habit or from obstruction to nasal breathing. The habit may be secondary to the obstruction in nasal breathing. This habit is not infrequently established from an inability to breathe through the nose because of enlarged adenoids, deviated septum, allergic rhinitis, frequent colds, polyps, or nocturnal and recumbent engorgement of the vessels of the nasal mucous membranes. All chronic mouth breathers should be evaluated by an otolaryngologist for possible nasal obstruction. Dental appliances for breaking the habit will not be of value unless the underlying cause is removed. The chronic gingivitis seen so frequently in the mouth breather cannot be treated effectively unless the mouth breathing is eliminated first.

Skin

The skin should be examined for abnormal texture (Fig. 30), color, pigmentation, scars, eruptions (Fig. 31), lesions (Fig. 32), and indications of local and

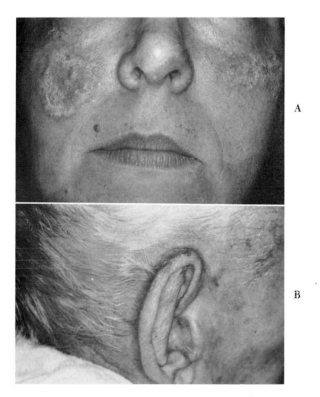

A

B

Fig. 30. A, Bilateral patches which are slightly elevated with violaceous center and scaly appearance at periphery and are typical both in character and location of chronic discoid lupus erythematosus. B, Senile keratosis and other changes typical of those occurring in skin of elderly people, especially those who have had constant exposure to sunlight. Note crustlike kerotic lesions on upper border of helix, pigmented areas in hair of temple, and atrophic changes in skin of face.

Fig. 31. A, Swelling of entire lateral aspect of face with multiple draining sinuses typical of actinomycosis. Sinus in lower right shows drop of pus at opening. Most of the other sinuses are closed at this time. **B,** Large bullae, some of which are intact and filled with fluid; others have ruptured and collapsed, leaving a wrinkled membrane over surface. These lesions are typical of those seen in epidermolysis bullosum.

systemic disease such as pallor, cyanosis, suborbital edema, and jaundice. It must be given careful consideration not only because it frequently reflects manifestations of systemic disease and the health of the individual, but also because it may be of considerable importance in the differential diagnosis of dermatologic lesions which appear only in the oral cavity or simultaneously on the skin and in the oral cavity (Figs. 33, 34, and 35). The texture of the skin of a normal healthy young individual has a certain degree of elasticity and thickness which causes it to quickly return to normal after it has been picked up in a fold between the thumb and index finger. In the older individual, as the skin loses some of its elasticity, there is some delay in the resumption of its former contour, when it is picked up and released. The elasticity generally decreases rapidly after the menopause, and in the senile person the skin is usually inelastic, thin, atrophic, and parchment-like. Such diseases as hypothyroidism, myxedema, and hyperthyroidism produce various changes in the texture of the skin. In hyperthyroidism the skin feels

Fig. 32. **A,** Xanthoma palpebrarum due to deposit of cholesterol in and about eyelids. Margin of upper lid is markedly thickened. Small nodules surround inner canthus. **B,** Numerous, varying-sized nodules covering face are adenomas of sebaceous gland origin.

smooth and silky and is generally moist and elastic. In hypothyroidism and myxedema, dryness and inelasticity are generally found. These changes may not be sufficiently clear-cut to be diagnostic, but such skin changes are highly suggestive of systemic diseases.

Color of the skin of the face may be compared with that of other areas of the body. However, since the dentist will be examining only the face and neck and exposed parts of the body, he must keep in mind that alterations of the color and texture may be physiologic in origin, e.g., the changes of "suntan" associated with constant exposure to the sun versus the lack of tanning or a sallow skin associated with an indoor life. The color of the skin is derived chiefly from its vascular bed and from the amount and distribution of its pigment. It may vary because of age, regional distribution of pigments, sex differences, and climatic differences.

In abnormal states the skin may be yellow, olive green, lemon-yellow tinted, red, bluish-red, light brown, or dark brown. Many factors control pigmentation, and one of the principles of the anterior pituitary gland appears to have considerable importance in the alteration of skin color, especially for protective purposes. In general, the underlying basis for alteration of skin color may be related to changes in the vascular bed, blood and bile pigments, metallic pigments,

A   B

C   D

Fig. 33. Child with chickenpox (varicella). Lesions are in vesicular stage. **A,** Characteristic vesicular lesions on palms. **B,** One of several palatal lesions. Other areas of oral mucosa
also are affected. **C,** Resolving lesions of varicella showing the pitlike character. **D,** Chronic lesion of same duration as those shown in **C** involving marginal gingiva between maxillary left
lateral incisor and cuspid.

and melanin pigments. Thus any physiologic and pathologic changes which
may affect these various factors may give rise to alterations.

Paleness or pallor cannot be considered as especially indicative of the
presence of an anemia; however, it is sometimes suggestive enough to warrant
this consideration. Pallor may be related to factors other than anemia such as
vasomotor phenomena. It must be differentiated from the sallow color of chronic
illnesses or the lack of exposure to sunlight. Pallor of the skin or mucous membrane may be due to a decreased flow of blood to these structures or to an actual
loss of hemoglobin. The color of an anemic patient varies with the factors responsible for the diminution of the hemoglobin; thus a combination of pallor
and jaundice may be produced in hemolytic anemia. If pallor is to be used
as a sign of anemia or as a sign of changes in the hemoglobin content of the
blood, then the areas to be observed should be those which are less well mela-

nized, nonkeratinized, and which contain a minimal stratum corneum, such as the lips, palpebral conjunctiva, and mucous membranes (the fingernail beds are also useful because of the translucency of the nails). Pallor or paleness, per se, is difficult to detect and, when it is thought to be present, the examiner should evaluate the possibility of its cause. It may be due to a decrease of hemoglobin pigment, a diminished flow of blood to the tissues, the presence of edema, or a

A   B

C   D

Fig. 34. *Scleroderma.* A, Loss of natural wrinkles, providing masklike appearance. Note also telangiectasia and reddish-purple blotches. B, Tense atrophic shiny skin with ulceration over the knuckle of ring finger. C, Atrophy of mucosa and loss of elasticity of skin resulting in limited oral opening. D, Changes in supporting tissues demonstrated radiographically by widening of periodontal space, finely trabeculated bone, and horizontal bone loss.

Fig. 35. *Herpes zoster.* **A,** Note vesicular lesions between eyebrow and hairline and beneath hair. **B,** Numerous crusted lesions on lip and ruptured lesions covered with fibrinous membrane on buccal mucosa.

decrease in melanin pigments. It must be remembered that melanin pigment can effectively screen out much of the color or lack of color due to altered hemoglobin or vascular changes. The detection of erythema, cyanosis, and pallor should be observed in those areas of the body which have a minimal or absent melanization.

An increased redness of the skin may be due to capillary dilatation, associated with blushing, fever, burns, exposure to sunlight, and telangiectasia due to x-ray therapy (Fig. 36). In rare instances generalized redness may be due to polycythemia vera. The tissues may be quite red in inflammatory changes. Areas of ulceration that allow the color of the underlying vessels to be readily seen may show an intensive red color. Where there is an increased desquamation of the skin or mucous membranes, such as may occur in the red beefy tongue of deficiency glossitis and desquamative gingivitis, the more superficial position of the capillary vessels may show more easily the color due to oxyhemoglobin. Vascular nevi give the skin involved a port-wine color; the gingivae may also be affected (Fig. 37).

Cyanosis is a term used to designate the predominance of reduced hemoglobin in the blood. It results when the absolute reduced hemoglobin in the blood reaches 5 grams per cent. The color of the tissues as a result of cyanosis varies considerably, depending upon the modifying factors. In general, it varies from a deep purplish-blue to heliotrope. Thus, the color produced by an alteration of the hemoglobin pigments may vary from the purplish-blue of cyanosis to the generalized redness of polycythemia vera.

Changes in the color of the skin or mucous membranes due to altered melanin pigmentation may be related to local changes such as prolonged irritation or to diseases of systemic origin such as Addison's disease. Most cases of

A   B

C   D

Fig. 36. *Changes in skin associated with irradiation.* **A,** Note atrophy, epilation, and telangiectasia. **B,** Note depigmentation and telangiectasia. **C,** Squamous cell carcinoma appearing as slightly elevated, ulcerated lesions covered by black crust and having rolled border with some desquamation. Changes in skin are due to irradiation. **D,** Multiple lesions on side of face. Uppermost is an elevated, crusted, indurated lesion—an advanced carcinoma of the skin. Lower lesion is an elevated, indurated slightly hyperkeratotic process—senile keratotic plaque. Two pigmented areas can be seen just below and anterior to the ear. The four lesions demonstrated by this patient are all reactions to exposure.

A   B

C   D

Fig. 37. *Discoloration due to hemangioma.* **A,** Port-wine stain of upper right lip, cheek, and nose. **B,** Gingival involvement in same patient. **C,** Very light red to pink, smooth, non-elevated discoloration of skin, over posterior lateral border and angle of mandible. **D,** Vascular nevi on neck.

altered skin color not due to hemoglobin, melanin, or metallic pigmentation are due to bile pigments which produce a yellow color. The most common cause of a yellow skin color is bilirubin pigment and is associated with prehepatic, hepatic, or obstructive jaundice. The skin may not be simply yellow in character but may also appear to be pale since, for example, in hemolytic anemia the combination of pallor and a yellow tint give the skin a lemon-yellow appearance. In other types of jaundice bile pigments may impart a fairly yellow tint to the skin and to all the other tissues except the teeth. As the disease or obstruction increases in severity the yellow color may become quite pronounced and may become greenish-yellow or darker. Jaundice associated with these disorders may be present generally throughout the skin areas and the scleras and the mucous membranes. Hyperpigmentation due to carotene such as may be seen in myxedema and carotenemia is more characteristically localized in the palms, soles, and face. Yellow pigmentation may also be due to drugs, chemicals, or chronic uremia. Thus mere discoloration of the skin must be differentiated from mere yellow discoloration of the skin due to exposure to certain chemicals such as Atabrine and carotene.

Melanin pigmentation is a normal component of the skin structure, and normally the degree of melanization varies from one individual to the next, depending upon their complexion, exposure to sunlight, or racial group. Alterations in the content of pigment are usually only of significance when the change is of recent origin. Melanosis or increased melanin pigmentation may result from external causes such as sunlight, mechanical irritation, wind, and heat. Systemic diseases, as well as many skin disorders, may produce melanosis. Melanosis may be seen in nutritional deficiency states such as pellagra or may be the result of hormone imbalance. Representative examples of the latter are pigmentation of the face in pregnancy (chloasma gravidarum) and the accentuation of the areas of primary melanization such as the nipples and areolae. Not infrequently in Addison's disease there is an increased melanin pigmentation of the buccal mucosa. The nature of the mechanism of melanosis in Addison's disease is not clear; however, it is well established that primary adrenal cortical insufficiency does cause melanosis, whereas adrenal cortical insufficiency secondary to hypopituitarism does so only rarely. In general, there is no characteristic pattern of melanosis aside from that produced from an increased number of melanoblasts. Melanosis is usually not uniform in character but is predisposed to certain areas of the body. Thus, it may occur in those areas of the body which are exposed to sunlight, in the so-called primary zones of melanization, and in association with localized external causes.

While many diseases do not produce an unequivocal clinical picture of melanosis that will allow a diagnosis on the basis of this picture alone, a few diseases show a melanotic skin picture which is suggestive of basic systemic diseases. The objective of the dentist is not to diagnose these diseases but to recognize that there is an alteration of the basic pattern of pigmentation. Inasmuch as the dentist sees his patients fairly frequently, he is in a position to notice changes or alterations in their normal pigmentation. (Fig. 38.)

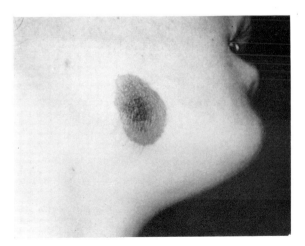

Fig. 38. Pigmented nevus over labial aspect of face bearing oval, dark brown, smooth patch with elevated black center. Black hairs originate from dark center.

Melanin pigmentation in the mouth is not usually seen in white persons of light complexion but is quite frequently observed in Negroes and in Caucasians with natural deposition of pigments. Melanin areas in the mouth are termed melanoplakia and are of diagnostic significance when seen in a person of light complexion or if known to be of recent origin. It is not known to what extent melanoblasts in the oral mucosa react to local physical factors such as irritation, heat, and chemical agents. In Negroes melanosis is detected more easily on the tongue than on the buccal mucosa. Of special interest to dentists is the increase in pigmented spots around the oral cavity and lips and mouth associated with intestinal polyposis.

Exogenous metallic pigments may be responsible for changes in the skin color, and the patient's occupation should be considered because of the possibility of metals and paints, insecticides, beverages, wallpaper, and electrotyping solutions being the causative factor. While most metallic pigments are exogenous in origin, an important exception to this is hemosiderin, an iron-containing pigment resulting from the destruction of blood or from a defect in iron metabolism.

The texture of the hair, as well as the amount present, may be suggestive of endocrine disturbances. In hyperpituitary disturbances the hair may be silky, of the lanugo type, and profuse on the cheeks. In hirsutism the distribution of hair is universal in extent, with a tendency for a masculine distribution; the hair is coarse and black and appears abundantly on the chin and upper lip (Fig. 22). This is especially noticeable in the female. In hypothyroidism there may be a diffuse loss of hair and what hair is present is harsh, dry, and brittle. Also, the skin is dry, and the nails are brittle. The reverse is true in hyperparathyroidism. These findings should not be confused with the increase in growth and change in color of hair which may be seen in women following removal of the ovaries or after menopause. Loss of the outer one-third of the eyebrows is seen at times as the result of hypothyroidism or syphilis.

A general survey of the patient should include a brief examination of the nails. This can be accomplished easily by a brief glance at the nails for obvious signs of disease; additional careful inspection may be made if indicated. The fingernails are important because they may show the presence of systemic disease. When disease is present in the nails of both the hands and feet, the disease is likely to be systemic in origin rather than local.

Onychophagia is of importance in dentistry because of its association with malocclusion, trauma to teeth, and gingivitis (Fig. 39, A). In the presence of diseases of the nails such as onychomycosis and mycotic paronychia, nail biting may spread the causative agent of the nail disease to the mouth. Nail changes due to roentgen rays include longitudinal ridging, slow growth, and brittleness. Koilonychia, or spoon nails, may be seen in association with anemia and is a part of the Plummer-Vinson syndrome. Chronic paronychia should be differentiated from the change of the nail base angle seen in clubbing of the fingers associated with hypertrophic osteoarthropathy (Fig. 39, B), which may be idiopathic in origin or result from atelectasis, bronchiectasis, heart failure, or other pulmonary disease. Excessive tobacco stain on the fingers is some indication of

A   B

Fig. 39. *Fingernails.* A, Nail biting. B, Hypertrophic osteoarthropathy.

mental unrest and is partially a quantitative estimate of the amount of smoking which the patient does. This may be related, if necessary, to cough, gingivitis, stomatitis, etc. Personal care of the fingernails gives some indication of what to expect in the way of care of the mouth. While not all patients who take care of their fingernails also take care of their mouth, they are more likely to do so than those who have no time for manicures and for other aspects of their personal hygiene.

It is not to be expected that the dentist should be able to make a diagnosis of diseases of the fingernails in general; however, he should have sufficient knowledge of changes to recognize a deviation from normal and in some instances to relate changes in the nails to systemic disorders and to disorders of the mouth. For example, he should correlate chronic nail biting with small fractures of the incisal edges of the anterior teeth and with gingivitis associated with the trauma from continual nail biting. It is necessary that the nail biting habit be eliminated before satisfactory periodontal therapy or restorative therapy can be undertaken. Furthermore, in some instances nail biting reflects psychologic unrest and this in itself may call for specialized therapy by a psychiatrist. It is not altogether easy at times to differentiate between a habit and that which is a compulsion to satisfy some psychic tension. Not infrequently the patient with bruxism, fingernail biting, excessive smoking, or other oral habits is emotionally disturbed to the extent that proper dental therapy cannot be accomplished.

Neck

An examination of the neck should be made for lesions, scars, lymph node enlargement, glandular enlargement (Fig. 40, A), deviations of the trachea, and the presence of developmental defects within the lateral aspects and the midline. Palpation should be done by comparison of both sides alternately or at the same time. Enlargement of lymph nodes may be due to local inflammation, neoplastic metastasis, or systemic disease. Examination should include palpation of the posterior auricular, submental, and anterior and posterior cervical nodes

A

B   C

Fig. 40. *Swellings of neck.* **A,** Endemic goiter in three members of same family. **B,** Bilateral enlargement of cervical lymph nodes typical of Hodgkin's disease. **C,** Chronic draining sinus due to tuberculous lymphadenitis.

and, when indicated, the supraclavicular, infraclavicular, epitrochlear, and axillary nodes. A differential diagnosis of swelling in the neck region makes necessary the differentiation of glandular elements, lymph nodes, fascial spaces, bones, and muscles.

Of special significance in the examination of the neck are the lymph nodes. In the normal individual very few lymph nodes are palpable even on careful clinical examination; however, their strategic location along the lymph channels makes them likely to be involved in a variety of infections and in various types of malignancies. Enlargement may be confined to small areas or may be widespread in nature and may be characterized by the cardinal signs of inflammation. Sequelae of involvement may be necrosis, rupture of the nodules, and the formation of a sinus. It is possible, however, for considerable enlargement to take place in the absence of any signs of inflammation. If the examiner discovers an enlargement or a mass in the usual location of lymph nodes, he should determine whether or not it is a solitary nodule or multiple masses. By bilateral palpation he should determine whether or not the process is unilateral or bilateral, whether the masses are discrete or matted together, and whether or not there is any tenderness present. The consistency must be noted to determine if the mass is hard, firm, or fluctuant. Palpation must be carried further to determine the presence of fixation to an underlying structure such as the mandible. The first evidence of lymph node enlargement may be pressure associated with the enlargement or signs of systemic involvement if the condition is inflammatory in character.

The most common causes of lymph node enlargement are acute and chronic infections of regional and/or systemic origin, so-called primary lymph node disease, such as Hodgkin's disease (Fig. 40, *B*), reticulum cell sarcoma, and lymphosarcoma, and the enlargement associated with leukemia and metastases from malignant disease. Lymphadenopathy associated with pulpal disease is most commonly found by the dentist. Tuberculosis (Fig. 40, *C*) and syphilis were formerly the most common causes of lymphadenopathy from specific infections.

The regional lymph nodes associated with the primary lesion of syphilis are characterized by a firm, painless swelling; in the secondary phase of syphilis, there is a generalized distribution of firm, shotty, nontender nodes. Enlargement due to metastasis of neoplastic lesions is characterized by being distinctly localized and very hard. The location of the lymphadenopathy may suggest the site of the origin of the disease since certain anatomic areas are drained by known groups of regional lymph nodes. The sequelae of any inflammation may leave the lymph node enlarged, firm, and easily palpable. Thus a differential diagnosis of enlargement must consider the possibility that previous injury or infection may be responsible for the enlargement which is felt at a later time. For example, in palpating enlargements in the neck such as a single mass in the midline just below the tip of the chin, the history and the physical characteristics of tumefaction, shape, size, consistency, attachment, and location must be determined. In this instance the physical characteristics are best defined by pressing the enlargement or node against the jaw bone or toward the floor of the mouth. If the enlargement is tender, has been present for only a short period of time, and is associated with a reactive lesion of the lower lip, the tip of the tongue, or the floor of the mouth, the diagnosis of metastatic carcinoma must be suspected. Lymphadenopathy in association with a metastatic carcinoma does not invariably mean that the lymph node enlargement is due to metastasis; enlargement secondary to ulcerating carcinoma may be the cause. When many of the lymph nodes of the neck are involved or multiple masses appear bilaterally in the neck rather suddenly in association with fever and malaise, the disease is usually of a general infectious nature,

In acute infectious diseases, the nodes may increase rapidly in size and become tender; they are usually discrete and firm but not hard and can be moved freely in their bed. When enlargement of the lymph glands of the neck begins insidiously in one area and spreads to other regions with a progressive increase in the size of the nodes, a chronic disease of the lymph nodes is usually present. In general, the glands are freely movable and are not tender. These are not characteristic findings of any specific chronic inflammatory process but may be seen in the specific infective granulomas, leukemias, Hodgkin's disease, lymphosarcoma, or malignant metastases.

Cervical lymphadenopathy may occur in Vincent's infection and in herpetic gingivostomatitis. Occasionally these two conditions may present diagnostic problems to the dentist, and a history of the time of onset of the lymphadenopathy is of importance in making the differential diagnosis. In herpetic gingivostomatitis the regional lymphadenopathy occurs prior to the lesions in the mouth, whereas in Vincent's disease the cervical adenopathy occurs after the lesions in the mouth. In acute infectious adenopathy the swelling usually subsides as soon as the primary lesions have healed; however, there may occasionally be suppuration with abscess formation. Infrequently the infection may break through the capsules of the gland and involve the surrounding glands. Where considerable scar tissue results, the lymph nodes may be palpable for many weeks and even months.

Lymphoid hyperplasia associated with many diseases is common in childhood, and adenopathy without any specific causative factor is also common. In the middle-aged or older individual the presence of localized and hard lymph nodes without obvious cause should direct the examiner's attention to the possibility of malignant metastasis. Lymph node enlargement from metastases may involve a single node or, in most instances, more than one node. At first the nodes which are involved are freely movable and do not exhibit tenderness when palpated. But as the disease progresses they become matted together and fixed to the surrounding structures; at this time they exhibit their characteristic hardness. Whenever such adenopathy is found in the neck region, especially in the submaxillary or superior deep cervical chains, carcinoma within the mouth, nasal pharynx, or nose should be suspected, and a diligent search should be made for a primary lesion in these regions. Occasionally malignant tumors may metastasize from distant parts of the body to the neck. Lesions involving the midline may involve the lymph chains on both sides. In the absence of sialolithiasis or a history of contact with epidemic parotitis or of a surgical procedure which might suggest operative parotitis, the examiner should direct his attention to the possibility of a neoplasm of the parotid gland. While radiographs with radiopaque fluid serve to assist in determining the extent and character of neoplasms of the parotid gland, it remains for the pathologist to make the precise diagnosis by studying a section of tissue from the gland.

An examination of the neck should include inspection of the veins of the neck. The position of the patient in the dental chair is such that congestion and pulsation of the jugular veins may sometimes be noticed in association with vascular hypertension, severe thyrotoxicosis, and congestive heart failure. Thus, in general, engorgement of the veins of the neck is suggestive of some obstructive process that prevents the return of blood flow or of right-sided congestive heart failure. When it is bilateral, the pathologic process may be of mediastinal or cardiac origin.

Swellings in the lateral aspect of the neck may be developmental, inflammatory, or neoplastic in origin. Branchial cleft cysts may be found along the anterior border of the sternocleidomastoid muscle, and Warthin's tumors may be found at the angle of the jaw. As in other masses found in this area, it may be necessary to perform a biopsy to determine the exact nature of the lesion. An adequate history and a complete examination of the mass are important in order to determine the true nature of the lesion. It is the history and the clinical examination which will determine whether or not a biopsy is to be performed.

The presence of a smooth, firm, solitary swelling along the anterior border of the sternocleidomastoid muscle that has been present since childhood and has not changed its characteristics is highly suggestive of a branchial cleft cyst. However, because of the presence of teratoma-like tumors in the area which have a tendency to become malignant in the fourth or fifth decade, a positive diagnosis of the swelling should be made. A doughy mass of cystic consistency found on the lateral aspects of the neck at birth or during early infancy is suggestive of hygroma colli (Fig. 41).

The examination of a patient with an enlargement or a mass in the neck should include an examination of the oral cavity for possible associated lesions. In the presence of a vague history and the absence of a contributing lesion in the oral cavity, the patient should be referred to a physician for consultation. When a lesion exists in the mouth, its exact nature should be determined.

Fig. 41. *Swelling of neck.* Hygroma colli (marked congenital enlargement of neck vessel).

Fig. 42. *Lesion of neck.* Scar from surgical removal of thyroglossal duct cyst.

In summary, an examination of the neck should be made for the presence of lesions, scars (Fig. 42), lymph node enlargement, enlargement of the salivary glands, deviation of the trachea, and developmental defects in both the lateral aspects and the midline. A mass in the neck should be regarded as neoplastic until proved otherwise. When a swelling in the neck exists and is attributed to a pathologic process in the jaws such as an abscessed tooth, the following should be determined: whether or not there is involvement of the fascia planes and potential spaces, whether or not the enlargement is firm or fluctuant, whether or not the overlying skin is red and fixed, whether or not the center of the mass is soft, and whether or not the patient has constitutional symptoms of malaise and fever. Localization of the suppuration and abscess formation is necessary in order that precise surgical intervention may be accomplished if necessary.

The parotid glands should be palpated for enlargements, and this may be done at the time that the neck is examined. It is difficult to palpate all of the parotid gland because of its extensive nature. It should be remembered that it extends posteriorly and upward to the lobe of the ear as well as below it and anteriorly to the anterior border of the masseter muscle. The dense fascia that surrounds the parotid glands does not permit any great amount of swelling to occur as a result of an inflammatory process without severe pain. The external features of the gland are palpated during the examination of the neck; however, the examination of the ducts and orifices is best accomplished by bimanual extraoral and intraoral palpation during the examination of the mouth. The external features may be altered by inflammatory processes, obstruction of the ducts, and neoplasms.

It should be pointed out again that the objective of this book is not to give a detailed descriptive review of all the diseases which produce swelling in these areas but is to present to the examiner a systematic approach for the detection of enlargements or masses in these areas. It is hoped that this will alert him to the cause of the enlargements so that he will more effectively utilize reference books containing a descriptive review of the lesions.

The technic of examination of the neck is based upon a knowledge of the location of anatomic structures most frequently involved by pathologic processes and a division of the structures into areas which are more easily covered by a systematic examination. In order for the examiner to carry out a thorough examination of the neck or lymphadenopathy, he must be aware of the anatomic location of the glands and the areas which they drain.

The *submental lymph glands* are located in the midline of the jaw just below the chin and between the attachments of the anterior digastric muscles. They drain the central portion of the lower lip, the tip of the tongue, and the anterior portion of the floor of the mouth. The *submaxillary lymph glands* are located below the midportion of the mandible about the submaxillary gland. This location can be best palpated by beginning at the anterior quarter of the masseter muscle and moving toward the midline. These glands drain the sides of the nose, the upper lip and lateral portions of the lower lip, the buccal mucosa and cheek, the midportions of the eyelids, and the anterolateral margins of the tongue. The *superficial cervical lymph* glands are located about the external jugular vein. They drain the external ear and the parotid gland and can be best palpated by manipulation of the tissues anterior to the sternocleidomastoid muscle. The deep superior and inferior cervical lymph glands are found along the course of the carotid artery and the internal jugular vein. These glands lie behind the sternocleidomastoid muscle and are especially numerous at the bifurcation of the common carotid artery. The deep superior cervical glands drain the back of the neck, the occipital region of the scalp, portions of the external ear, and the posterior and central portions of the tongue, palate, nasopharynx, nose, larynx, and upper part of the esophagus. The deep inferior cervical glands drain the back of the neck and the lower portion of the occipital scalp and superior anterior chest wall.

The examination of the neck and adjacent structures is one of the most important elements of the clinical examination of structures outside the mouth. This anatomic region is not only important to disease of the mouth and contiguous tissues, but also is often related to disease distant from the neck, especially disease of the chest. As previously mentioned, cardiac and pulmonary diseases are prime examples.

Examination Procedure.—Of initial importance is the correct seating of the patient in a relaxed unstrained position in the dental chair, preferably without head support. The examiner should be able to move the patient's head freely to relax muscle tension so as to facilitate palpation (Fig. 43). Depending upon the site to be examined, palpation is bilateral or unilateral. The position of the examiner depends upon the particular procedure used. Bilateral palpation is usually best accomplished with the examiner standing behind the patient, whereas unilateral palpation can usually be best accomplished with the examiner standing in front of the patient.

The first step in the examination is inspection of the neck for changes in contour and symmetry, changes in color and texture of the skin, scars, and dilatation and pulsation of the neck veins. The inspection should be systematic, and

Fig. 43. *Palpation of neck.* Note head position to facilitate relaxation of muscles.

like areas should be compared. Inspection should follow a definite procedure beginning with the parotid gland area. It should then proceed to the areas at the angles of the mandible, the borders and base of the mandible, the submandibular areas, the submental region, the midline of the neck, the anterior triangles of the neck, and along the borders of the sternocleidomastoid muscles. After inspection of these areas and while the patient is still facing the examiner, an inspection of general contours should be made while the patient moves his head slowly from side to side. This procedure may serve to bring out masses or demonstrate a lack of mobility.

Palpation of the neck and contiguous structures should be carried out with a definite procedure in mind. After the initial inspection, the examiner should start the palpation procedure standing behind the patient. The muscles should be completely relaxed. The examiner should begin by placing the flat surfaces of the finger tips at the same position on both sides of the neck and bilaterally palpating the parotid region and the tissue between the ascending ramus of the mandible and the sternocleidomastoid muscle. The head should be moved from side to side sufficiently to allow free access to the structures beneath the areas.

The examiner then should palpate bilaterally down the angles of the jaw, along the bases of the mandible, and below the mandible to the midline (Fig. 45). In the midline, the tissues and nodes in the submental region should be palpated by pressing them upward against the symphysis of the jaw. Later, during the examination of the floor of the mouth, bimanual palpation serves to retest some of the structures present in this area. Any deviation of contour that is abnormal in itself or different from the other side of the jaw should be noted. The midline of the neck should be examined, and the hyoid bone and thyroid cartilage should be palpated while the patient is at rest and while he is swallowing. The thyroid gland is attached to the larynx and trachea and will ascend during the swallowing act. Unless a pathologic process associated with the thyroid gland has caused fixation of the surrounding structures, any such lesion will ascend with the thyroid gland when the patient swallows (Fig. 44). The examiner should extend the palpation to the lateral areas of the neck by passing the closed fingers along the anterior and posterior borders of the sternocleidomastoid muscles while the patient is in a forward position and during rotation and lateral bending of the neck. The palpation should extend the length of the sternocleidomastoid muscles and upward to behind the ears (Fig. 46).

During the examination the examiner should be alert to rigidity of muscles, tenderness, induration, and solitary or multiple masses. In many instances the history will serve to enhance the physical examination procedure. The possible relationship to disease in the oral region or elsewhere must be recognized.

A brief review of the lesions found in the several areas of the neck seems in order at this time. Single masses which appear in the midline may be related to lymphadenopathy, thyroid disease, developmental disturbances such as thyroglossal duct anomalies, and cellulitis. Single masses in the submaxillary region may be cellulitis, sialolithiasis of Wharton's duct, neoplasms of the submaxillary and sublingual glands, and regional lymphadenopathy associated with inflammatory lesions of the oral cavity. Palpation of this area is overlapped by intraoral and extraoral palpation of the floor of the mouth. Single masses in the lateral aspects of the neck may be developmental anomalies such as branchial cleft cysts and hygroma colli cysticum, regional lymphadenopathy, and neoplastic disease. Multiple masses in the neck are most usually the result of lymph node involvement. This may be due to hyperplasia associated with infectious disease, secondary inflammatory hyperplasia associated with acute or chronic oral lesions, or neoplasia.

A   B

Fig. 44. *Thyroid adenoma.* **A,** Note apparent absence of lesion in area of suprasternal notch prior to swallowing. **B,** Enlargement due to adenoma may be seen as patient swallows.

Fig. 45. *Palpation.* **A,** Parotid gland. **B,** Submaxillary gland. **C** and **D,** Submaxillary lymph nodes. **E,** Submental lymph nodes.

Fig. 46. *Palpation.* **A-E,** Cervical lymph nodes. Note position of head and displacement of muscle to facilitate palpation.

Jaws

In the examination of the jaws, the functional movement of the mandible and the temporomandibular joints with the jaws separated, the anteroposterior relationship of the mandible and maxilla, the symmetry of the jaws, the presence of "clicking" and "snapping" of the joints, and the presence of swelling and tenderness of the jaws and joints should be considered. Further evaluation of the temporomandibular joints in relation to occlusion should be carried out in the analysis of the occlusion and masticatory system.

The examination should be routinely carried out for the sake of thoroughness and is a necessity whenever the chief complaint and related symptoms are referred to this area. All of the principles of the physical examination may be used.

Inspection should be carried out with the examiner standing directly in front of the patient. The symmetry of size and functional lateral movements of the jaws (with the teeth apart) should be noted. The patient should be able to move the mandible equally well from side to side. The joints and muscles attached to the mandible should be observed during movement. The movements should be carried out easily without muscle spasms or undue strains of the facial muscles. The patient should be instructed to carry out protrusive movements of the mandible with the teeth separated. The examiner should pay special attention to deviation of the jaw from the midline and to jerky movements. The presence of abnormal, nonsymmetrical, and jerky movements suggest the possibility of joint or muscle disorders. Traumatic injury of the joints, infections of the joints, muscle hypertonicity or hypotonicity, and fractures of the jaw are common causes of abnormal jaw movements. Abnormal movements may also be related to neuromuscular disease.

Palpation of the muscles and joints is best accomplished with the examiner standing behind the patient. Bilateral palpation is the method of choice since movements of the joints demand contralateral action of the joints and muscles (Fig. 47). The examiner should feel for smoothness in the function of the joints. With the closed fingers of both hands placed on the temporomandibular joint areas, the examiner should ask the patient to make opening movements from rest position, right and left lateral movements with the teeth apart and then together, protrusive movements with the teeth together and then apart, and closing movements from rest position to initial contact of the teeth and maximum occlusal contact. The movements of the joints should be smooth and free from jerky and abnormal action. In lateral movements there is a slight lateral shift or movement of the joint on the side toward which the movement is being made. The opposite joint will move forward and somewhat medially. The possibility of conditioning and training the patient's muscles should be considered before the examiner unequivocally states that abnormal function exists or that there is loss of function. Even so, conditioned movements are important findings since they have important relationships to the muscles, joints, and occlusion. Occasionally ankylosis of the joint may produce abnormal findings on palpation of the joints. Occlusal interferences will also produce jerky and abnormal movements of the joints. This will be discussed in greater detail in Chapter 5. The joints should also be palpated for swelling and tenderness.

A B

C D

Fig. 47. *Palpation of temporomandibular joint.* **A-D,** Note various positions of mandible.

The muscles responsible for movement of the mandible should be palpated for signs of tenderness, enlargement, muscle spasm, and tonicity. This should be done while movements of the type just described are carried out. Those muscles which are suitably located for palpation are the anterior, middle, and posterior portions of the temporalis and masseter muscles. The digastic muscles are less effectively palpated, and the external and internal pterygoid muscles cannot be palpated. The known functions of the pterygoid muscles allow their action to be grossly evaluated.

Auscultation of the joints can be accomplished simply by listening for any abnormal sounds of "snapping," "grating," or "clicking" that may occur during the movements just described. A stethoscope has limited use but may be of value to one trained in its use for the temporomandibular joint sounds.

Percussion of the jaws may be of value when cavities, fractures, or reflex movements of the mandible are to be evaluated. Percussion should be indirect when percussing for cavities and fractures of the bone and direct when testing for reflex action of the mandible.

REFERENCES

Draper, G., Dupertuis, C. W., and Caughey, J. L.: Human Constitution in Clinical Medicine, New York, 1944, Paul B. Hoeber, Inc.

Jeghers, H.: Pigmentation of the Skin, New England J. Med. **231**:88-100, 122-136, 181-189, 1944.

Kampmeier, R. H.: Physical Examination in Health and Disease, Philadelphia, 1954, F. A. Davis Co.

MacBryde, C. M. (editor): Signs and Symptoms. Applied Pathologic Physiology and Clinical Interpretation, ed. 3, Philadelphia, 1957, J. B. Lippincott Co.

Monash, S.: Normal Pigmentation of the Oral Mucosa, Arch. Dermat. & Syph. **26**:139, 1932.

Pullen, R. L. (editor): Medical Diagnosis. Applied Physical Diagnosis, ed. 2, Philadelphia, 1950, W. B. Saunders Co.

Clinical examination–oral

After a general survey of the patient's health, the examiner should carry out a detailed and systematic examination of the mouth. The order begins with the lips and traverses the buccal mucosa and contiguous structures, the hard and soft palates, the tonsillar region, the floor of the mouth, the tongue, the gingivae, and the teeth. The examination should be carried out systematically and routinely in this manner so that no portion will be missed.

The plan to be followed here is based on the concept that the examiner should learn how to examine the mouth, know what to expect in the normal mouth, and know what variations of the normal to consider. It is only logical to assume that he will not be able to detect the abnormal unless he is aware of the normal and its variations. It is suggested that the student should make a record of his examination findings regardless of the presence or absence of pathologic conditions. After he has acquired skill in the procedures of the examination and has developed an appreciation for the normal findings, he may eliminate the inclusion of such negative findings except in those instances in which the absence of pathologic conditions is of significance. Thus it may be necessary to make a positive statement regarding the absence of certain features of a disease in order to provide the negative and positive correlative data necessary for a diagnosis. It is best not to write "negative" in recording the absence of disease; it is better to remove any doubts about the area having been examined by a positive statement as to the regions covered. When no disease is present, the student examiner should give a description of the normal. If diagnosis is to be complete and if obscure lesions are to be noted, the technic of oral examination must be careful and exacting and should include more than a "checkup" of the teeth. The order of the examination procedure should be organized in a logical sequence.

GENERAL APPRAISAL OF ORAL HEALTH

Lips

Inspection and palpation of the physiologic and anatomic features of the lips in health and disease—form, position, function, color, texture

Labial and Buccal Mucosa

Inspection and palpation of the physiologic and anatomic features of the labial and buccal mucosa in health and disease—color, texture, glands, ductal orifices, attachments of the frenula

159

Palate

Inspection and palpation of the physiologic and anatomic features of the hard and soft palates in health and disease—color, texture, glands, ductal orifices, density, rugae, function

Oropharynx

Inspection of the physiologic and anatomic features of the tonsils and throat in health and disease—color, size, form

Floor of the Mouth

Inspection and palpation of the physiologic and anatomic features of the floor of the mouth in health and disease—sublingual and submaxillary glands and ductal orifices, lymph nodes, sublingual sulcus, lingual aspects of the mandible

Tongue

Inspection and palpation of the physiologic and anatomic features of the tongue in health and disease—color, papillae, lymphoid tissue, glands, attachment, position, function, size, texture

Gingiva

Inspection of the physiologic and anatomic features of normal and healthy gingiva—color, form, density, level of epithelial attachment, depth of gingival crevice

Findings in disease—alteration of normal color, form, density, and attachment

Examination procedures

Charting—free gingival margin, depth of gingival crevice, level of epithelial attachment, mobility of teeth

Teeth

Inspection, exploration, and percussion of the physiologic and anatomic features of the teeth in health and disease—color, size, form, structure, number, erosion, abrasion, fractures, functional contours, carious lesions, contact relationship of the teeth

Charting—caries, decalcification, vitality, missing teeth

Occlusion

Inspection, palpation, and analysis of the physiologic and anatomic features of the dentofacial structures in health and disease—facial form analysis, primary dentition analysis, mixed dentition analysis, adult occlusion analysis, functional analysis of the masticatory system

Edentulous Mouth

Partially Edentulous Mouth

CLINICAL EXAMINATION OF THE MOUTH
General Appraisal

The clinical examination of the mouth should begin with a general appraisal of the patient's oral health. The appraisal should include a brief survey of the patient's oral hygiene, state of the teeth, presence of lesions of the soft tissues, presence of acute or chronic distress, presence or absence of prosthetic appliances, presence of edentulous areas, presence of calculus, presence of stains on the teeth, and presence of halitosis. Thus the general survey may be recorded in the following manner: "This is a partially edentulous patient wearing a maxillary full and a mandibular partial denture which appear to be functioning adequately and not causing the patient any distress; the teeth are in good alignment and the color is normal for the patient's age; the oral hygiene is good and there is no evidence of halitosis; there are no lesions of the soft tissues or obvious signs of gross dental decay." In another instance the summary might be as follows: "This is a patient with multiple edentulous spaces without restoration; the remaining teeth show rampant decay, excessive attrition, and a lack of adequate dental care; the oral hygiene is poor and the breath presents an offensive odor; there is evidence of periodontal disease and extensive ulceration of the gingiva which is causing the patient acute distress."

A general appraisal of a patient's mouth serves to inform the examiner how extensive the examination will be and how much time will be required to perform it. It may also indicate what instruments will be needed for the examination and may suggest the necessity for special examination aids. It may also serve to establish a general outline of the areas which should be given special consideration. This part of the examination may be done prior to the rest and thus allow the examiner to make another appointment with the patient at a time when the complete examination can be given more time. It may serve to point out immediately the necessity for referral and consultation.

Obvious signs of rampant dental decay, especially in young patients, should alert the examiner to the necessity for caries control as well as restoration of the teeth. The possibility of control and prevention of decay can be best accomplished through the use and evaluation of carious activity tests. The examiner may elect to carry out these tests at the time of the general appraisal and have their results at hand for the remainder of the examination and for the diagnosis, prognosis, and treatment plan.

The examiner may also wish to have the radiographs taken at this time, including any special radiographs that might be considered necessary. Thus he may elect to carry out the history, the general examination of the patient, and the general appraisal of the patient's mouth and then schedule an appointment for a time after the radiographs are ready to be read.

It is not unusual nor does it lack rationale for an examiner to make a general appraisal of the mouth before any history is obtained or the examination procedure carried out. The procedure has merit when used correctly and does not exclude a more thorough examination. It is usually only justifiable for screening purposes or for evaluating emergency complaints. The latter purpose serves to orient the examiner as to the parts of the history and examination that may be omitted temporarily until relief of acute symptoms can be accomplished.

Under ordinary circumstances the breath of a patient with a normal healthy mouth does not attract the attention of the examiner. The odor of garlic, onions, alcohol, and tobacco may be readily recognized on the breath. Disagreeable odors which are sometimes considered to be somewhat characteristic may be found in association with poor oral hygiene, periodontal disease, rhinitis, sinusitis, tonsillitis, and necrotizing gingivitis. Vincent's or necrotizing gingivitis is considered to have a characteristic fetid odor. Foul breath may also accompany bronchiectasis, lung abscesses, and gastrointestinal upset. Occasionally the fruity odor of acetone can be recognized on the breath of an individual with diabetes mellitus. It is not necessarily, however, a constant finding and may be found only when the patient is in diabetic coma. The appraisal of breath odors may remind the examiner that certain features of the patient's general health history have been overlooked. It is not unusual for a patient to be concerned with halitosis; its evaluation at this time in the examination will generally help to remind the examiner of the necessity for a detailed examination for its cause.

The general appraisal helps to establish rapport and reminds the patient that his complaints will not become lost in the intricacies of the examination procedures. Many patients are impatient to learn of the evaluation of their oral health before an adequate examination can be accomplished. A brief review and discussion of their oral problems will aid in establishing the need for more extended examination procedures.

Thus, in many instances, it may be rational and even a necessity to make the general appraisal before any history is taken or any other examination procedure carried out. After the initial survey the examiner may then continue with the detailed examination of the mouth, using all the necessary principles of the physical examination—inspection, palpation, percussion, and auscultation. Once again it must be stated that the patient must be made aware of the necessity for a complete examination even though the examination procedure does not appear at times to concern immediately those areas he considers important. It is probably a good practice to enlighten the patient along these lines before beginning the detailed clinical examination.

The instruments and materials necessary for the examination need not be extensive; the following are suggested as basic requirements (Fig. 48).

Mouth mirrors No. 5, No. 7	Finger cots
Explorers No. 3, No. 6, No. 17	Dental floss—silk or nylon
Periodontal pocket measuring probe,	Chip syringe or air-jet
U. Mich. No. 0	Water syringe
Cotton pliers	Articulating paper
Cotton	Disclosing solution
Sponges—2 by 2 inches	Tongue depressor

Fig. 48. *Examination.* Instruments and their arrangement for the examination.

Good illumination is a primary prerequisite for a thorough examination of the teeth. The patient should be seated properly and comfortably for proper instrumentation and access to all areas of the mouth.

Lips

The lips should be inspected and palpated for variations of the normal and for evidence of disease. Inspection is directed toward changes in color, form,

Fig. 49. *Lips.* **A** and **B**, Children. **C** and **D**, Adolescents. **E**, Young adult. **F**, Senile person. Note relation of the teeth to the position of lips.

texture, and obvious lesions. Palpation is carried out bidigitally to determine the texture, pliability, and firmness of the underlying and surface tissues. Induration, hyperkeratosis, and glandular involvement can be determined by this procedure.

The actual examination of the mouth begins with an inspection of the lips with the mouth unopened. Inspection of the lips is performed first because these are the first structures to attract attention in approaching the examination of the mouth. Normally they are smooth and pink in color, and in the younger individual fissuring is minimal. (Fig. 49.) With advancing age a curl develops in the corner of the mouth medial to the lower end of the mesiolabial sulcus. This is known as the labiomarginal sulcus. It becomes more prominent as the individual becomes older because of the loss of tissue tone and the decrease of fat in the tissues (Fig. 50). Various patterns of facial expression and loss of teeth tend to accentuate these grooves.

The patient should be requested to open his lips just slightly, and the line represented by the lower edge of the upper lip should be noted for its relationship to the teeth. The line which the lower border of the upper lip makes with the teeth may vary normally from an approximation to the incisal edges of the lower teeth to the cervical one-third of the maxillary teeth. The patient should also be asked to smile or to show his teeth so that the examiner can note what portion of the teeth may be seen readily; this may be an important consideration in dental restorations. The portion of the tooth structure and gingiva which can be observed when the subject speaks varies normally from a complete exposure of the mandibular incisors and cuspids to a complete blocking of the maxillary teeth by the upper lip. In others it may vary from a complete blocking of the lower incisors by the lower lip to a complete exposure of the maxillary teeth and gingiva.

The integrity of the seventh cranial nerve can be tested by instructing the patient to show his teeth or to smile (Fig. 24). Normally these movements will show a symmetrical position of the lips and the angles of the mouth. The posture of the upper and lower lips is related to the anatomic contours of the jaws and

Fig. 50. *Lips.* Changes associated with age and loss of teeth; note development of prominent lateral labial sulcus.

Fig. 51. *Lips.* **A,** Senile cheilitis; atrophy and hyperkeratosis associated with age and exposure to weather. **B,** Loss of all normal fissures of lower lip due to atrophy. Clean, shallow ulcer with very thin border suggests delayed healing and is typical of ulcers which result from acute exposure of lip showing solar cheilitis.

teeth, tonicity of the muscles, and the size of the lips. When the mandible is in the tonus rest position, the lips should just be in approximation without undue strain on the lip muscles.

Usually the color of the upper and lower lip is the same, except in individuals exposed to sunlight and wind. In these instances the color of the lower lip may be masked by some scaling and desquamation. Prolonged exposure to the elements, as occurs in farmers, cowboys, and sailors, may cause permanent changes in the lips (Fig. 51). Though these changes are variations of the normal and are not the result of disease, they are of considerable importance in the etiology of leukoplakia and carcinoma. In prolonged exposure to the elements the mucous membrane becomes thickened and is of a bluish to purplish color. A histologic section of the lip of an individual exposed to wind and sun may show scarring and chronic inflammation due to the effects of ultraviolet rays and dehydration. In these instances the capillary routes become prominent and are seen clinically as red dots over the lips.

When the individual is a mouth breather, the lower lip may be chapped and dry. This, too, will alter the coloration since the flaking and desquamation of the epithelium tend to mask the underlying red color of the lips. Therefore, when the upper and lower lips are compared, the upper one appears to be brighter in color. Children, and sometimes adults, have a peculiar habit of sucking or chewing on their upper or lower lip (Fig. 52). This causes excessive desquamation of the epithelium and increased circulation of that particular lip. In these instances the lip which is being manipulated is more red in color than the other lip.

The color of the lips is often more significant than the color of other areas because of their thin epithelial covering and their capillary supply. Any disease which affects the number of red blood cells, the amount of reduced hemogloblin, or the oxygen-carrying capacity of the blood may cause various changes in the normal color of the lips. In cardiac failure the lips may have a bluish tint, and in congenital shunts the color may be almost purple. Emphysema, increased blood volume, increased viscosity of the blood, and disturbances of the hemoglobin molecule may produce varying degrees of the blue color of cyanosis.

Palpation of the lips may be done at this time or during the inspection of the labial mucosa. The presence of external lesions suggests the earlier time. The lips should be palpated between the index finger and the thumb while the muscles are relaxed and then while they are pursed. When the lips are relaxed, they are soft and resilient throughout the outer surfaces, and the bands of the orbicularis oris muscle can be felt in the body of the lips. When the lips are pursed or tensed, occasionally a secondary fold of soft tissue may be felt just inside the lip and has frequently been called a second lip (Fig. 53). While this is a fairly common occurrence, it may be extensive enough to present an esthetic problem. This is especially true when the individuals are public speakers or singers. Ectopic sebaceous glands are seen so frequently on the vermilion border of the upper lip that they may be considered to be a variation of normal. They are of little significance except in those instances in which they are very extensive and cause esthetic problems. Changes in the lip due to habits or exposure to wind and

A   B

Fig. 52. *Lips*. Roughness and hyperkeratinization associated with chewing of lips.

A   B

Fig. 53. *Lips.* Double lip. **A**, Minor. **B**, Marked.

A   B

Fig. 54. *Lips.* Mouth breathing; note the difference in shade, texture, form, and position of the lips and the position of the tongue.

sunlight are not in themselves pathologic conditions, but they may be of significance in the diagnosis of orthodontic and periodontal problems. Thus the posture, color, form, texture, tonus, and activity of the lips may relate to mouth breathing or undue pressure on the teeth; these are of significance often in the diagnosis of malocclusion and gingivitis (Fig. 54).

Findings in Disease.—The size and form of the lips should be examined for evidence of disease. Large lips may be an expression of a variation of normal or may be due to angio-edema or neoplasms. The lips are frequently thickened in cretinism, and they appear to be protruded in acromegaly. Swelling of the lips is most commonly due to edema associated with injury or exposure to an offending allergen. In the latter instance a history of reaction to dental agents such as oil of cloves and other dental drugs, systemic therapeutic agents, and cosmetic agents will provide the clue to the cause of the edema. In these instances the response to elimination of the suspected agent and to the use of antihistamines should be noted. (Remember that an individual may be sensitive to antihista-

Fig. 55. *Lips.* Marked and sudden swelling of one or both lips, especially accompanied by swelling of the eyelids, is indicative of angioneurotic edema. This is usually an allergic response.

mines, too.) Generally, an enlargement of the lips of sudden onset suggests an allergic etiologic agent (Fig. 55). The size and form as well as texture and tonicity of the lip vary within normal limits with age, sex, race, and exposure to the weather.

Obvious signs of disease such as primary and secondary lesions can best be evaluated on the basis of the type of lesion present and the history of the lesion (Figs. 56 to 59). The first step in the diagnosis of any lesion of the lip is to determine whether or not the history and the signs and symptoms presented are suggestive of a developmental, dermatologic, traumatic, metabolic, allergic, or neoplastic disease. In general the history and location of the lesion will be the primary evidence for the diagnosis of a developmental disease. Traumatic lesions can best be related to their history of occurrence; however, occasionally a biopsy may be necessary to make a differential diagnosis from neoplastic disease.

Fissuring at the corners of the mouth (Fig. 60) should direct the examiner's attention to vitamin deficiencies and/or in elderly patients (in whom the labiomarginal sulcus is deep and excessive salivation or xerostomia is present) toward ulceration of the sulcus and infections with yeast or bacteria. The contiguousness produced by the accentuation of the labiomarginal sulcus results in an extension of the commissures of the upper and lower lips into skin areas which are not suited to continuous wetting or drying; these areas are then prone to cheilitis. Fissuring may also occur from extensive stretching of the mouth; this may be seen in association with dental procedures. The secondary ulcerative lesions of herpes simplex are also seen frequently at the commissures following dental procedures. Longitudinal fissuring of the lower lip should direct the examiner's attention toward the possibility of actinic cheilitis, dehydration, and mouth breathing. Fissures which have been present for a long period of time, have a tendency to bleed, and are indurated should be evaluated for neoplastic disease.

A   B

Fig. 56. *Lips.* **A,** White, thin plaque of vermilion mucosa called "smoker's patch." This is an example of focal hyperkeratosis produced by mechanical, chemical, and thermal injury. **B,** Typical picture of "smoker's cancer." Let lateral one-third of vermilion is covered by thin, opaque, keratinized plaque. The most lateral zone has recently become thicker, whiter, and more firm, and there is slight rolling of the most lateral border.

A   B

Fig. 57. *Lips.* **A,** Small elevated, crusted lesion on vermilion border of lip—early squamous cell carcinoma. **B,** Crusted, verrucal-appearing, 1 cm. lesion, slightly elevated above the surface, on the middle one-third of the left vermilion. The lesion is indurated. This type of squamous cell carcinoma is frequently mistaken for a "cold sore."

Fig. 58. *Lips.* Two vesicular, crusted lesions, one involving upper lip and one involving left nares; note the well-demonstrated conglomerate character so typical of herpetic lesions.

A   B

Fig. 59. *Lips.* **A,** Lesion involving mucocutaneous junction in midline of upper lip, with elevated border about depressed center. Rolled border is feature of neoplasia; the lesion is a basal cell carcinoma. **B,** Some deformity of lip produced by slightly craterous ulcer of vermilion with rolled, white border—moderately advanced squamous cell carcinoma.

Fig. 60. *Lips.* **A,** Angular fissure, traumatic in origin; note change in shape of lower lip associated with lip biting. **B,** Vermilion of lip and vestibular mucosa demonstrating irregularly contoured, elevated, yellowish adherent, soft membrane. This succulent, yellowish membrane is composed of fibrin which has exuded from area of traumatized mucosa.

Ulceration characterized by chronicity, failure to heal, induration, and lymphadenopathy suggests neoplastic disease (Fig. 59). Hyperpigmentation of rather recent onset accompanied by other signs and symptoms of a systemic nature should suggest the possibility of metabolic disorders such as Addison's disease.

The foregoing discussion is not meant to be an extensive categorization of all the diseases which may affect the lips, and when a more descriptive account of lesions of the lip is needed for a final diagnosis, the examiner is referred to textbooks of oral pathology or dental medicine.

Labial and Buccal Mucosa

The examination of the mucosa should begin with reflection of the upper and lower lips and inspection of the color and texture of the labial surfaces (Fig. 61). The lips should be palpated in a systematic manner, and this should be a routine part of the examination. The presence of unsuspected mucous retention cysts is not an uncommon finding when the routine practice of bidigital palpation is carried out. Palpation should start with the outer edge of the lip and proceed to the vestibule. It may be bilateral as well as bidigital (Fig. 62).

Inspection and palpation of the labial surfaces of the lip will show varying

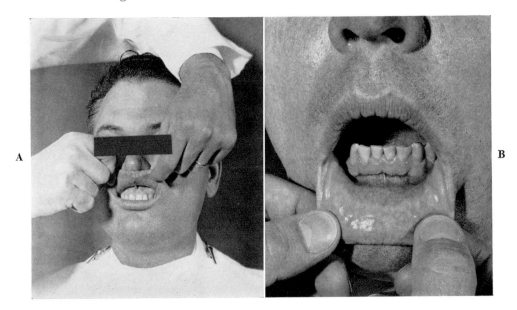

Fig. 61. *Lips.* Inspection of lips and vestibular mucosa.

degrees of nodularity associated with numerous mucous glands which are situated in the submucous tissue (Fig. 63). These glands have a granular feeling somewhat analogous to tapioca. The degree of nodularity may be increased by chronic irritation, especially the use of tobacco.

Several folds of tissue, called frena or frenula, traverse the vestibular fornix (Fig. 64). In the midline, sagittal folds connect the alveolar process with the upper and lower lips. In children, before the eruption of the teeth, the superior labial frenulum is attached to the crest of the alveolar process and forms a raphe that may reach to the palatal papilla. With the eruption of the teeth and vertical growth of the alveolar process, the attachment migrates superiorly and can be found normally on the attached gingiva or may be restricted to the alevolar mucosa of the vestibule. Most frequently in the adult it is found at the junction of the attached gingiva and alveolar mucosa. The inferior labial frenulum is found most often attached at the junction of the alveolar mucosa and the attached gingiva. However, it may extend for some distance onto the attached gingiva. The position of the attachment is related to the eruption of the teeth and vertical growth of the alveolar process. The lateral frenula are present in the area of the cuspids and bicuspids. They are usually more prominent in the lower arch than in the upper. The position of the attachment of the lower lateral frenulum varies considerably and may be attached high on the attached gingiva or in the alveolar mucosa of the vestibule. Inspection and palpation of these frenula are best accomplished when the lips and cheeks are retracted. (Fig. 64.) Their position and attachment may be studied on stone models when function impressions are taken. As will be pointed out later, the attachments are of significance in periodontics, orthodontics, and prosthodontics.

A   B

C   D

Fig. 52. *Lips.* **A,** Inspection. **B,** Bidigital palpation. **C** and **D,** Bilateral and bidigital palpation.

A   B

Fig. 63. *Labial mucosa.* **A,** Vestibular glands. **B,** Developmental pit at commissure.

A   B

C   D

Fig. 64. *Frenula.* **A,** In primary dentition. **B,** In young adult. **C,** Maxillary lateral and midline mandibular frenula. **D,** Mandibular lateral frenula.

The cheek should be reflected and the buccal mucosa inspected for color, texture, and lesions (Fig. 65). The cheeks should be retracted sufficiently to give the examiner a clear view of their entire mucosal surface. The examiner should then traverse the buccal mucosa from the vestibular reflection of the mucous membrane to the alevolar processes and posteriorly to the fornix of the vestibule opposite the maxillary tuberosity. The mucous membrane is normally pink in members of the Caucasian race, while in the Negro it is more bluish or bluish-gray. This bluish color may have an uneven or patchy distribution. Brown pigmentation may be normally present in buccal mucosa in the Negro.

Quite commonly isolated or confluent ectopic sebaceous glands are present adjacent to the corner of the mouth and extending to the molar region. In front of the anterior border of the masseter muscle, there may be a rounded eminence containing fat tissue. This is called the buccal fat pad of Bichat. The eminence is variable in size and is seen most prominently in the newborn infant. However, pronounced residual eminences of this fat pad may be seen in the adult (Fig. 66, *E*).

At the occlusal line in most individuals there is a longitudinal fold of tissue

A   B

Fig. 65. *Buccal mucosa.* Reflection and inspection; note position of examiner's fingers and manipulation of lip for an adequate field of vision.

which extends from a point near the angle of the mouth to just anterior to the fold created by the elevation of the pterygomandibular raphe (Fig. 66, *A*). This may appear as a thin white line or as a rather thickened elevation and has been called the linea alba buccalis or torus buccalis. It may be seen infrequently in young children, but it is seen most commonly in adults. It is a thickening of the mucosa resulting from pressure of the cheek into the line of occlusion. It may become accentuated from trauma of biting (Fig. 66, *B*). The white color is due to surface keratinization. Near the anterior termination of the linea alba buccalis there is often found a projection of the mucosa called the caliculus angularis (Fig. 66, *C*). The linea alba buccalis and the caliculis angularis are not important except in the presence of injury and irritation.

The cheek should be examined also by bimanual palpation (Fig. 67, *A*). By this method both the underlying structures and the surface of the mucosa can be felt. The examiner should be especially careful in his palpation of the deep structures in the cheek because lesions may be present in this type of loose tissue without showing externally or being noticed by the patient.

Opposite the second maxillary molar is an eminence of the mucous membrane called the parotid papilla which marks the opening of Stensen's duct (Fig. 67, *B*). The size of the papilla varies considerably and in some instances may extend into the interproximal surfaces of the molar teeth. Many persons (even dental students) seeing this papilla for the first time view it with alarm, believing it to be a tumor of some kind (Fig. 67, *C*).

The parotid papilla is soft in consistency on palpation, and if the parotid

Fig. 66. *Buccal mucosa.* **A,** Linea alba buccalis. **B,** Intensification of linea alba by cheek chewing. **C,** Caliculus angularis. **D,** Fordyce spots. **E,** Persistent bilateral buccal fat pads.

A

B   C

Fig. 67. *Buccal mucosa.* **A,** Bimanual palpation of cheek. **B,** Parotid papilla. **C,** Hemangioma anterior to pendulous parotid papilla.

Fig. 68. *Inspection of parotid papilla.* **A,** Drying of mucosa in order to observe flow and character of saliva. **B,** Note drop of saliva at orifice of duct.

Fig. 69. *Buccal mucosa.* Note sharp demarcation of color at junction of alveolar mucosa and gingiva.

gland is manipulated, a quantity of serous, somewhat clear fluid may be expressed from the papilla (Fig. 68). Careful bimanual palpation may serve to demonstrate the hard firm cordlike Stensen's duct just in front of the anterior border of the masseter muscle (Fig. 67, A).

The mucous membrane in the fornix of the vestibule is thin, and the many small venules which traverse this tissue are easily seen. It is not unusual for students who see these vessels for the first time to be unnecessarily concerned. The reflection of the cheek tissue onto the alveolar process is characterized by a change in the consistency and attachment of the mucous membrane. The alveolar mucosa covering the alveolar process is attached loosely to the underlying bone. The juncture of the alveolar mucosa and the gingiva is indicated by a sharp scalloped line which vaguely parallels the free margin of the gingiva. The alveolar mucosa appears dark red in color when compared to the normal pale pink color of the gingiva. The sharpness of the color contrast between the two tissues varies considerably from one individual to another. In general, the more pale the gingival tissues, the greater is the contrast in color (Fig. 69).

Behind the distal molars of the upper and lower arches are soft tissue prominences which are called retromolar papillae. In the maxilla these papillae are continuous with the gingiva which covers the termination of the maxillary tuberosity and alveolar tubercle. In the mandible the retromolar papilla is an accentuation of the free gingival margin and is continuous with the retromolar pad. The reflection of the attached gingiva and the cheek mucosa in this region is the site of an aggregation of buccal glands. The prominence caused by the glands gives the tissue a padlike appearance and has been called the retromolar pad, although more commonly the term has been used to designate collectively the prominence caused by both the retromolar papilla and the retromolar pad. The retromolar papillae and the retromolar pads are of significance in periodontal therapy and in the placement and wearing of dentures. Considerable normal variation exists in the form and consistency of the retromolar papilla and the retromolar pad. The form of the retromolar papilla is dependent to a certain extent upon the position and the eruption of the most distal molar teeth and the form of the alveolar process. In older individuals there is a tendency for atrophy of the mucous glands in the retromolar pad so that this prominence becomes more firm than in younger individuals and, as a result, the color appears to be more pale pink or white than previously. With the extraction of the most distal molars there is a new retromolar papilla established behind the remaining molars, but the retromolar pad remains in its original position. With the loss of the most distal molar teeth, movement of the pad under palpation is generally found. This is especially true when the pad is located somewhat to the lingual aspect of the mandible.

Findings in Disease.—Inspection and palpation of the labial and buccal mucosa, frenula, retromolar papilla, and retromolar pad should be routine procedure in the examination of the mouth. The oral cavity is the special field of the dentist and more often than not patients with disease in a portion of this area will consult their dentist before they consult a physician. While the dentist may direct his attention to the diagnosis, prevention, and treatment of diseases of the teeth in an adequate manner, he has a tendency to view passively other areas of the mouth even when confronted with signs and symptoms of disease. It must be remembered that many diseases show their symptoms in the labial and buccal mucosae. (Fig. 70.) All too often signs of disease, whether related to the teeth or not, are simply overlooked in the routine dental examination. This is unfortunate because most patients and physicians, who generally observe the mouth only when they are looking at the tonsils or the throat, are aware that the dentist is better equipped by training to evaluate abnormalities in any part of the oral cavity.

The *color* of the labial and buccal mucosae may be altered by keratinization, pigmentation, scarring, inflammatory changes, and changes in the amount of reduced hemoglobin and red blood cells and their hemoglobin content. Thus the examiner's attention during an inspection of this tissue may be directed toward

Fig. 70. *Buccal mucosa.* Thick, opaque, and somewhat firm folds involving much of buccal and vestibular mucosa throughout mouth. Opacity is not due to hyperkeratosis but to deposition of amyloid in submucosa.

any of these factors whenever changes in color are noted. Inasmuch as the labial and buccal mucosae normally are not generally keratinized, localized, or diffused, keratinization may be detected by gray-white or silver-appearing lesions. The most frequent deviation from the normal pink color is related to varying degrees of white associated with lichen planus, focal hyperkeratosis, chronic cheek biting, chemical burns, and leukoplakia. Therefore, when white-appearing lesions with varying degrees of hyperkeratinization are found in these areas, the examiner should be prepared to use his knowledge of the history of the lesion and his findings in the examination as to size, location, distribution, and other characteristics, and relate these findings to a descriptive knowledge of such lesions. Illustrative cases demonstrating the technic of making a differential diagnosis can be found in Chapter 8.

The pallor of anemia and the yellow tint of jaundice may be noted in the labial and buccal mucosae and may be used as positive correlative data. However, it must be remembered that pallor and yellow pigmentation are only symptoms of disease and when present should suggest the need for evaluation and for a search for their cause. When the examiner notes pallor of the mucous membranes, he should search for pallor in other areas and should also rely on other positive correlative findings before making a presumptive diagnosis of anemia. Pallor of the lips and oral mucosa is not sufficient evidence in itself to refer a patient for blood studies, nor is the report of 13.8 mg. per cent hemoglobin in the blood sufficient evidence to suggest any type of anemia, let alone start that patient on iron therapy. Thus, pallor of the mucosa, lips, fingernail beds, and conjunctiva is only suggestive of anemia, whereas the additional findings of papillary atrophy of the tongue, exacerbations and remissions of burning and tingling sensations of the tongue, paresthesias of taste, systemic symptoms of dyspnea, palpitation, irritability, abdominal discomfort, dysmenorrhea, and a low-grade fever all strongly suggest the tentative diagnosis of some type of anemia. Even so, the final diagnosis cannot be rendered until the patient has had a complete study of the blood and a complete examination of the body.

Hyperpigmentation of the labial or buccal mucosa should be evaluated for recent onset, distribution, change in intensity, and relationship to pigmentation elsewhere in the mouth and the body. Melanin pigmentation, which may vary in intensity from a light brown to a dark blue-black and be localized to very small islands or be diffuse through large areas, is especially significant when it is of recent onset in normally blond individuals. Increased pigmentation may be exogenous or endogenous in character and systemic or local in origin. Normal physiologic pigmentation increases in intensity with age. In Addison's disease brown to brownish-black dots of pigment or a diffuse bluish-black pigmentation may occur on the buccal and labial mucosae, palate, lips, gums, and/or tongue. Heavy metal intoxication may also cause pigmentation in these areas.

It is not unusual for the petechiae of emboli in subacute bacterial endocarditis to be present here as well as on the inferior surfaces of the tongue and in the conjunctiva. The labial and buccal mucosae may also show the petechial hemorrhages and ecchymoses of purpuras and leukemias (Fig. 71). It is not uncommon for trauma to produce ulcerations, traumatic fibromas, and mucous retention cysts (Fig. 72). A tentative diagnosis of the nature of the lesion may be based upon the clinical history and the appearance and consistency of the lesion. In many instances the history and the clinical examination of the lesion are sufficient to make an adequate diagnosis. However, the final diagnosis of those lesions whose diagnoses are not obvious should be based upon a biopsy. Indications for biopsy are reviewed in Chapter 7. Where a tentative diagnosis of a

Fig. 71. *Vestibular mucosa.* Dark spots in lower vestibular mucosa which are petechial hemorrhages due to idiopathic thrombocytopenic purpura.

A   B

Fig. 72. *Labial mucosa.* **A,** Smooth, nodular vestibular swellings of vestibular areas which may be produced by salivary gland tumors, lipoma, or mucous retention cysts. Palpation and other information determined that this was salivary gland tumor. **B,** Smooth, elevated, translucent, fluctuant swelling in lower vestibular mucosa which arises on erythematous base. Mucoceles of this type frequently are demonstrated in this location.

traumatic ulcer is made in light of the clinical examination and history of the lesion, the examiner should recall the patient three or four days after the source of the trauma has been removed for a re-evaluation of the lesion. This is a mandatory procedure in view of the tendency of many lesions to show later neoplastic change. If the ulcerative lesion fails to heal within a reasonable length of time after the traumatic agent is removed, then the examiner should do a biopsy. While ulceration of the labial and buccal mucosae may be due to chronic irritation such as sharp edges of teeth, rough dental fillings, or ill-fitting dentures, traumatic ulcers may also have a superimposed malignancy present.

The orifices of the parotid ducts should be inspected and palpated. Palpation of the parotid papilla and Stensen's duct should be carried out by palpation between the index finger of one hand placed inside of the mouth and the index finger of the other hand which is placed on the outside of the cheek. Inflammation of the incisive papilla, expression of a purulent type of saliva, and the presence of a hard mass in Stensen's duct suggest the presence of a stone or sialolith in the duct (Fig. 73, A). Inflammation of the parotid papillae, coupled with a purulent type of saliva expressed from the ducts, and the signs and symptoms of swelling and pain of the parotid region suggest inflammation of the parotid gland. Enlargement of the gland with or without visible signs or symptoms of changes of the saliva or of the parotid papillae, especially in the absence of systemic symptoms, suggests the possibility of a tumor or neoplasm.

Changes in the flow of saliva as evidenced by a dry mouth or excessive salivation should direct the examiner's attention to the cause of the changes. Xerostomia, or dry mouth, may be local or systemic in origin. Sialorrhea, or excessive salivation, may be psychogenic, systemic, or local in origin. Generally an obstruction of only one of the ducts of the parotid glands is not sufficient to cause obvious signs of dry mouth. Dry mouth may be related to fear, dehydration, drugs, dentures, etc. Excessive salivation may be associated with faulty dentures, pain in the mouth, metal intoxications, substances giving an unpleasant taste, etc. To evaluate the sign of dry mouth, the examiner should determine the duration and degree of incapacitation and review the history, which might reveal the etiologic

A   B

Fig. 73. *Parotid papilla.* **A,** Stone in orifice of parotid duct. **B,** Recurrent herptic ulcers, one involving parotid papilla.

agent. Ordinarily an excessive flow of saliva is normal for anyone undergoing dental procedures; however, the amount varies from one individual to another. Sialorrhea is of significance to the operator since it tends to slow down dental procedures since a dry field for working and vision is necessary. Sialorrhea coupled with a metallic taste should be evaluated for the possibility of metal intoxication. Xerostomia and sialorrhea are only symptoms of disease, and they must be evaluated the same as other symptoms of disease. Therefore, the time and mode of onset, character of the dysfunction, presence or absence of contributory signs and symptoms, and the etiologic factors producing the symptoms must be determined before an attempt is made to make a diagnosis by a comparsion with a description of the diseases either known by the examiner or which may be located in reference material. Thus, the examiner should collect his facts and evaluate his findings and then compare them with a descriptive knowledge of the disease before attempting to make a diagnosis.

Occasionally the persistence of a large buccal fat pad may be of significance to the dentist (Fig. 66). While it cannot be considered as pathologic and is within the range of normal, in many instances its prominence does affect dental procedures. It is of concern to the prosthodontist in the placement and the wearing of dentures, inasmuch as it tends to be chronically irritated by cheek biting. This is especially true in the natural dentition where extractions without replacements have occurred with drifting and extrusion of the remaining teeth. A loss of alignment and an overjet of the maxillary teeth and the presence of sharp edges from abnormal wear or carious lesions, together with a persistent large buccal fat pad, predisposes to chronic irritation of the mucosa overlying the buccal fat pad. Thus the diagnosis of chronic cheek chewing must take into consideration not only the alignment of the teeth, the correct amount of maxillary overjet, and sharp edges of the teeth, but also the prominence of a persistent buccal fat pad.

The position of the attachment of the labial and lateral frenula may be of pathologic significance when the position of the frenula interferes with the normal eruption of the teeth or when the relative position of attachment is changed because of periodontal disease. Occasionally a space will exist between the maxillary central incisors which is associated with a persistence of the tectolabial frenulum. In these instances the superior labial frenulum is not reduced to a vestige but remains as a large fibrous band of tissue which may extend even across the free border of the gingiva to the palatine or incisal papilla (Fig. 74). This is of significance to the orthodontist when the fibrous band is not eliminated and prevents the closure of the diastema between the central incisors even after the lateral incisors and cuspids have erupted. It is also possible that the abnormally large and attached frenulum does not in itself cause or maintain the diastema between the central incisors but may be secondary to other factors such as congenital absence of lateral incisors and to various types of bone patterns in the midline of the maxilla that are of genetic and familial origin.

An attachment of the inferior labial frenulm above the junction of the alevolar mucosa and the attached gingiva becomes of significance when periodontal disease and recession of the gingiva involves the attachment of the frenulum. When there is a deep labial or inteproximal pocket between the two lower central in-

A

B   C

Fig. 74. *Labial frenula.* **A,** Persistent labial frenulum in deciduous dentition. **B** and **C,** Persistence of labial frenulum attached to incisive papilla with associated spacing of permanent teeth.

cisors and the attachment of the labial frenulum is in or near the marginal edge of the gingiva, stretching and movement of the lip cause an extension of the margin of the pocket and correct toothbrushing is impossible (Fig. 75, *A*). This arrangement of the margin of the periodontal pocket and the attachment of the labial frenulum makes proper deflection of food impossible and prevents the proper stimulation of the tissues by toothbrushing. This may also occur in the maxillary midline frenulum and in the lateral frenula (Fig. 75, *B*). The presence and location of the lateral frenula are also of significance in the preparation of the mouth for partial and full dentures.

The retromolar papilla of the mandibular arch is of significance to the periodontist when the most distal molar is only partially erupted and the pericoronal tissues fail to completely obliterate with the formation of a normal retromolar papilla. In other instances, the most distal molar may be fully erupted yet the gingival crevice around the distal aspect of the molar be greater than 2 to 3 mm.

A   B

Fig. 75. *Frenula.* **A,** Inferior labial frenulum attached to gingival margin of mandibular incisor, producing gingival recession. **B,** Superior buccal frenulum attached to gingival margin of maxillary bicuspid; note associated recession.

Fig. 76. *Mandibular third molar pericoronal flap.*

in depth because of hyperplasia of the retromolar papilla. Abnormal pericoronal flaps and a hyperplastic retromolar papilla are conducive to pathologic processes (Fig. 76). The pericoronal flap is especially prone to the production of a pericoronitis and acute necrotizing inflammation. The hyperplastic retromolar papilla is conducive to the production of a periodontal pocket on the distal aspect of the most distal molar because the increased depth of the gingival crevice precludes the possibility for adequate cleansing of the area.

Palate

After inspecting and palpating the lips and labial and buccal mucosae, the examiner should examine the hard and soft palates. The mucous membrane of the hard palate is firmly attached to the underlying bone and presents some degree of keratinization; these factors give it a pale pink color often with a bluish-gray hue. The peripheral zone of the hard palate is firm but somewhat resilient and connects the tissue of the palate proper to the teeth; this tissue makes up the palatine gingiva and is firmly attached to the underlying bone and teeth. In the midline of the palate there is a narrow whitish streak which is termed the palatine raphe (Fig. 77, A). It extends from a small projection, the incisive papilla, and extends posteriorly over the entire length of the hard palate. It is often ridgelike in shape in the anterior portion and may take the form of a groove posteriorly. Radiating from the incisal papilla and the anterior portions of the palatine raphe are irregular branching ridges termed the palatine rugae (Fig. 77, B). On each side of the raphe, at the junction of the hard and soft palates, frequently a small depression is visible; these are the palatine foveas, into which merge the openings of the excretory ducts of the palatine glands (Fig. 77, C). In the lateral portions of the tissue between the palatine raphe and the alveolar gingiva are palatal glands, nerves, and blood vessels; these elements are fairly extensive between the periosteum and the submucosa in the molar region but much less extensive anteriorly.

The compressibility of these tissues is of significance in the design of dentures, and their compression when taking an impression is to be avoided; otherwise errors in the impression will result. This is the only area in the hard palate

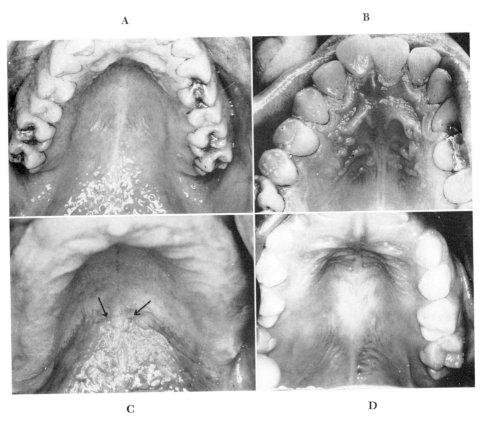

Fig. 77. *Palate.* **A,** Palatine raphe. **B,** Palatine rugae. **C,** Fovea palatinae. **D,** Incisive papilla; note fovea palatinae.

A   B

C

Fig. 78. *Palate.* A-C, Gingivopalatal groove associated with prominent tuberosity and pterygomandibular raphe.

into which a large amount of fluid can be injected without causing tissue damage. Palpation of the tissues in this region shows them to be softer and more resilient than the adjacent alveolar mucosa or the medial portion of the hard palate. A rather thick band of firm tissue, continuous with the maxillary retromolar papilla, may sweep across the alevolar tubercle and give the distal termination of the gingiva a cleft appearance where it meets the hard palate (Fig. 78). This cleft is especially prominent where the pterygomandibular raphe fits into the groove when the mouth is opened. On palpation this band of gingiva is firm but somewhat movable. With the extraction of the adjacent molars this tissue may become less pronounced or may increase in size. It is significant in the treatment of periodontal disease and in the placement of partial or full dentures. This hyperplastic tissue prevents adequate treatment of deepened gingival crevices around the maxillary molars by conservative means. Surgical removal of the tissues is usually necessary for proper treatment and removal of periodontal pockets even when shallow. The form of this tissue in relation to the crown of

Fig. 79. *Examination of palate.* **A,** Palpation of posterior border of hard palate; note position of head and approach to the area to be examined. **B,** Palpation of incisive papilla. **C,** Palpation of palatine suture. **D,** Palpation of lateral palatine space. **E,** Inspection of soft palate.

the teeth prevents adequate passage of food over the tissues, and not infrequently the gingival crevice accumulates debris. Occasionally the eminence is primarily dense fibrous tissue. After removal of the teeth the persistence of this band of fibrous tissue may cause complications with the adequate adaptation of dentures. Not infrequently the tissue becomes flabby and even more hyperplastic than originally; this further complicates the proper seating of the dentures.

The soft palate is covered with mucous membrane which is thin compared to that of the hard palate; no cornified epithelium is normally present. Numerous mucous glands and blood vessels are present in the soft palate; their structural arrangement gives the soft palate a darker red color than the hard palate. The boundary between the hard and soft palates may be readily seen by noting the change in position of the soft palate when the patient says "ahhh." This boundary is extremely important in the proper retention of dentures. Bilateral elevation of the soft palate occurs when the patient says "ahhh" or when the palatal reflex is elicited by touching the soft palate and causing the patient to "gag."

The palate should be palpated and inspected for changes in color, density, and texture and for variations in the form which may present problems in denture construction (Fig. 79). The junction of the hard and soft palates and the location of the loose mucous membranes should be determined since the design of full dentures and palatal bars is directly related to so-called denture-bearing areas where there is firm and dense attachment of the mucosa.

Findings in Disease.—The color of the hard and soft palates may be changed by a localized or diffuse increase in pigmentation, a change in the integrity and the permeability of the blood vessels, a change in the hemoglobin content of the blood or an increase in the amount of reduced hemoglobin present, a change in the character of the epithelium of the mucosa, and changes in the density and attachment of these tissues (Fig. 81). The most common change in color is associated with the process of inflammation from traumatic agents. This may be localized or may involve the whole soft and hard palates. Pressure from full dentures or palatal bars may be seen frequently (Fig. 81) and may produce color changes from bluish-white to brilliant red.

The color of the soft palate may show varying degrees of red resulting from engorgement of the blood vessels that traverse it. This active hyperemia, frequently accompanied by petechiae and ecchymosis (Fig. 1, A), is seen quite often in association with colds and coughing episodes and allergic manifestations. The soft palate is also a common site for traumatic injuries, herpetic ulcers, and purpuric manifestations, and a large ulcer may be found on it (Fig. 12, D) in Vincent's angina.

Excessive smoking may produce hyperkeratinization of the palatal mucosa and metaplasia of the ducts of the mucous glands. The palatal appearance is characterized by a diffuse silver-white color from the hyperkeratinization and scattered punctate red areas indicating the orifices of the ducts of the mucous glands. A brown staining of the keratinized surfaces may occur, especially in the area in which a pipestem or a cigar rests. This has been called the smoker's patch. The extensive keratinization of the palate with involvement of the orifices of the mucous glands is called nicotine stomatitis (Fig. 8). The areas of hyper-

A   B

C   D

Fig. 80. *Examination of palate.* **A,** Plaque of white, verrucal tissue covering large part of denture-bearing area of palate—low-grade squamous cell carcinoma. **B,** Purpura secondary to myelogenous leukemia. **C,** Lobulated, elevated, soft, purplish lesion in posterior hard palate and anterior soft palate having a history of progressive enlargement; lesion is typical of salivary gland tumors which arise from palatal glands. **D,** Perforating lesion of hard palate, which may be produced by gummas, squamous cell carcinoma, or salivary gland tumors. This one is a squamous cell carcinoma.

A   B

Fig. 81. *Palate.* **A** and **B,** Hyperemia associated with wearing of partial denture and complete denture.

keratinization feel somewhat less resilient and are coarser textured than the surrounding tissues. When there is marked involvement of the orifices of the mucous glands, they may be felt on palpation.

Fairly frequently the middle portion of the palatine raphe will show a firm bony enlargement. The color of the mucosa on the surface of this enlargement is usually pale pink to white unless inflammation from trauma is present. The size and form of the enlargement may vary from a slight flat elevation of the median portion of the palatine raphe (this is usually considered to be a variation of normal) to a large nodular mass which may reach the proportions of a walnut (Fig. 6). On palpation, the mass is hard, firm, bonelike in consistency, and nonmovable. This is a torus palatinus and is of clinical significance because of its relationship to the construction of full dentures and palatal bars on partial dentures and because of its blastomatoid characteristics. It is not a neoplasm and is only of significance to the patient when it interferes with mastication, speaking, and swallowing or when the patient has a cancer phobia. All types of primary and secondary lesions may occur in the palate as elsewhere in the mouth; however, the most frequent type of lesion is ulceration, and it is generally the result of traumatic injury. The most frequently offending etiologic agents appear to be hard toast, chicken bones, and toothbrush bristles. Inflammatory changes of the incisive papilla are fairly frequent and may be associated with any of the traumatic agents previously mentioned. The extensive enlargement of the incisive papilla may result from a cyst (Fig. 82). In these cases there is no radiographic evidence of bone involvement. Not infrequently malocclusion of the anterior teeth may result in impingement of food and of the mandibular central incisors upon the incisive papilla. Chronic trauma of this nature may give rise to a hyperplastic enlargement of this tissue.

In many instances of partial denture and full denture construction and periodontal disease, the significance of hyperplastic tissue in the anterior palatine region is overlooked. Deep gingival crevices and periodontal pockets are difficult to treat by conservative means because of the tendency of this tissue to persist. The construction of dentures over tissue which is soft and edematous, and pre-

Fig. 82. *Cyst of incisive papilla.*

sents some degree of inflammatory hyperplasia may well lead to additional in-flammatory hyperplasia when patients attempt to wear dentures irrespective of how well the prosthesis may have fit originally. Inspection and palpation of these tissues prior to denture construction will avoid this complication.

Occasionally an ill-fitting denture will produce an inflammatory hyperplasia of the palate which is characterized by localized or diffuse small red nodular-like elevations of the mucosa. These lesions are within the boundaries or at the periphery of the denture (Fig. 83). The elevations may be polypoid or papil-lomatous in form. This has been termed palatal papillomatosis or polypoid hyperplasia of the palate. Many inflammatory and neoplastic diseases may involve the palate, and it is suggested that the student consult reference works for a comprehensive description of them. The underlying principles governing the approach to the diagnosis of abnormalities of the hard and soft palates are the same as apply elsewhere in the mouth except in instances in which the anatomic and functional relationships present may, in themselves, orient the examiner's attention toward specific items of diagnostic interest. The movement of the soft palate is dependent on the function of the ninth and tenth cranial nerves. In the presence of paralysis, the soft palate will sag on the affected side, and the uvula will be pulled to the unaffected side. It is not uncommon for people with unilateral paralysis of the soft palate to have difficulty in swallowing food, and in some instances water and food may enter the nose upon deglutition. The absence of a palatal reflex is common in hysteria, paralysis of the palate, and in anesthesia due to disease of the second division of the fifth cranial nerve. The degree of gagging which accompanies the palatal reflex varies considerably from one individual to another. The palatal reflex is of significance in the construction of full dentures and in many other dental procedures. There are many individuals in whom the palatal reflex is so hypersensitive that the least manipulation of the tissues in the posterior portion of the mouth, especially those adjacent to the soft palate, will produce gagging. In such persons only a few dental pro-cedures can be accomplished without topical anesthetics.

Fig. 83. *Palatal papillomatosis* associated with wearing of ill-fitting dentures.

Fig. 84. *Cleft palate.* Complete cleft with surgical closure of lip and ridge tissue.

A   B

Fig. 85. *Soft palate.* **A,** Absence of uvula; post-tonsillectomy. **B,** Bifid uvula.

Clefts of the roof of the mouth and the lip may present serious phonetic, esthetic, and functional problems. While the diagnosis of cleft palate does not present a problem in itself, the evaluation of functional incapacitation and of the structures involved may require an extensive physical and radiographic examination. These procedures are outside the scope of this book. Of significant importance to the general practitioner is the early referral of the patient to the proper specialist for consultation. The treatment of clefts requires the close cooperation of the prosthodontist and the oral surgeon. Of equal importance is the periodic examination and maintenance of the teeth and supporting structures which may be involved in the retention and stabilization of extensive prosthetic appliances required to cover a cleft. Fig. 84 shows an extensive cleft of the soft and hard palates; the maxilla and lip have been surgically closed. A cleft of this magnitude requires all the dental support that can be gained. A loss of teeth in the patient shown would make it very difficult to provide an adequate prosthetic appliance.

The uvula may vary considerably in size from one individual to another. It may be barely present or may extend almost to the tongue. It may be congenitally absent or lost by surgical removal (generally an accident); rarely it may be bifid and represent a mild form of cleft palate (Fig. 85).

Oropharynx

The tonsillar area and the oropharynx (Fig. 86) usually must be inspected by the use of a tongue depressor. Since there is a tendency for the tongue to retract and obscure the examiner's vision, it is necessary that the depressor be applied properly. Its tip should be placed back of the junction of the horizontal and vertical portions of the tongue; by using this point as a fulcrum to maintain a constant forward and downward pressure, the examiner can hold the tongue out of the line of vision. Unless this technic is followed, gagging will result, and the oropharynx will be obscured.

Tonsils may vary greatly in size; in children they tend to be large and to project toward the midline of the tonsillar fossa. If they have not been removed, they tend to atrophy during the latter part of the third and fourth decades so that in older age the lymphoid tissue may have regressed to such a degree as to appear as if a tonsillectomy had been done. In the plane with the soft palate and on the posterior wall of the pharynx is a ridge of tissue called Passavant's ridge. This functional landmark is of significance in the closing off of the nasal cavity during deglutition. In the presence of a cleft palate, the location of this ridge is of significance to the prosthodontist in the construction of obturator bulbs.

The size and form of the oral cavity and the oropharynx may vary considerably and are often related to the character of the facies. A broad-faced child usually has a broad and rather large oropharynx, while the narrow-faced child has a narrow and small oropharynx. Anatomic variations of the form and size are great. Though the normal appearance of the pharynx is hard to define, in general it is moist and bright pink, and a few dilated veins and nodular promi-

Fig. 86. *Inspection of soft palate and posterior pharyngeal wall.* Note lymphoid tissue on posterior pharyngeal wall and paralysis of left side of soft palate.

nences are present. The true size and form of the normal oropharynx is difficult to establish because of the variation in the quantity of the lymphoid tissue
which surrounds the pharynx in the area designated as Waldeyer's ring. In general there is a physiologic enlargement in childhood and a diminution in adults.
Normal age changes are not well known, and a clinical standard for normal
lymphoid tissue is difficult to establish. The tonsils in healthy children may en-
large considerably in the absence of disease, presumably in response to unknown
demands.

Findings in Disease.—It has been said that enlarged pharyngeal and palatine
tonsils cause mouth breathing by blocking the nasal pharynx and that this may
give rise to an acquired swallowing reflex, causing an undesirable thrusting of
the tongue. It must be remembered that mouth breathing is related not only to
obstruction of the pharyngeal air passages by hypertrophied pharyngeal lymphoid
tissue, but also to paranasal sinus infection, engorged turbinates, and septal deviations. It is obvious that nasal obstruction, resulting in difficult nasal breathing, may induce habitual mouth breathing which continually dries out the gingival tissues and contributes to gingival disease. It has been suggested also that
chronic mouth breathing interferes with normal development of the dental arches
and face in susceptible individuals because of the influence of malfunctioning
muscles. Further, it has been suggested that inflamed and enlarged tonsils produce an involuntary and reflex muscle action of the tongue and adjacent muscles,
whereby the mandible and/or tongue is moved forward (tongue thrusting) to
increase the space around the inflamed tonsil and give relief from pressure upon
it. Thus chronic tongue thrusting, resulting either from enlarged tonsils or reflex
muscle action, can produce malocclusion of the teeth in susceptible individuals.

Since the palatine tonsils are those most easily observed by the dentist, gross
enlargement is usually used as a criterion for the diagnosis of encroachment upon
the oropharyngeal space (Fig. 87). However, the diagnosis of inflamed and in-

Fig. 87. *Fauces.* Tonsils appearing as two oval structures on lateral aspect of fauces showing intense lymphoid hyperplasia. In children this enlargement is due to repetitious and persistent upper respiratory infections.

fected tonsils should not be made on the basis of enlargement alone. The chief characteristics of a chronically infected tonsil are persistent redness of the tonsil and adjacent mucosa with repeated attacks of tonsillitis and the presence of lymphadenopathy of lymph nodes draining the tonsils. The diagnosis of infected or inflamed tonsils and a rationale for the removal of tonsils and adenoid tissue when related to the prevention or treatment of malocclusion require considerable rapport and understanding between the dentist and the physician. The referral of a patient to a physician for evaluation and treatment of mouth breathing or tonsil abnormality should not be predicated with a diagnosis of the abnormality; rather, the referral should be based on the dental examiner's findings and its significance to the patient's oral health.

Floor of the Mouth

The structures which occupy the floor of the mouth include the sublingual glands and ducts, the superior part of the submaxillary glands and ducts, the lingual nerves and branches, and various lymph nodes along the inferior border of the mandible. The sublingual sulcus is traversed in the midline by the lingual frenulum which attaches to the inferior surface of the tongue and reaches forward to the mandibular alveolar process. Close to the lingual frenulum and on each side of it lies a small round nodule called the sublingual caruncle. This papilla contains the openings of the submaxillary gland duct and often those of the sublingual gland duct. Sublingual folds containing the sublingual glands extend posteriorly and laterally in the floor of the mouth from the vicinity of the sublingual caruncle to the molar region (Fig. 88). The ridges over the sublingual glands contain the openings of the minor sublingual ducts.

Examination of the floor of the mouth can be best accomplished by inspection and palpation. The former is carried out by having the patient elevate his tongue while the examiner retracts the tissues away from the mandible with a mouth mirror (Fig. 89). The examination should start with inspection of the

Fig. 88. *Floor of mouth.* Sublingual caruncle indicated by arrow; note bilateral retrocuspid papillae indicated by arrows.

Fig. 89. *Inspection of floor of mouth.* **A,** Retraction of tongue. **B,** Reflection of light into floor of mouth.

color of the tissues and observation of the position of the structures in the floor of the mouth during functional movements of the tongue. Any inflammatory changes about the caruncle or enlargements of the sublingual ridges should be noted. The position of the attachment of the lingual frenulum on the mandibular alveolar process, best observed when the patient places the tip of the tongue on the palate or the lingual aspects of the maxillary incisors and pushes against them, should also be noted, especially if partial dentures or full dentures are con-templated. This same maneuver allows the examiner to determine the relation-ship of the floor of the mouth to the alveolar ridge and to note any encroachment of the tissues of the floor of the mouth into edentulous spaces.

Palpation of the floor of the mouth is best done bimanually. The examiner should face the patient, who should be in an upright position with the head and jaw turned slightly downward in order to get maximum relaxation of the muscles of the floor of the mouth. When possible the examiner should use the first finger of his left hand for intraoral palpation of the left side and the first finger of his right hand for the right side. The structures should be palpated against the examiner's other fingers which are placed extraorally and, where nec-essary, against the mandible (Fig. 90). The lingual aspects of the mandible can be best palpated when the floor of the mouth is being examined. In order for the examination to be successful, it is necessary that the patient remain relaxed.

Palpation of the floor of the mouth should begin in the midline and traverse the soft tissues posteriorly as far as the examiner can go without causing undue discomfort to the patient. At the same time he should palpate the lingual surface

A   B

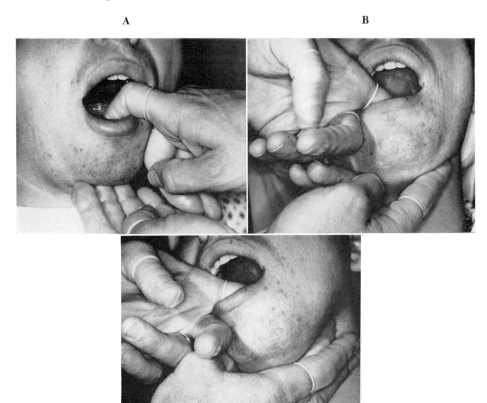

C

Fig. 90. *Bimanual palpation of floor of mouth.* **A-C,** Note altered head position to facilitate examination of each area.

of the mandible for the presence of exostoses, areas of tenderness, and loss of
firmness. In a normal mouth he should be able to feel the soft nodular tissue of
the sublingual glands and the submaxillary duct. He should also be able to feel
the firm mass of the muscles in the floor of the mouth and occasionally the mental
spine. The contents of the sublingual fossa and the submaxillary fossa should be
palpated (Fig. 91). The examiner can usually follow the external oblique line
of the mandible from the area of the bicuspid teeth to the ascending ramus. The
bony prominence on the lingual aspect of the mandible made by the bone over
the apices of the molar teeth, as well as the mylohyoid muscle attachment, should
be palpated. In this area just posterior to the last mandibular molar, the lingual
nerve can occasionally be palpated just beneath the mucosa as it enters the floor
of the mouth in the posterior lingual region.

Findings in Disease.—Changes in the color of the floor of the mouth are
unusual, but they may be present in association with inflammatory changes, hyperkeratotic changes, and retention cysts. Not infrequently ulcerations will occur

as a result of trauma or in association with primary or secondary herpes. A swelling in the floor of the mouth should be palpated to determine its consistency and its extent. Soft fluctuant masses are probably cystic in nature, and hard boardlike manifestations may be associated with cellulitis of the sublingual space; hard, firmly attached enlargement associated with the sublingual glands may be inflammatory or neoplastic in origin. Neoplastic change may involve the mucosal surface or the glandular structures. Occlusal type radiographs are sometimes helpful in determining the presence or absence of stones in Wharton's duct. It must be remembered, however, that stones are not always associated with the formation of cysts in the floor of the mouth (Fig. 92). Enlargements of the floor of the mouth associated with cystic lesions may often be associated with periods

Fig. 91. *Bimanual palpation* of contents of sublingual and submaxillary fossae. Note retraction of tongue from the mandible to gain access to the fossae.

Fig. 92. *Ranula.* Note enlargement of floor of mouth and displacement of tongue.

of remission, related to an increased flow of saliva which generally occurs at mealtime. Cellulitis of the floor of the mouth is usually associated with pulp disease.

Lesions of the floor of the mouth which present enlargement, induration, and infiltration but do not involve the mucosa are difficult to evaluate without an adequate history and biopsy. In general, cystic lesions of the floor of the mouth present sufficient evidence in the history and in the examination to strongly suggest their character. However, it is not infrequent that neoplastic diseases of the floor of the mouth, especially those involving the salivary glands, show the signs and symptoms of a cystic structure as well as those of a neoplasm. Therefore, it is necessary to palpate completely the floor of the mouth for the presence of disease in the glandular structures as well as the ducts. In the presence of neoplastic disease, the examiner should be able to feel the loss of the normal contour of the gland, its hard, firm, nodular consistency, and its attachment to surrounding structures if invasion has occurred. If the examiner has had sufficient experience in palpation of a normal gland, he should have no difficulty in determining whether the consistency, form, character, and function are abnormal. In those cases where marked inflammation has produced fibrosis, scarring, and an obliteration of many of the glandular elements, the changes presented may be sufficiently confusing to require a biopsy for an adequate evaluation. Any hyperkeratotic lesion, persistent ulcerative lesion, or enlargement of the floor of the mouth should be biopsied. Recent induration and swelling of the floor of the mouth associated with the signs of inflammation, especially pain and tenderness, should direct the examiner's attention to a history of pulp disease and the possibility of an alveolar abscess draining into the sublingual space.

Tongue

In the past, many indications of health and disease have been attributed to the tongue. However, it cannot be said that all were based on sound principles. This structure was considered especially sensitive to gastrointestinal disturbances, but, since the development of the fluoroscope, electrocardiography, and other forms of diagnostic aids, the use of the tongue as an indicator of general systemic health has been largely dropped. Thus, due to lack of scientific evidence, the idea that a coated tongue represents constipation and other gastrointestinal disturbances should be considered misleading and of no significance. A certain degree of coating is normal; the amount may vary from day to day and from morning to afternoon in the same individual. Probably of more significance is the absence of any coating. However, even this finding is a rather nonspecific manifestation.

Clinical examination of the tongue should include visual inspection of as much of the surface as is possible to see. The tongue should be observed in its normal position in the mouth and in an extended position. To ensure as much inspection of the surface as possible, the tip should be grasped in a piece of gauze between the examiner's index finger and thumb and gently pulled forward so that the lateral surface, base, and dorsal surface can be inspected (Fig. 93). The anatomic landmarks to be considered are the papillae (filiform, fungiform,

A   B

Fig. 93. *Inspection of tongue.* **A,** Lateral border. **B,** Dorsum.

circumvallate, and foliate) the foramen cecum, the lingual tonsil or tissue, the lingual veins, and the anterior lingual glands and ducts (Fig. 94).

The largest of the papillae are the circumvallate. They number from six to sixteen and are situated almost parallel to and in front of the terminal sulcus, forming a V or Y. Their size and number vary considerably from one individual to another and may cause the student some apprehension when he sees them for the first time. The foramen cecum is usually a small depression at the junction of the terminal sulcus; it is located just behind the circumvallate papillae at the apex of the V formed by these papillae.

The lingual tonsils are accumulations of lymphoid tissue on the root of the tongue. They may extend as far back as the epiglottis and laterally through the palatine tonsil. Lymphoid tissue is seen commonly on the posterolateral borders of the tongue associated with the foliate papillae (Fig. 94). Patients may complain of soreness of these areas. Generally the soreness is on one side, and the patient attributes it to rubbing the tongue against sharp tooth surfaces. While sharp teeth may aggravate this tissue, inflammatory lymphoid hyperplasia is the main factor. Because the soreness may last for from several days to a week, many patients become concerned with the possibility of cancer. Most are unaware of the existence of lymphoid tissue in this area and do not associate the soreness with a cold or sore throat that they may have at the time or have had in the immediate past.

The anterior lingual gland (gland of Blandin and Nuhn) lies close to the inferior surface and the tip of the tongue. Its ducts, of which there are from

A   B

C   D

Fig. 94. *Tongue.* **A,** Fungiform papillae. **B,** Circumvallate papillae. **C,** Foliate papillae. **D,** Varicosity of sublingual vein.

five to seven, open on small protuberances of the mucous membrane under the tongue on the plica fimbriata. The glands occasionally give rise to mucoceles. On the inferior surface of the tongue in the median plane and extending from the inferior surface of the tongue to the gums or the alveolar ridge, there is a fold of tissue called the lingual frenulum. An abnormally broad lingual frenulum may result in tonguetie (ankyloglossia).

Generally in the median plane of the tongue, there can be seen on the dorsal surface a shallow groove called the median lingual sulcus. Occasionally the tongue is furrowed on its dorsal surface. The furrow may vary in extent from an exaggeration of the median lingual sulcus to a network of irregular grooves. A furrowed tongue is generally of no clinical significance. It is considered to be of developmental origin, but the grooves appear to be more pronounced with advancing age. Infrequently, deep grooves may accumulate food debris and produce unpleasant odors and inflammation (Fig. 95, A).

Two other rather common variations of the tongue which may be seen are

A   B

Fig. 95. *Tongue.* **A,** Furrowed tongue with glossitis migrans. **B,** Median rhomboid glossitis; note absence of papillae but no inflammatory changes.

phlebectasia linguae and median rhomboid glossitis. The former is merely a dilatation of the lingual veins seen on the inferior surface of the tongue. Some forms of these blood vessel varices may be seen in the skin and mucous membranes as a hereditary hemorrhagic telangiectasia; lingual varicosities may be related to this defect provided there are other areas of involvement. However, in general, lingual varicosities are quite common in older individuals, are of local origin, and are of no particular significance. Median rhomboid glossitis is a term used to describe a minor developmental disturbance of the tongue located just anterior to the foramen cecum in the middle third of the dorsal third of the tongue (Fig. 95, B). It has a rhomboidal and red appearance and is often mammillated on its surface. It differs from the surrounding surface of the tongue in color and in surface appearance. The appearance is related to the absence of papillae. This disturbance is of no clinical significance, is not an inflammatory lesion as the term implies, is seen infrequently, and is considered within the range of normal. It may be mistaken for carcinoma; however, carcinoma is rare in this location.

The tongue should be palpated as well as visually inspected. Since most of it is muscle, it should have the resilient characteristics of muscle tissue and, depending upon the thickness at the particular area of palpation, should have a uniform consistency. The position of the tongue in its normal position in the mouth is of special clinical significance to the orthodontist and the prosthodontist. At rest, the tip of the tongue and its lateral borders approximate the edges of the teeth. Though indentations of the teeth may be seen on the tongue, this does not necessarily mean undue pressure nor is it characteristic of any particular disease. However, when the tongue appears to more than fill the area allotted it and extends over the surfaces of the teeth, it should be evaluated for macroglossia or displacement by such factors as enlarged tonsillar tissues. An extremely large tongue or one which is habitually placed forward of its normal position to compensate for an air passage which has been encroached upon by enlarged tonsils may cause generalized diastemas of the anterior teeth or undue labially directed force on them.

The tongue should be examined during its action to determine whether or not there are asymmetrical functions; it should also be studied during swallowing to determine whether or not abnormal swallowing habits are present. The normal position of the tongue and its functional movements are important for the stability of both partial and full dentures. The size, shape, and control of the tongue is especially important to the stability of lower dentures. When much of the posterior alveolar ridge has been lost, there is a tendency for the tongue and the sublingual fold, which runs from the lingual frenulum to the glossopalatinus arc, to overflow onto the remaining alveolar ridge. This tissue may prevent the taking of an adequate impression unless it is recognized and the impression tray altered to block it out.

The normal position of the tongue is such that it lies lax in the floor of the mouth. The apex lies slightly below the incisal edges of the mandibular incisors, and the dorsal surface is visible above the teeth in all parts of the mouth. Some tongues appear to assume a low level and some a high level. The edges in the low-level position tend to rest on the posterior mandibular teeth while in the high-level position they rest on the maxillary teeth. A retraction of the apex of the tongue downward and backward or upward, and a depression of the tongue into the floor of the mouth, represents an unfavorable position during function and is undesirable for denture stability (Wright). Many tongues assume upward retracted positions in response to encroachment upon the normal tongue space.

A   B

Fig. 96. *Tongue.* **A,** Smooth, oval, craterform ulcer arising on anterior dorsum of tongue that shows atrophy and hyperkeratosis; changes are secondary to previous x-ray therapy. Biopsy verified that ulcer had undergone malignant change. **B,** Tongue which is thick and bound to floor of mouth as evidenced by limited displacement produced by tongue blade; note ulcer under nodule on left side where the tongue contacts sharp teeth. These findings frequently exist in advanced carcinoma of the tongue.

Findings in Disease.—The clinical examination of the tongue should include inspection and palpation for size, function, and lesions. Disturbances may be congenital, traumatic (Fig. 96), infectious, metabolic, hormonal (Fig. 97), allergic, hematologic, neuromuscular, and neoplastic (Fig. 98) in origin. Of these, trauma is the one most common cause of lesions. It must be remembered that in order to effectively diagnose any lesion of the tongue, a history must be taken first in a systematic way so as to uncover all existing symptoms of the disease. This history cannot be limited merely to a review of the tongue itself; it must be an entire systems review since the presenting lesions may be oral manifestations of a systemic disease. A thorough history of the tongue should be taken, and those salient features of the history which might orient the direction of the examination should be kept in mind during the examination procedure.

The examiner who is aware of the normal size, texture, and resiliency of the tongue and has a knowledge of the normal anatomy of the tongue and its

A

B

Fig. 97. *Pigmentation.* **A,** Intense Addisonian pigmentation of tongue; note that pigment shows symmetrical bilateral distribution. **B,** Pigmentation of lip associated with Addison's disease. (Courtesy Dr. Stefan Fajans.)

Fig. 98. *Carcinoma of tongue.* **A,** Marked enlargement of tongue due to squamous cell carcinoma developing in a syphilitic glossitis. Secondary infection is superimposed with development of abscesses; note lateral indentations on tip and left border of tongue. **B,** Exophytic, lobulated, sessile, white lesion attached to lateral border and extending onto inferior surface. Appearance of lesion plus induration indicates a squamous cell carcinoma.

variations should be able to detect any disturbances of this organ. It must be remembered that the tongue goes through an intricate developmental period, and occasionally growth disturbances will be found. The history and duration of the disturbance and the absence of traumatic agents will serve to orient the examiner toward a developmental disturbance. The most common are bifid tongue, tonguetie, furrowed tongue (Fig. 95, *A*), median rhomboid glossitis (Fig. 95, *B*), thyroglossal duct cysts, and macroglossia. Macroglossia, in the absence of systemic disease such as cretinism and infantile myxedema, may be considered to be developmental in origin if there is no change in the resiliency and texture of the tongue. Macroglossia associated with neoplastic, inflammatory, or retrogressive changes will usually show changes in resiliency, texture, function, and sensation.

Changes involving the surface of the tongue and papillae but not involving deep-seated lesions or induration should alert the examiner's attention to drug reactions, vitamin deficiency manifestations, anemias, dermatologic diseases, or geographic tongue. Chronic infective granulomas, traumatic lesions, and neoplasms usually produce marked changes in the consistency, function, and sensations of the tongue. Rarely are the manifestations of dermatologic disease confined to the tongue, and the examiner can usually orient his diagnostic thinking in the direction of a dermatologic disease when he finds lesions present in the mouth and also on the skin. This does not mean that lesions of the mouth and skin have to be related; however, the relationship should be evaluated. Traumatic lesions are usually painful on palpation, and a positive history of trauma can be obtained. Lesions associated with infective granulomas are usually deep seated, change the consistency of the tongue, give rise to functional problems, and are likely to be of long duration. Primary lesions of the chronic infective granulomas such as syphilis are of short duration, produce little change in sensation of the tongue unless the lesion is in an advanced stage, and the patient has a history of contact with syphilis (Fig. 98, A).

Of special significance to the dentist are the mucous patches of secondary syphilis. These may occur on the tongue as well as other areas of the mucous membranes. The patch may arise as a macule, papule, or vesicle which frequently may ulcerate to form a lesion not unlike a canker sore except for the absence of an erythematous halo and pain. Most often it appears as a grayish-white, slightly elevated lesion comparable to the papule of the skin (Fig. 99). The membranelike surface can be removed easily. The mucous patch is highly infective.

In order to make a diagnosis of any lesion of the tongue, it is necessary to have an adequate history, the results of the clinical examination showing the character and extent of the lesion, and a descriptive knowledge of the disease which may be producing the lesions. In general, it is possible to classify the particular zone of pathology to which the examiner must orient his thinking simply by determining the general characteristics of the lesions which are present.

A   B

Fig. 99. *Tongue.* **A,** Tuberculous ulcer. **B,** Mucous patch of syphilis.

Developmental disturbances are fairly characteristic because of their location (such as the lines of fusion), failure of parts to obliterate, and uncomplicated anomalies of size. Traumatic lesions tend to be recognized because of a positive history of trauma. However, chronic traumatic ulcers can be a diagnostic problem because of their tendency to resemble carcinoma, and biopsy may be necessary. Dermatologic lesions generally have skin manifestations, and the diagnosis usually can be made on the basis of skin involvement. Single lesions are usually of traumatic or local neoplastic origin whereas multiple lesions are more likely to be manifestations of systemic disease, dermatoses, or allergic disorders. Changes in the resiliency, density, function, and sensation of the tongue should suggest to the examiner the possibility of chronic infective granulomas and neoplasms. The history and system review are significant prerequisites for making a diagnosis of this type of lesion. When there is no positive history of trauma or disease to account for a lesion, a neoplasm of the tongue should be suspected, especially if the lesion is deep seated and of long duration and there is a positive history of progressive growth.

Superficial lesions of the tongue that are either localized or diffuse in nature, accompanied by changes in the papillae and changes in the size and consistency of the tongue due to edema, suggest the possibility of anemias, vitamin deficiencies, and drug reactions. A review of the history or inquiry into the patient's use of drugs may serve to orient the diagnosis of the lesions. Sensitivity reactions can arise from antibiotic therapy. The manifestations of drug sensitivity can arise from ingestion of the drug or contact with the drug. Drug reactions, vitamin deficiency, and anemias all produce some degree of change in the tongue sensations.

Sensitivity changes of the tongue may vary from a mild burning sensation to deep pain. The pain may be localized, diffuse, deep seated, or superficial. A burning sensation is the most commonly encountered pain of the tongue. This generally involves the lateral borders and the tip; however, it may be general in coverage or even vague in localization. Inability to localize pain is common when neurosis is a factor. The examiner must be careful not to classify readily those patients with obscure tongue pain as psychoneurotic individuals. The most common cause of pain of the tongue is traumatic injury such as biting. Traumatic injuries are easily determined because of their history. Burning tongue may be associated with dentures, anemias, or menopause, and the burning is generally intensified by irritation. Occasionally occlusal disharmony will result in a burning sensation and hyperesthesia of the tongue. The mechanism for this is unknown, but this relationship should be investigated. An occlusal adjustment will relieve many of these patients, especially when the pain also involves the face and ear region.

In macrocytic anemia the tongue may be painful and red. The whole tongue or just the lateral borders, may be affected. The papillae are atrophic or absent, with the result that the tongue has a bald, glassy, slick, or glazed appearance (Fig. 100). These changes may also reflect some form of anemia which is a secondary expression of some other state such as sprue, Plummer-Vinson syndrome, pregnancy, and vitamin B deficiency. It should be pointed out that the tongue manifestations seen in some of the diseases just mentioned are not particularly characteristic; the diagnosis of anemia certainly cannot be made on the basis of tongue changes alone. Such changes should alert the examiner to the possibility of the presence of concomitant systemic disease and the need for additional positive correlative data. The same reasoning applies to the so-called magenta-colored tongue of riboflavin deficiency and the red, beefy, painful, swollen tongue of pellagra (Fig. 100).

The two most common ulcerative lesions of the tongue are traumatic ulcers from biting and the shallow, painful lesions associated with primary and secondary herpetic stomatitis (canker sores). There is generally no difficulty in making a differential diagnosis of these lesions. The history of onset, the char-

A   B

C

Fig. 100. *Tongue.* **A,** Pellagra. **B,** Cheilitis and glossitis of vitamin B deficiency. **C,** Pernicious anemia.

acter of the lesion, and the multiplicity of the herpetic lesions tend to make their recognition relatively easy.

Another fairly common disturbance of the tongue is the so-called geographic tongue. It is also commonly called glossitis migrans and wandering rash of the tongue. It is a chronic and transient more or less circinate mucosal atrophy or desquamation of the superficial epithelium of the tongue. The lesions are red in those areas in which atrophy of the papillae has occurred and white in those areas in which hyperplasia of the filiform papillae has occurred prior to their atrophy and loss. In general, the degree of redness depends on the relative color of normal areas and the degree of desquamation. In many instances no white elliptic borders will be present. Not infrequently the areas will appear as small areas of red depapillated islands, especially if the tongue is heavily coated or the filiform papillae are hyperplastic (Fig. 101). The character and location of these lesions change from day to day. The cause is unknown. They are of no significance except to apprehensive persons.

A   B

C

Fig. 101. *Geographic tongue.* A-C, Same tongue at one-week intervals showing so-called migration of lesion.

Fig. 102. *Black hairy tongue.*

An overgrowth of the filiform papillae in the presence of pigment-producing mold or fungus gives the appearance of a hairy tongue. This condition is usually caused by the use of hydrogen peroxide, sodium perborate or, in some instances, antibiotics. A positive history of prolonged use of these drugs in the presence of an overgrowth of the filiform papillae suggests a diagnosis of black hairy tongue (Fig. 102).

Gingiva

The gingival tissues should be examined for color, form, density, level of attachment, and depth of crevice. The examination should be systematic and should start with the gingiva in the third molar region and extend around the buccolabial and lingual surfaces of the arches to the opposite side. It should consider both the attached and free gingivae. An appreciation for normal gingivae at different ages is necessary (Figs. 103 to 105).

The normal and healthy attached and free gingivae are uniformly coral pink in color throughout the mouth. The color of the gingiva is dependent upon the vascularity of the mucosa, the hemoglobin content of the blood, the amount of reduced hemoglobin in the blood, the density and attachment of the connective tissue, the width of the epithelium, the degree of keratinization and pigmentation of the epithelium, and the presence or absence of inflammation. The shade and intensity of the normal color varies from one individual to another. The gingiva in the primary dentition period is usually uniformly pale pink throughout the mouth but tends to show more the vascular pattern of the subpapillary venous plexus. This is probably true because of the absence of keratinization and chronic inflammation.

Physiologic pigmentation, either diffuse or localized in character, may alter the shade and uniformity of the color of both the primary and adult dentitions (Fig. 1). Localized pigmentation may cause a variation of from light brown to dark blue. Diffuse or generalized pigmentation modifies the shade of the gingiva in direct proportion to the color of the skin. In general the gingiva of the primary and mixed dentition periods will show less diffuse or generalized pigmentation than the adult dentition. This follows the normal physiologic development of pigmentation with age. The gingiva is usually a pale coral pink in the primary dentition but may show areas of whiteness (blanching) and redness (erythema) associated with eruption of teeth during the mixed dentition period. While one of the signs of a healthy gingiva is a coral pink color, this color may be present even though there is a hyperplastic alteration of the form of the gingiva associated with inflammation deep in the gingival crevice. It is also pale pink with gingival fibromatosis. In general, however, the pale pink color which turns to white on pressure (blanching) denotes a healthy gingiva.

The form or contour of the interdental papillae, free gingival margin, and the attached gingivae is related to the morphology of the crown of the tooth, the spacing of the teeth, the contour of the roots of the teeth, and the presence or absence of disease. In a normal healthy mouth the gingiva fills the interproximal spaces and ends in a knifelike edge and is closely adapted to the surfaces of the teeth. The form of the interproximal space is especially significant to the form of the interdental papilla. Where the width of the crown of the tooth at the

A   B

C   D

Fig. 103. *Normal gingivae.* **A** and **B**, Note form of gingiva and uniform shade in primary dentition. **C** and **D**, Changes in form and uniform shade in mixed dentition.

A   B

C   D

Fig. 104. *Normal gingivae.* **A** and **B**, 20 years of age. **C** and **D**, 35 years of age.

cervical area is not much less than that at the contact area, the height of the interproximal papilla will be shorter than in those instances where the width at the cervical portion of the crown is considerably less than that of the width at the contact area. It is to be expected that attrition of the contact areas, physiologic atrophy of the gingiva, and passive eruption will give rise to variations in the form of the gingiva. The contact areas between adjacent teeth are subject to wear, and the consequent loss of tooth structure brings about a movement of the teeth in a mesial direction (mesial drift) which compensates for the decrease in mesiodistal width of the teeth. Thus, the space below the contact area (interproximal space) varies with the type of tooth, the position of the tooth, and the position of the adjacent tooth. The form of the gingival tissue which fills this space is thus related to these factors and to the presence or absence of disease. Where diastemas are present, the interdental papilla will follow the contour of the alveolar ridge (Fig. 106). Where the diastema is large or where there is absence of teeth, there will be little suggestion of a papillary contour in the usual sense; however, a modified type of papilla may be found on the mesial or distal proximal aspect of the teeth. This can be readily observed on the distal aspect of the mandibular bicuspids and mesial aspect of the mandibular molars where intervening teeth have been lost. While this condition cannot be considered as normal, it can be considered as healthy when the relative con-

A

B

C

Fig. 105. *Normal gingivae.* **A** and **B**, 45 years of age. **C**, 55 years of age; note uniform shade, stippling, and adaptation of gingiva to the teeth.

Fig. 106. *Gingival contour* associated with diastema and spacing of the lower incisors.

tour of the gingiva is favorably related to the contour of the crowns of the teeth. In these instances the gingiva should be closely adapted to the surface of the tooth and end in a knifelike edge.

The surface of the attached gingiva, including the interdental papilla, is generally stippled, while that of the free gingival margin and the borders of the interdental papilla is smooth. The texture of the surface can be more readily appreciated when the gingiva is dry. There is considerable variation in the degree of stippling even in the absence of disease. The surface may vary from a light stippling to that not unlike velvet and somewhat analogous to that of the surface of an orange. Stippling and keratinization of the gingiva are generally considered to be a protective adaptation to function. They are not well developed in the primary or mixed dentition but become more prominent in the young adult and progressively more apparent in the older adult. In older persons there appears to be a decrease in gingival keratinization with advancing age associated with atrophy of the oral epithelium and concomitantly a decrease of gingival stippling. This is difficult to evaluate because of the difficulty of separating those changes due to aging from those due to disease of the periodontium which is almost universal in patients of the older age group. A small papule is often present on the lingual aspect of the gingiva adjacent to the mandibular cuspid. It is called the retrocuspid papilla and is of no pathologic significance (Figs. 88 and 107).

The density or consistency of the gingiva depends upon its location, its attachment, and the presence or absence of disease. Normally it is firm and resilient and tightly bound down to the alveolar process and teeth except at the free gingival margin and the borders of the interdental papilla. On palpation of the attached gingiva, the examiner should be able to feel primarily the contour of the underlying bone and only slight movement or resiliency of the interposed attached gingiva. Palpation of the free margin should yield slightly more to pressure and should give a sense of slight movement. Surface palpation and light rubbing will reveal the degree of stippling and to some extent the degree of keratinization. Palpation of the attached and free gingivae will be found especially helpful in relating their contour to the underlying bone and tooth structure. Thus, palpation of the gingiva and the underlying bone and tooth structure will

Fig. 107. *Retrocuspid papilla.*

serve to determine the true size and form of the gingiva and will relate the form to bony prominences.

The depth of the gingival crevice or sulcus in the adult is considered to be normal if it does not exceed 1.5 to 2 mm. The position of the gingival margin on the crown of the tooth varies with the age of the individual and with the degree of eruption of the tooth. The depth of the crevice may vary considerably during the active eruption of the teeth. This may be readily appreciated by probing it in the mixed dentition. Quite often the crevice of the erupting permanent maxillary incisors will be very deep, especially where the free gingival margin is located high on the enamel. This usually represents a transitory stage, and with the completion of the eruption of these teeth and the completion of the growth of the alveolar bone the depth of the gingival crevice reaches normal limits.

In the normal adult mouth the level of the epithelial attachment should be on the enamel or at the cementoenamel junction. In the presence of simultaneous atrophy of the alveolar crest and marginal gingiva, without an increase in the depth of the crevice, migration of the attachment apical to the cementoenamel junction is considered to be physiologic. However, this recession of the gingiva probably does not occur in the mouth that has been free of disease. The position of the epithelial attachment in the young adult is usually on the cervical one-third of the teeth. Since the establishment of occlusion cannot be considered to be final at this time, changes in the position of the gingival margin and epithelial attachment are to be expected. Within certain limits the compensatory eruption of the teeth for wear or physiologic attrition will, to a certain extent, determine the later position of the gingival margin and the epithelial attachment.

Inasmuch as the form of the gingiva is intimately related to the form of the teeth, this relationship is best served for the protection and stimulation of gingiva and supporting structures when the epithelial attachment is at or above the cementoenamel junction. Any recession below this level must be considered as abnormal. It is possible, however, for the gingiva to be healthy even though it is attached below the cementoenamel junction. This is frequently seen in elderly individuals, but the problem of maintaining the health of the gingival tissues and of the exposed cementum is exceedingly more difficult than when the gingival tissue and attachment are in their normal positions. The main difficulty arises because of the loss of the normal and physiologic relationship between the gingivae and the contours of the teeth. When the teeth and gingiva are in the normal position, the convexity of the labial, lingual, and buccal surfaces of the teeth prevents food from being forced into the crevice and at the same time allows the food to pass over the gingiva and provides stimulation and massage of the tissues.

CLINICAL SIGNS OF NORMAL GINGIVA

1. Color—uniform pale pink except for physiologic pigmentation when present
2. Form—should fill the interproximal space and end in a knifelike edge closely adapted to the surfaces of the teeth
3. Density—interdental papillae and free and attached gingivae should be firm and dense in all areas

4. Crevice—should not exceed 2 mm. in adults
5. Attachment—the epithelial attachment should be on the enamel or at the cemento-enamel junction in children and adults; may be on the cementum in elderly individuals; however, it should not be more than 1 mm. below the cementoenamel junction

The difference between normal and healthy gingiva is important for the recognition of normal tissue in contrast to that which is abnormal in form and attachment but healthy. This distinction becomes important in the recognition of the effects of past disease and in evaluating the success of periodontal therapy. The color and density of healthy gingiva are the same as for normal gingiva; however, the form and level of the epithelial attachment are not the same. The depth of the gingival crevice is the same for both normal and healthy gingivae. Gingivectomy, necrotizing gingivitis, periodontitis, gingivitis, and gingival recession may permanently alter the form of the gingiva; therefore, the gingiva is no longer normal. However, if the gingival tissue is free of inflammatory and other abnormal changes of color, form, and density, and the gingival crevice does not exceed 2 mm., the gingiva may be considered to be healthy although not normal.

CLINICAL CRITERIA FOR A HEALTHY TISSUE
1. Uniform pale pink color except where physiologic pigmentation exists
2. Contour and relationship of the gingivae to the teeth functional
3. Tissues firm and dense
4. Depth of gingival crevice should be less than 2 mm.
5. Level of the epithelial attachment irrelevant

Findings in Disease.—Changes in the color of the gingiva may result from any alteration of those factors which are responsible for its normal pink color. Changes may be related to the mucosa of the rest of the mouth or may be localized to particular areas of the gingiva. Thus the alteration of color may involve simply the free gingival margin of one or more teeth or involve all the attached gingiva and extend into the alveolar mucosa. The examiner should determine the areas which show the alteration of color and make a record of these findings.

The significance of the change in color from the normal is important not only for a diagnosis of disease in these tissues, but also for an evaluation of periodontal therapy. The changes may be transitory or of long duration. When observing an abnormal color, it must be remembered that the color which is seen at that particular time may not be the same as that which existed at a prior time. Where a color other than pale coral pink exists throughout all of the gingiva, the examiner should relate this apparent change in color to the rest of the oral mucosa and the skin since an alteration of the color may be associated with a more generalized disease (Fig. 108). For example, a paleness of the gingiva, buccal mucosa, palate, lips, conjunctiva, and fingernail beds may be related to an anemia; a generalized redness of the gingiva, buccal mucosa, palate, and tongue may be related to a sensitivity manifestation or, when this redness also includes the face, hands, and neck, may indicate the presence of such a condition as polycythemia; a melanosis of the gingiva, buccal mucosa, and palate may indicate Addison's disease; or a bluish cast to the gingiva, buccal mucosa, palate, tongue, hands, and face may indicate the presence of a central or peripheral

Fig. 108. *Gingival pallor* associated with severe anemia. **A,** Note absence of the change in color (shade) that exists normally at the junction of the alveolar and gingival mucosa. **B,** Hemorrhage about center of incisor and bicuspid secondary to leukemia.

cyanosis. Therefore, the examiner in his inspection of the gingiva for changes in color must consider the possibility of changes also existing elsewhere.

The most frequent change in the color is associated with chronic inflammation. The alteration of the normal color as the result of inflammation is related to the chronicity of the injurious agent and to the response of the tissues to this irritation. Inflammation is a physiologic response of the tissues to injury and is accompanied by changes in the vascular bed, maturation of the epithelium, pigmentation of the gingiva, and alteration of the activity of the connective tissue of the submucosa. Changes in the vascular bed which alter the color of the gingiva are capillary dilatation and active hyperemia, increased capillary permeability with exudation, hemorrhage per diapedesis, passive congestion with a reduction in the rate of capillary flow, and a reduction in lymph flow. Active hyperemia with capillary dilatation and engorgement of the vessels, especially associated with acute inflammation, gives rise to a bright red erythematous discoloration. Where the capillary bed is obvious and where the epithelium is thin, as in the alveolar mucosa, buccal mucosa, soft palate, and pharyngeal wall, the examiner may see evidence of a relative increase in number of capillaries; this effect is from a complete utilization of the capillary reserve. The engorgement of an increased number of capillaries tends to give the tissues an erythematous discoloration with a netlike appearance. This is seldom seen in the gingiva proper because of the masking of the changes by hyperplastic epithelium and the depth of the subpapillary venous plexus. However, it may be readily observed where the epithelium is atrophic, ulcerated, and thin and where the inflammatory reaction extends to the alveolar mucosa.

While an initial bright red erythematous discoloration usually signifies active hyperemia and acute inflammation, such a discoloration may also be present in chronic inflammation where the epithelium is thin and atrophic and the underlying capillaries are near the surface (Fig. 109). In general, however, in the presence of chronic inflammation and where the surface epithelium is intact, an excessive amount of reduced hemoglobin in the vessels will give the tissues a bluish-red discoloration. Increased permeability of the vessels in inflammation results in an edema with the result that fluid in the tissues tends to mask the discoloration present. The loss of red blood cells from the capillaries either by diapedesis or rhexis into the connective tissue results in a breakdown of the hemoglobin into hemosiderin and other pigments. Where the amount of pigment in the gingiva is significant, a brownish-blue to bluish-black discoloration will be present. Passive hyperemia or congestion of the venules results in a localized accumulation of excessive reduced hemoglobin and gives the tissues a bluish hue. This bluish hue superimposed upon a redness is the most common finding in chronic inflammation.

The thickness of the epithelium and the maturation of the epithelium may be altered as the result of injury or irritation and allow the underlying vascular changes to be more apparent to the observer. This is true in acute inflammation and is especially prominent where there is ulceration of the epithelium, although the formation of a pseudomembrane may completely cover the area of ulceration so that none of the underlying vascular changes may be readily observed. However, the border of the ulcerative lesion may well show the bright red erythematous character of acute inflammation. Active chronic inflammation tends to stimulate the proliferation of the epithelium and of the connective tissue. In these instances, there is usually an increase in the width of the epithelium and the underlying connective tissues. As a reparative phase of the inflammatory

Fig. 109. *Localized intense redness* (indicated by dark shade) around the maxillary central and lateral incisors. This is a response to the materia alba present.

reaction becomes significant, the proliferation of the connective tissue and epithelium may completely mask the presence of deeper inflammatory changes, especially in the gingival crevice or periodontal pocket. Thus the color associated with active chronic inflammation in a deep gingival crevice may be completely masked by the attached gingiva and free gingival margin where the inflammation has subsided and the color has returned to normal. In such instances the gingiva is not without signs of abnormality since gingival enlargement and loss of adaptation to the teeth is evident.

Accretions, films, plaques, and necrotic tissue may also alter the color of the gingiva. Certain tooth pastes may give the gingiva a whitish cast; drugs and therapeutic agents may give rise to rather characteristic discolorations. The presence of a serpiginous grayish slough that may be easily removed to show an area of ulceration suggests necrosis with the formation of a pseudomembrane. This is characteristic of necrotizing gingivitis (Vincent's infection) (Fig. 110). The presence of a white filmlike plaque on the surface which can be easily removed to show intact gingiva is found frequently in association with the accumulation of food debris and filamentous organisms in the mouths of those with poor oral hygiene. These light films may form overnight but may be readily brushed aside with a toothbrush.

Granulation tissue associated with either initial injury or repeated trauma is quite vascular and gives the gingiva a red coloration. If this tissue subsides and forms avascular scar tissue, it will give the gingiva a white discoloration. The white color is also partly due to the reduced amount of melanin and hemoglobin normally present. Its optical characteristics resemble edematous tissue and tend to reflect white light.

The desquamation of the epithelium of the gingiva in those areas which are pigmented, either diffuse or locally, will allow the color from the papillary and subpapillary vascular network to be more readily seen. In darker races, melanosis of the tongue would appear to be more significant than melanosis of the

Fig. 110. *Necrotizing ulcerative gingivitis* (Vincent's); note pseudomembrane and destruction of interdental papillae and intense marginal redness in maxillary and mandibular anterior region.

buccal mucosa or gingiva. Aside from the physiologic pigmentation associated with the darker racial groups, probably the most common discoloration of the gingiva is due to metallic pigmentation arising from impregnated amalgam. It is found most frequently in the area of an extraction site or adjacent to a large silver amalgam restoration in the free gingival margin or interdental papilla. Impregnation of amalgam occurs as the result of fracturing of amalgam during the extraction of the tooth, with fragments of the amalgam becoming embedded in the gingival tissues. With the organization and repair of the wounded area, the only evidence of the remaining amalgam may be that of a bluish-black discoloration. Similar discolorations resulting from impregnated amalgam and carborundum particles may be found in the gingival tissues from grinding and contouring of the amalgam restorations. Not infrequently large deposits of darkly stained calculus may show through the free gingival margin and produce a dark blue or bluish-black discoloration of this tissue. Removal of the calculus or insertion of paper between the calculus and the free gingival margin will serve to show whether or not the discoloration is due to calculus or to pigmentation within the gingival tissue itself. Other metallic pigmentations associated with heavy metals such as bismuth, arsenic, mercury, or silver are usually more widespread, and the patient will usually give a history of the therapeutic use of these heavy metals.

An examination for discoloration must take into consideration local, systemic, and exogenous factors capable of producing color changes in the gingiva. It is necessary that the examiner have an appreciation of the range of normal for the various racial groups. In order for him to effectively utilize descriptive reference material concerning gingival and other mucosal discolorations he must obtain an adequate history of the time of onset and possible relation to exogenous, systemic, and local factors; inspect the discoloration to determine its extent, its color, its location and distribution; and palpate the discoloration to determine its consistency and surface texture and to determine the presence or absence of enlargement or tenderness.

It is necessary that the examiner recognize not only conspicuous deviations from the normal contour and form of the gingiva, but also the initial signs of disease. Other than in association with acute traumatic injuries, changes in color may be the first manifestations of disease of the gingival tissues; afterward, hyperplastic or atrophic changes in the form of the gingiva may be observed. In the prevention of periodontal disease, it is necessary that the early and initial signs and symptoms be recognized; after the disease is already present, the signs and symptoms of alterations of color, form, and density are important for the recognition, classification, and diagnosis of periodontal disease.

Alteration of gingival form may result from changes within the gingiva itself of local or systemic origin; from changes in the form and/or position of the teeth resulting from dental decay, traumatic occlusion, dental abrasion, or extrusion and pathologic migration; or from changes in the bony supporting structures. Changes in form may be localized to the gingiva of single teeth or generalized to involve the gingiva throughout the mouth; may be limited to the gingival margin or to the interdental papilla; or may be diffuse in character and involve both the free and attached gingivae. An alteration of the form from changes within the gingiva itself may be expressed clinically by gingival enlargement, gingival atrophy, loss of gingival tissue, characteristic festooning, clefting, loss of attachment, and lack of adaptation to the teeth.

Changes are most often caused by local factors. Thus, most periodontal disturbances are inflammatory in nature since inflammation is the reaction of the tissues to injury. Systemic factors may alter the form, but most often they only modify the response of the tissue to local injury. In the presence of chronic irritation, such as calculus and soft debris, the gingiva may be enlarged, causing

Fig. 111. *Alteration of gingival form.* **A,** Rolled gingival margins. **B,** Hyperplastic interdental papillae. **C** and **D,** Enlargement of gingiva produced by pericemental abscess. **E** and **F,** Discrete gingival enlargement. **E,** Granuloma gravidarum. **F,** Traumatic fibroma.

the free margin to be blunt and rolled and the interdental papilla to be swollen and to overfill the interproximal spaces (Fig. 111). Acute inflammation associated with a periodontal abscess gives rise to gingival enlargement localized to one or two teeth (Fig. 111). Circumscribed or discrete enlargements of the gingiva may be reactive or neoplastic in origin (Fig. 111).

Changes in the form of the gingiva are common during the mixed dentition when eruption of the teeth and superimposed inflammatory changes give rise to enlargement of the gingiva and alterations of the gingival contour (Figs. 112 and 116). While these changes are generally transitory in nature, the effect on the adult periodontium cannot be underestimated. Thus, alterations of the gingival form during the mixed dentition cannot be considered entirely physiologic in nature, and while a certain amount of inflammatory reaction is to be expected during the eruption and positioning of the teeth, chronic inflammatory hyperplasia with alteration of the form and contour of the gingiva over long periods of time may result in permanent deformity of these tissues.

Rather specific morphologic changes in the gingival contour may be encountered in Stillman's clefts and McCall's festoons (Fig. 112). Clefting may range from V-shaped notches to thin slits extending from the edge of the free gingival margin and along the exposed surface of the root of a tooth. These clefts

A   B

C

Fig. 112. *Alteration of gingival form.* **A,** Eruption cyst. **B,** Stillman's cleft. **C,** McCall's festoons; note extreme toothbrush abrasion.

may be seen in any area of the mouth but are seen most frequently in association with the lower anterior teeth. McCall's festoons are an exaggeration of the normal gingival festoon. Inflammatory changes may be superimposed upon these changes. It is thought that Stillman's clefts and McCall's festoons are directly related to traumatic occlusion. However, it seems likely that additional factors are also responsible for the production of these alterations of the normal contour, viz., large roots with inadequate base bone.

Loss of gingival tissue as evidenced clinically by exposure of the interproximal spaces, exposure of the cementum, and recession of the gingiva should be evaluated for the presence or history of necrotizing gingivitis and chronic periodontitis, for a history of gingivectomy, and for those local factors which may produce recession of the gingiva. Necrotizing gingivitis (Vincent's infection) and chronic periodontitis are the primary causes for the loss of interdental papillae. Traumatic occlusion, improper toothbrushing, and orthodontic movement of the teeth may produce gingival recession. It must be remembered that the alignment and form of the teeth and the form of the alveolar arches may in themselves predispose to gingival recession (Fig. 113).

A systematic appraisal of the form of the gingiva is necessary for the formulation of a diagnosis since the descriptive knowledge of specific diseases of the

Fig. 113. *Alteration of gingival form.* **A,** Gingival recession and McCall's festoons associated with traumatic occlusion. **B,** Gingival recession resulting from improper toothbrushing. **C,** Gingival recession associated with orthodontic movement. **D,** Change in gingival contour produced by recurrent Vincent's infection.

periodontium is based upon alteration of the color, attachment, density, and form of this tissue. A generalized bluish cyanotic discoloration, together with a generalized soft and spongy enlargement of the tissues, should direct the examiner's attention toward those factors which produce local or generalized gingival hyperplasia. These factors may be local, dysfunctional, or systemic in origin. Simple hyperplasia is generally related to local irritants such as calculus, soft debris, poorly adapted margins of restorations, and mouth breathing. The enlargement may be associated with a modification of the normal inflammatory response of the tissues to irritants because of hormonal imbalance in puberty and pregnancy, and because of therapeutic agents such as Dilantin sodium.

Clinical manifestations of changes in the consistency of the gingiva can be best evaluated by digital palpation. The examiner should differentiate changes of the gingiva itself from those arising from changes in its surface texture and underlying bone. The changes in consistency are usually related to the alteration in form. Palpation with slight pressure may be utilized to discover edema, pitting, fluctuance, induration, and friability of the tissues.

Soft spongy gingival tissues which pit on slight pressure may be associated with an accumulation of intercellular fluid in the mucosa and submucosa. Localized edema of the gingival tissues may be found due to an obstruction of the venous or lymphatic return either by tumors or inflammation; it also may be mechanical or allergic in origin. By far the most common cause of edema is that associated with chronic inflammation. This local type is produced by those factors which favor filtration, such as increased capillary permeability and obstruction of the venous return. Exaggerated sponginess and pitting edema are seen frequently in certain types of leukemia. Neoplastic disease, such as carcinoma, may result in tissues which are extremely soft and friable. Fluctuance may be associated with intercellular and intracellular edema of the mucous membranes of the gingiva and may also be found with periodontal abscesses. When palpation reveals fluctuance, the examiner must be sure to rule out crepitus and changes in the underlying bony structure. Fluctuance involving the surface of the gingiva may be associated with bullae and vesicles whose margins are well defined. Fluctuance associated with periodontal abscesses is of a somewhat different character than that associated with vesicles or bullae because of the nature of the fluid present. Vesicles and bullae have a rather thin covering and tend to rupture easily. Tenderness is a prominent feature of periodontal abscess and a thick serosanguineous purulent material may be expressed provided there is a drainage site.

Palpation of an enlarged gingiva which is characterized by a firm, hard, and leathery consistency should suggest fibrosis associated with chronic inflammation, gingival fibromatosis, or neoplasia. Firm, smooth, nodular circumscribed lesions of the gingiva may be related to bony protuberances or exostoses (Fig. 114). Localized enlargements may be reactive (inflammatory) or neoplastic in origin. The final diagnosis of this type of lesion is best made by a gingival biopsy. Occasionally a small, firm, movable, discrete yellowish-white lesion may be found on the attached gingiva, especially in the area of the mucobuccal fold in the posterior part of the mouth. Such lesions are generally confluent ectopic

Fig. 114. *Alteration in gingival contour.* Exostoses.

Fig. 115. *Gingival texture.* Persistent stippling in the presence of periodontal disease.

sebaceous glands and their true identity may be established by a gingival biopsy if necessary.

Changes in the texture of the surface of the gingiva is a common finding in gingival disease. The loss of the normal stippled surface results in a smooth glossy surface. A smooth surface may be presented when there is atrophy of the gingival epithelium, desquamation of the superficial layers of the epithelium, and stretching of the epithelium from underlying edema or scar tissue. While stippling is utilized as one of the criteria for a healthy gingiva, it may be present in chronic periodontal disease. It is related to superficial tissues and not necessarily to deeper portions of the periodontium. Thus, with gingival massage, it may exist in the presence of deep intrabony periodontal pockets (Fig. 115).

The surface texture of the gingiva associated with hyperkeratosis may vary from a slightly rough or pebbly texture to an elevated circumscribed verrucous nodular leathery texture. A verrucous texture is generally related to the degree of hyperkeratosis. Friability, ulceration, and induration are important features of hyperkeratosis to be evaluated by inspection and palpation. The differential diagnosis of hyperkeratotic lesions includes leukoplakia, focal hyperkeratosis, and lichen planus. Although all of these lesions appear clinically as white, lichen planus does not present the rough nodular surface texture that leukoplakia and focal hyperkeratosis do. It is possible, however, that these lesions may present a diagnostic clinical problem in their early stages because of the slight degree of hyperkeratinization. In these instances a history and clinical examination may not be sufficient to arrive at a diagnosis, and a biopsy is indicated. Focal hyperkeratosis, beginning leukoplakia, erosive lichen planus, and desquamative gingivitis frequently present diagnostic problems even to clinicians who are well versed in examination procedures and oral diagnosis. However, such problems may be minimized by proper attention to the history and by understanding the characteristics of these lesions and the principles and indications for biopsy. Thus, focal areas of hyperkeratosis associated with chronic trauma alone may suggest to the examiner the tentative diagnosis. However, in view of the tendency for leukoplakia and focal hyperkeratosis to break down into malignancies, a clinical diagnosis without microscopic examination is of doubtful value, especially in older individuals.

The clinical evaluation and diagnosis of lichen planus of the gingiva depends to a large extent upon the configuration of this lesion and the texture of its surface (Fig. 7, A). The surface of lichen planus is usually only slightly rough and hyperkeratotic. Its borders may be well defined by inspection because of its white color, but it may be difficult to palpate because of the absence of a well-defined elevation and lack of roughness of the surface. When present, linear striations, nodule points, and involvement of other areas such as the tongue, buccal mucosa, and flexor surfaces of the extremities aid in making the clinical diagnosis of lichen planus. The history is of considerable significance here since lichen planus may be somewhat transitory in nature; the history of onset is usually vague and not usually related to traumatic agents.

The location of the epithelial attachment and the depth of the gingival crevice should be determined in all areas of the mouth since alteration of the normal level of attachment and depth of gingival crevice is a positive sign of gingivitis and periodontitis. An increase in the depth of the crevice and associated apical migration of the epithelial attachment and resorption of alveolar bone are signs of a periodontal pocket. An increase in depth may be related to gingival hyperplasia. In this instance the level of attachment is on the enamel or at the cementoenamel junction, and there is no loss of bone.

Any increase in depth over 2 mm. must be considered as a sign of disease. Usually other signs of disease such as altered color, form, and density will also be present. In some instances a significant increase in depth will be present without apparent signs of inflammation; however, the deeper portions of the crevice will be involved. Thus the active inflammatory reaction of the surface tissues may subside, leaving these tissues to appear clinically as relatively healthy. However, the inflammatory process deep in the crevice still has active chronic inflammation present. This may be easily overlooked if inspection and palpation of all the gingival crevices are not carried out routinely by probing.

When the epithelial attachment is located on the cementum, disease is then present or has been present. This means that the presence of the epithelial attachment on the cementum is a positive sign of present or past disease. In either case it is an abnormal position. If the disease has been arrested and the color, form, and density reflect good function, the gingiva is healthy even though it cannot be considered normal.

Excessive mobility of the teeth may be due to loss of bone support, root resorption, or traumatic occlusion. In chronic destructive periodontal disease the loss of bone may allow the teeth to become so mobile that movements of 1 to 2 mm. or more are possible. In other instances the same quantitative loss will show no increase in the mobility of the teeth. Resorption of the roots of teeth from orthodontic movement, occlusal trauma, or unknown cause may increase the mobility of the teeth so involved. Here again the teeth may show no excessive mobility. Teeth in traumatic occlusion may show extreme mobility without an increase in the width of the periodontal membrane space.

Increased mobility of the teeth is an important sign of periodontal disease, and the examination should include palpation of all the teeth for evidence of this condition. The prognosis of treatment and treatment planning may depend to a large degree on the amount of mobility present, the cause of the mobility, and the possibility of its limitation.

One of the most significant findings in periodontitis is the presence of periodontal pockets involving bifurcation and trifurcation areas. Such areas cannot be kept free of irritants in most instances and are prone to the formation of periodontal abscesses. Actual pocket formation into these areas generally spells a poor prognosis for the teeth so involved. Treatment is difficult, if not impossible, because of the anatomic form of the areas. The presence of periodontal pockets involving bifurcation and trifurcation areas cannot be determined adequately without the use of a periodontal probe. Radiographic evidence is not conclusive—only suggestive. In many instances involvement may be present without radiographic evidence of their presence. The radiographic signs of periodontal disease will be found in Chapter 6.

It is important not only to recognize that disease exists, but also to determine the cause of the disease. By far the most important causes of periodontal disease are local factors. These consist of local irritants such as bacterial plaques, soft debris, calculus, overhanging margins on restorations, food impaction, and carious lesions. Dysfunctional factors such as unilateral mastication, lack of stimulation of the tissues, malposed teeth, mouth breathing, traumatic occlusion, and lack of function are also important in the etiology of periodontal disease. Systemic disease such as diabetes mellitus may affect the resistance of the individual to local irritants; it does not in itself produce periodontal disease. The response of the tissues may be modified or adversely affected by pregnancy, puberty, and leukemia. Thus periodontal disease is largely inflammatory in nature and the result of local injury. The following outline of periodontal disease may serve to summarize the clinical findings in the examination of the periodontium.

CLASSIFICATION OF PERIODONTAL DISEASE

1. **Simple gingivitis**

   This is an acute or chronic inflammation due to poor oral hygiene or local irritants. Alteration of color, form, and density of the tissues is related to response of the tissue to injury. Some degree of gingival enlargement is present but is not extensive. The changes may involve only a few areas of the free gingival margins. (Fig. 116.)

2. **Infective gingivitis**

   A. **Vincent's infection (necrotizing ulcerative, ulceromembranous)**

   The color, form, density and attachment of the gingivae may be significantly altered. Alteration is characterized by necrosis of the gingival margins and interdental papillae which leaves punched-out craterlike depressions. The surfaces of the lesions are covered with a gray or grayish-yellow pseudomembrane which is easily removed, leaving a bleeding ulcerated surface. The margins of the lesions present a pronounced erythematous appearance. The lesions may involve only a few areas on all the teeth. Symptoms include pain of varying degrees, sialorrhea, wedging sensation of the teeth, and foul breath. Local lymphadenopathy is likely to be present. Fever, malaise, anorexia, and other systemic manifestations may be present. (Figs. 12, 111, and 117.)

   B. **Herpetic gingivostomatitis**

   This is an acute process due to the initial invasion of any or all of the oral mucosa by the herpes simplex virus. Early features include regional lymphadenopathy, fever,

| A | B |

Fig. 116. *Gingival disease.* **A,** Eruption gingivitis. **B,** Simple marginal gingivitis.

Fig. 117. *Gingival disease.* Acute necrotizing ulcerative gingivitis (acute Vincent's infection).

malaise, and "sore throat." The latter is generally dysphagia rather than typical sore throat. There are generalized gingival hyperemia, tenderness, and usually vesicles. The lesions generally follow the initial systemic phase; they arise as vesicles which soon rupture to form shallow ulcers with an erythematous halo. Lesions may involve only the gingiva but generally involve all of the oral mucosa. The disease is self-limiting, lasting from about a week to ten days. (Figs. 118 and 13, *C.*)

Fig. 118. *Gingival disease.* Acute herpetic gingivostomatitis; note lesions on free gingival margins of all maxillary incisors.

A   B

Fig. 119. *Gingival disease.* **A,** Simple hyperplastic gingivitis; mild. **B,** Severe.

Fig. 120. *Gingival disease.* Hereditary gingival fibromatosis.

3. **Hyperplastic gingivitis**
   A. **Simple hyperplastic gingivitis**
      This is a simple enlargement of the gingival tissues, especially the free gingival margin and the interdental papillae, due to chronic irritation. Alteration of color, form, and density is related to the inflammatory response of the gingiva. The proliferative response of the tissues is more marked than in simple gingivitis. Thus, altered form is a constant and characteristic finding. The chronicity of the irritant is also an important factor. The tissue is soft and spongy. The color is bluish-red. (Fig. 119.)
   B. **Hereditary gingival fibromatosis**
      This is a progressive proliferative process in which the normal contour and form of the gingiva are altered. The tissue is generally pale pink, firm, and very dense. The enlargement may be so pronounced as to completely cover the teeth. Local irritation may be superimposed. The tissues tend to return progressively after surgical removal even in the absence of local irritation. (Fig. 120.)
   C. **Gingivitis modified by systemic factors**
      (1) **Dilantin hyperplasia**
          This is a progressive proliferation of the gingiva associated with Dilantin therapy. Clinical signs and symptoms are the same as those of simple hyperplastic gingivitis. To make the diagnosis of Dilantin gingivitis, it is necessary to know the patient is taking Dilantin sodium. Local irritants cause the inflammatory response; Dilantin only exaggerates this response, with resultant gingival enlargement. (Fig. 121.)
      (2) **Pubertal gingivitis**
          This is gingival enlargement which is thought to be associated with hormonal imbalance at the time of puberty. The color, form, and density changes are the

Fig. 121. *Gingival disease.* Marked Dilantin hyperplasia.

A   B

Fig. 122. *Gingival disease.* Pubertal gingivitis.

same as in simple hyperplastic gingivitis. The color is intense, and the gingiva tends to bleed readily. This is a nonspecific inflammatory hyperplasia. Local irritation is the cause of the inflammatory response; the hormonal imbalance appears only to modify the response. (Fig. 122.)

(3) **Pregnancy gingivitis**

This is gingival enlargement showing all the signs and symptoms of simple hyperplastic gingivitis plus a greater tendency to bleed. It is a nonspecific inflammatory response of the tissues to local irritants; the response is modified by hormonal imbalance that occurs during pregnancy. Unless the physical state of pregnancy exists, the diagnosis relative to the signs and symptoms present would be simple hyperplastic gingivitis. (Fig. 123.)

(4) **Leukemic gingivitis**

This type of gingivitis is characterized frequently by marked gingival enlargement. The enlargement is due primarily to the infiltration of the gingival tissues by neoplastic blood cells which produces a peculiar thickening of the gingival margins which have a tendency to stand away from the teeth. The color may be bluishred to pink. The tissues are generally soft and spongy. Spontaneous and persistent hemorrhage occurs frequently. The gingival enlargement in some forms of the disease may cover the surface of the teeth. Regional lymphadenopathy may be present. A complete history and examination are necessities. Areas of ulceration suggestive of Vincent's infection may be present. (Fig. 124.)

Fig. 123. *Gingival disease.* Pregnancy gingivitis.

A   B

Fig. 124. *Gingival disease.* **A,** Leukemic gingivitis (granulocytic). **B,** Leukemic gingivitis (monocytic).

4. **Hormonal gingivitis**
   A. **Chronic desquamative gingivitis**
      A type of gingivitis associated with altered premenopausal hormonal stimulation. It is occasionally seen in males. Desquamation of the epithelium is the most constant feature; this may be limited or diffuse throughout the gingiva. The color of the gingiva varies from one location to another from grayish-blue to brilliant red. The over-all appearance of the gingiva may show a patch of speckled discoloration. In some forms the entire gingiva may be erythematous. The density of the gingiva is soft, and digital palpation may be attended by peeling of the epithelium. Stippling is absent, and the gingiva is not tightly bound down to the underlying tissues. Some degree of hyperplasia is present, and the surface of the epithelium is easily stripped or peeled off in severely affected areas. Pain is a common symptom and varies in intensity according to the severity of the process. (Fig. 125.)
   B. **Chronic atrophic senile gingivitis**
      This type of gingivitis is related to postmenopausal hormonal stimulation. It also is occasionally seen in males. The gingival tissues are thin and atrophic and are easily traumatized. Thus many of the changes seen are secondary to the lack of protective adaptation of the gingiva to trauma. Not infrequently even well-fitting dentures cannot be tolerated. Clinically the cheek mucosa may have a milky appearance and irregular grayish-white areas that can be mistaken for leukoplakia. In general, the tissues are pale and grayish-white. In some areas a mild degree of hyperkeratinization may be present. (Fig. 126.)

A   B

Fig. 125. *Gingival disease.* Chronic desquamative gingivitis.

A   B

Fig. 126. *Gingival disease.* Chronic atrophic gingivitis.

Fig. 127. *Gingival disease.* Atrophic gingivitis due to trauma.

Fig. 128. *Periodontitis.* Gingival appearance with periodontitis of varying severity.

C. **Atrophic gingivitis**

This refers to gingival recession excessive for age. The gingiva is usually free of in-flammation unless the exposed cementum is hypersensitive and for this reason is not kept clean. The soft tissue recedes at an equal rate with the loss of alveolar bone. Atrophy may be due to poor toothbrushing habits, hyperfunction, bruxism, or hypo-function. Generalized recession in young individuals may be related at times to large teeth and an inadequate bony support. (Fig. 127.)

5. **Periodontitis**

This is an inflammatory disease, usually the sequela of untreated gingivitis, characterized by an extension of the inflammatory process into the deeper structures of the periodontium. The color, form, and density are all expressions of chronic inflammation. Periodontal pockets are present, and the teeth may or may not show hypermobility. Clinically the gingiva is red or bluish-red and soft and spongy, and the margins are thick and rolled. The interdental papillae are soft and spongy and may overfill the interproximal spaces. There is generally supragingival and subgingival calculus present throughout the mouth. (Fig. 128.)

The clinical evaluation of color, form, density, and attachment is an important step in the formulation of a diagnosis, and careful collection of the facts will serve to orient the examiner to the proper field of reference. It is impossible for the student or general practitioner to know all the ramifications of periodontal disease or to have the descriptive knowledge necessary to make a diagnosis of obscure or differential diagnostic problems. He must remember, however, that his reference to the literature must be based upon his orientation to the correct field and his ability to relate his findings to those descriptions in the reference material which are couched in terms of abnormalities of color, form, density, epithelial attachment, and depth of the gingival crevice.

Examination Procedure.—The examination of the gingiva should begin with a systematic inspection from the junction of the alveolar mucosa to the free gingival margin. Any alteration of the normal color should be recorded. The location, extent, and coloration should be given in detail. An attempt should be made to determine the cause of the alteration, viz., pigmentation, cyanosis, desquamation, etc. All information should become a part of the patient's permanent record, since it is valuable in making the ultimate diagnosis and in determining the progress of therapy. The inspection should also include observation of the signs of altered form. The form may be altered by disease or past therapy. Gingival enlargement may be diffuse or localized; the areas involved should be recorded. For example, the gingival form may be described thusly: "The free gingival margins of the maxillary central incisors are blunt, rolled, and enlarged; the interdental papillae of this area are swollen and overfill the interproximal spaces; the gingiva is enlarged sufficiently to cover half of the labial surface of these teeth."

The teeth should be examined for the presence of soft debris, plaques, stains, and calculus. The type, location, and amount should be noted and recorded. This should be done prior to the examination of the teeth for dental caries since it is necessary to clean the teeth thoroughly before effective evaluation of the presence of carious lesions can be accomplished. Discoloration of the teeth from exogenous causes can be evaluated best before the teeth have been cleaned, while discoloration associated with endogenous causes can be best appreciated after the cleaning.

Many colored substances which are introduced into the mouth or substances which are broken down in the mouth may stain the teeth or produce soft plaques upon them (Fig. 129). Such extrinsic stains may be green, yellow, orange, brown, or black. The origin of many of these colors is not well understood, but they probably arise from sulfides formed in oral putrefaction and/or from pigment-

Fig. 129. *Stains.* A and B, Green stain. C and D, "Metabolic" black stain. E and F, Tobacco stains.

producing bacteria. A green stain frequently appears on the necks of children's teeth, especially on the maxillary incisors. This appears to be associated with the remains of Nasmyth's membrane but may also be associated with penetration of the surface of the enamel beneath the membrane. A thin line of black pigment, "mesenteric line," may occur about the necks of the teeth of individuals, usually females, who often exhibit very good oral hygiene. It is most often seen on the lingual aspects of the maxillary teeth in the form of a fine black line fol-

Fig. 130. *Examination of gingiva.* **A,** Palpation of free and attached gingiva over eminences produced by roots of central incisors. **B,** Palpation of gingiva over the roots of molar teeth. **C,** Palpation of gingiva over tuberosity. **D,** Inspection of the alveolar and gingival mucosa of the tuberosity. **E,** Inspection of retromolar papilla, pads, and flaps. **F,** Palpation of retromolar area.

Fig. 131. *Charting.* **A-R,** Location of free gingival margin in relation to the cemento-enamel junction and recording it on the chart. The drawings to the left are schematic representations of measuring the free gingival margin in relation to the cementoenamel junction. The pictures in the center show the measurement clinically. The schematic drawings to the right show the measurement recorded on the chart (Fig. 137). **S** and **T** show completion of the free gingival margin on chart. **W-Z,** After the free gingival margin has been determined in relation to the cementoenamel junction and recorded on the chart, the location and depth of gingival sulci over 3 mm. are recorded. The drawings to the left are schematic representations of the probe in periodontal pockets. The pictures in the center indicate the position of the probe clinically. The schematic drawings on the right show the depth of the pocket on the chart as measured from the free gingival margin. The depth of the periodontal pocket is measured from the free gingival margin to the base of the pocket. This measurement is indicated by a vertical line placed on the involved side of the tooth drawn apically from the free gingival margin to the measured depth of the pocket. **ZZ,** Completed chart showing free gingival margin and location and depth of periodontal pockets; chart indicates pockets on distal surface of incisor and mesial surface of the cuspid.

M-O

P-R

S-T

U-W

X-Z

ZZ

Fig. 131 (cont'd). For legend see opposite page.

lowing the gingival margin (Fig. 129, *C* and *D*). It can be removed but tends to recur in a few days despite adequate home care. The etiology of this stain is not known. It appears to be of no pathologic significance and cannot be used as an indication of the patient's oral hygiene. Orange to orange-red stains may be seen either as thin lines or diffuse plaques around the necks of the teeth, and their etiology has been attributed to the action of chromogenic bacteria. These stains are of no pathologic significance, but they do give some indication of the oral hygiene of the patient. Tobacco stains may either be deposited upon the surfaces of the teeth or penetrate into the substance of the enamel and dentin. This type of staining is dependent primarily upon the presence of mucinous plaques on the teeth. It is not necessarily dependent upon the amount of tobacco used. Persons who chew tobacco or smoke cigars appear to be more prone to have penetration of tobacco juices into the pits and fissures of the teeth. The amount of staining which occurs is directly proportional to the presence of lamellae, cracks, and poorly calcified areas.

Palpation of the gingiva (Fig. 130) should be systematically carried out to determine the resiliency, texture, and status of the underlying tissues. Areas of tenderness, friable tissues, loss of normal texture, exuded pus, and soft spongy tissue should be noted.

Charting.—The level of the attachment and the position of the free gingival margin should be measured relative to the cementoenamel junction and a record made of these measurements. The initial measurements are made by ascertaining the cementoenamel junction and measuring the height of the gingival margin from this position (Fig. 131). This procedure is followed throughout the mouth, and these measurements should be made at four points: the mesial and distal aspects of the buccal or labial surfaces and the mesial and distal aspects of the lingual surfaces of each tooth. The free gingival margin is then drawn on a dental chart which has been ruled with 1 mm. gradations. When this has been accomplished, the examiner then should probe the depth of all the gingival crevices to determine where the crevices exceed the normal limits of 2 to 3 mm. in depth. This will serve to determine the position of the epithelial attachment relative to the cementoenamel junction. The actual measurement is made from the free gingival margin to the base of the crevice or periodontal pocket. This measurement of the depth of periodontal pockets is recorded on the chart as demonstrated in Fig. 131.

Though certain clinically evident changes in the color, form, and density of the gingiva and radiographic evidence of bone resorption may suggest the presence of periodontal pockets, the only reliable method for detecting their presence and extent is to probe the gingival crevices with a suitable periodontal instrument. The most suitable for measuring the depth of periodontal pockets is a very thin calibrated probe. It should be straight, resilient, and marked at 3, 6, and 8 mm. (Fig. 132). From a practical standpoint, probes which are marked for every millimeter are somewhat confusing. The probe must be carefully inserted to gain the deepest penetration possible without penetrating the gingival tissue or epithelial attachment. The examiner must know the anatomy of the root surfaces of the teeth well and must be able to detect alterations in the surfaces of

Fig. 132. *Gingival probing.* Gingival probe with 3, 6, and 8 mm. markings.

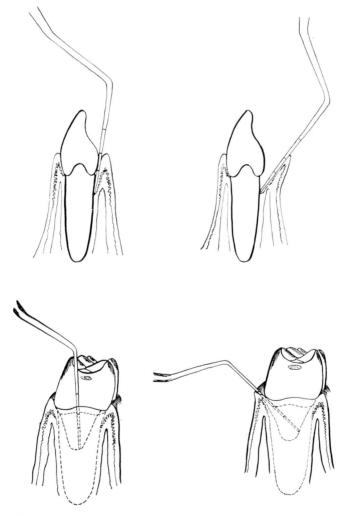

Fig. 133. *Gingival probing.* Correct method on left; incorrect on right.

the roots in order that the probing can be accurately accomplished. Calculus, enamel pearls, variations in the cementoenamel junction, and interradicular areas require special attention.

Full delineation of periodontal pockets may at times be difficult because of malpositioned teeth, overhanging restorations, carious lesions, tortuous pockets, tender gingiva, hypersensitive cementum, and gingival bleeding. Because of the convexity of the anatomic crown, the examiner should attempt to measure the depth of the pockets always at the same angle and as nearly parallel to the long axis of the tooth as possible (Fig. 133). Pockets involving interradicular areas are at times difficult to measure because of the relationship between the roots and crowns of the teeth. The measurement of the depth of pockets involving bifurcation and trifurcation areas is not so important as establishing that the involvement of these areas does exist. Probing for bifurcation areas of the mandibular molars does not present too much difficulty, especially when a "cowhorn" explorer is used. While this explorer cannot be used to measure the depth of periodontal pockets, it is of considerable aid in determining the extent of bifurcation involvement (Fig. 134). The area in which it is most difficult to ascertain the extent of periodontal pockets is the trifurcation area of the maxillary

A   B

C   D

Fig. 134. *Clinical probing.* Examination of bifurcation area with "cowhorn" explorer.

A   B

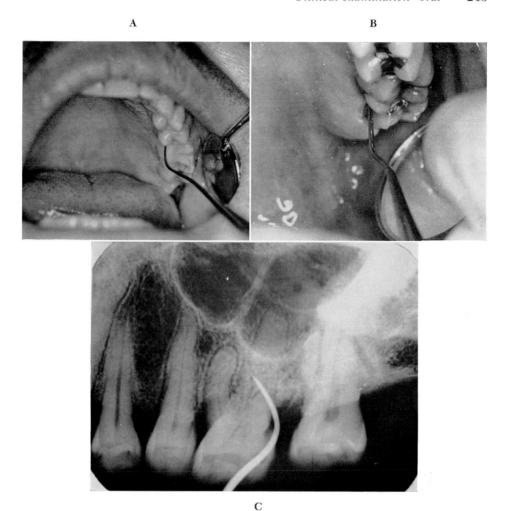

C

135. *Gingival probing.* Examination of trifurcation area with periodontal probe.

molars. Because of the anatomic arrangement of the roots, the convexity of the distal aspect of the crowns, and the angle at which the probe must be inserted, the probing of intrabony pockets involving the trifurcation area on the distal aspect of maxillary molars may be quite difficult (Fig. 135). Radiographs are especially helpful for determining the anatomic features of the interradicular area and help the examiner to probe these areas more effectively. It is important to record the depth of the periodontal pockets in these areas; however, it is more important to know whether or not actual involvement of the interradicular area has occurred. The examiner must fully delineate the extent and depth of the periodontal pockets and determine how much alveolar process has been lost on the mesial and distal aspects of the teeth and on the lingual, buccal, or labial aspects.

Periodontal pockets involving long fused roots of molars are usually of less significance than those involving teeth with divergent roots. Thus it is very important that the examiner not only attempt to measure carefully the extent and depth of periodontal pockets, but also to relate the morphology of the pocket to the length and form of the roots. Information relative to the morphology of the root will not only aid in more efficient probing of the periodontal pockets, but will also be useful in determining the prognosis and treatment of the teeth involved.

The mobility of all the teeth should be tested and the degree of mobility indicated in terms of a numerical reference (Fig. 136). The use of 1, 2, 3, and 4 will facilitate recording the degree of mobility; 1 may be used to indicate minimal lateral movement and 4 to indicate extensive lateral and intrusive movement of the teeth. Excessive mobility of the teeth may not be associated with periodontal pockets, and conversely periodontal pockets involving trifurcation and bifurcation areas will not necessarily cause increased mobility. Although bifurcation and trifurcation exposure and excessive mobility of the teeth are common clinical features of periodontal disease which are used in making a diagnosis, their significance to the prognosis and treatment planning varies considerably with individual cases. This is discussed in further detail in Chapter 8. Inasmuch as the treatment of periodontal disease is based upon the history and findings of the clinical examination, it is necessary that the examination of the periodontal structures be as complete as possible.

A clinical chart for recording periodontal as well as other dental findings is shown in Fig. 137. The charting shown represents most of the periodontal facts which might be recorded in a given case. The ruled lines are representative of 1 mm. The symbols which may be used on the chart are not necessarily exhaustive; however, the ones given are those which are used most often. The chart represents a complete record of the location of gingival margins, epithelial attachment, and the location of periodontal pockets. Symbols for missing teeth,

Fig. 136. *Detection of mobility.* Note placement of finger on lingual aspects of tooth to detect displacement caused by handle of explorer.

SYMBOLS FOR CHARTING

1. Missing		5. Open Contact	‖	9. Bridge
2. Cavity	●	6. Mobility	M 1-2-3-4	10. Periapical Area
3. Decalcified Area	✳	7. Bifurcation Exposed	V	11. Hypoplasia
4. Food Impaction	✝	8. Drifted, Extrusion	D→	12. Overhang
				13. Extract

Fig. 137. *Charting.* Completion of periodontal charting in a typical case; numbered boxes are to record vitality measurements.

caries, periodontal pockets, interradicular involvement, periapical involvement, and teeth to be extracted are presented; their positions and meanings are given.

Teeth

Examination of the teeth should be preceded by a careful prophylaxis so that calculus, stains, and soft debris will not interfere with exploration and inspection. For this reason stains, oral hygiene, and the location and character of calculus should be considered during the examination of the gingivae.

The examination should be systematic and always begin and end in a definite locality. Methods of examination include inspection with the naked eye using a mouth mirror, exploration with suitable sharp explorers, and percussion using the end of the handle of the mouth mirror or single-ended explorer.

Radiographic examination and vitality testing should also be considered part of a thorough examination.

The examiner should remove any debris and dry the teeth before attempting to examine them for carious lesions. The use of a saliva ejector will facilitate the examination procedure. The patient should be instructed to rinse the mouth thoroughly before the examination is begun. A mouthwash of water containing a few drops of 28 per cent ammonia may be provided to aid in removing thick mucous saliva from the mouth.

The following should be considered in the examination of the teeth: color and stains; size, form, structure, and number; erosion, abrasion, and fractures; vitality; functional contours; carious lesions; contact relationship.

Color and Stains.—The color of the teeth may show considerable normal variation; the primary teeth are generally bluish-white, while the permanent teeth are generally more opaque and show variations of gray and yellow hues as the individual becomes older. The inherent color is determined by the translucency and thickness of the enamel and by the thickness and color of the underlying dentin. Alteration may be physiologic or pathologic and intrinsic or extrinsic in origin. As the individual grows older the enamel becomes worn and thinner, and unless it is lost entirely and wear of the dentin takes place, the dentin becomes thicker because of the deposition of secondary dentin. Because of the thinness of the enamel and the thickness of the dentin, the teeth of older persons are generally more yellowish or grayish-yellow in color than those of younger persons.

Discoloration may result from developmental disturbances whereby the normal pattern of enamel prisms and dental tubules are disturbed. Examples of this type may be seen in amelogenesis imperfecta, dentinogenesis imperfecta, brown hereditary teeth, and dental fluorosis or mottling.

Discoloration can also result from intrinsic pigments formed at the time of the development of the teeth or after the teeth have fully formed (Fig. 138). Pigments arising from hemolysis of blood cells or associated with jaundice may discolor the teeth. Discoloration associated with blood-borne endogenous pigments usually disappears with the termination of the disease process. The color of the teeth in these conditions may be markedly green, yellow-brown, or orange-yellow in appearance. With the death of the pulp, degeneration and decomposition products from the iron and proteins in the pulp tissue may diffuse into dentin, and the teeth will be stained gray, yellow-brown, or black. A dark gray color may indicate devitalization; however, this finding should be supplemented with vitality tests before the final diagnosis is made (Fig. 138, *B*). Internal resorption of the dentin may produce a pink or black discoloration of the teeth. These teeth give a positive response to vitality tests.

Discolorations may arise from the introduction of medicaments into the root canals and pulp chambers during endodontic therapy. Staining may also occur from permeation of medicaments into the dental tubules when sterilizing a cavity preparation. Metallic staining may arise from the ingestion or inhalation of metals or their salts. This occurs most often from the use of drugs but may be an occupational hazard. In most instances these metals or their salts are de-

A   B

C

Fig. 138. *Teeth—altered color.* **A,** Discoloration associated with porphyrinuria. **B,** Devital tooth. **C,** Pigmented teeth which vary in both degree and distribution of pigment. The pigmentation is complete in the anterior teeth but involves only the cervical areas of the molars. The color in the anterior teeth is purplish-brown; in the posterior teeth it is a canary yellow. This is the type of pigmentation produced by tetracycline.

posited in plaques or films upon the teeth; however, they may penetrate the enamel and dentin. This is especially true of teeth that are porous and have extensive cracks and lamellae. A history of the patient's occupation is extremely important in making a differential diagnosis of stains of the teeth. The use of tobacco is the most frequent cause of staining. This is especially true when abrasion has exposed dentin and the patient chews tobacco. In general, cleaning will only remove the external tobacco stains, and tobacco stains of dentin, fissures, pits, and lamellae will be difficult, if not impossible, to remove.

From the foregoing description of exogenous and endogenous stains it is apparent that the diagnosis is dependent upon an adequate history and a descriptive knowledge of a few characteristic stains. The diagnosis of most of the stains is dependent upon a history of the conditions which may be responsible for the staining such as occupation (e.g., an industrial worker may be inhaling copper, brass, or bronze particles), developmental disturbances associated with defects in the dentin and enamel, serious diseases such as hepatitis or erythroblastosis fetalis, restorative or endodontic procedures, use of drugs containing iron, mercury, or other staining elements, use of colored dentifrices, use of tobacco, and a history of pulp disease. The rather characteristic location and color of green stain, black linear stain, and red-orange stains associated with chromogenic bacteria make their diagnosis more dependent upon a descriptive knowledge than upon the history. However, the history is of value in the sense of negative correlation.

Size, Form, Structure, and Number.—The examiner should pay particular attention to the size, form, structure, and number of teeth, since developmental disturbances are frequently manifested by an alteration of these factors. This is especially true of the developing dentition because the size of the teeth play an important role in occlusion. The size of the crowns, the length and configuration of the roots, and the space presented by absence of teeth are all important to restorative procedures. Edentulous area should be evaluated for the presence of impacted or unerupted teeth.

Anomalies of size include macrodontia and microdontia. Anomalies of number include supernumerary teeth and complete or partial anodontia. Developmental disturbances of form include geminated teeth, fused teeth, concrescence, enamel pearls, dens in dente, Turner's teeth, odontomas, Hutchinson's teeth, mulberry molars, accessory cusps and roots, and hypoplastic defects (Fig. 139). Hereditary alteration of form includes hypoplasias, dentinogenesis imperfecta, dentin dysplasia, and amelogenesis imperfecta. Both hereditary and developmental defects show an alteration of structure. Extrinsic or environmental alterations that are responsible for variation in form after the teeth have fully formed may be manifest as erosion, abrasion, caries, or excessive attrition.

Enamel dysplasia refers to hypoplasia and hypomaturation of the enamel. Enamel hypoplasia is a defect that occurs as a result of any disturbance in the formation of the enamel matrix. Enamel hypocalcification occurs as a result of any disturbance which interferes with normal deposition of calcium, while hypomaturation occurs from incomplete crystallization of the enamel. These types of enamel dysplasia can result from local, systemic, or hereditary disease.

Local factors that can produce defects in the teeth include periapical inflammation, trauma, and surgical procedures. Periapical inflammation of a

A   B

Fig. 139. *Teeth—altered form.* **A**, Fusion. **B**, Hypoplasia of central incisor (Turner's tooth).

A   B

Fig. 140. *Teeth—altered form.* **A** and **B**, Hypoplasia; note rhythmic character of defects.

deciduous tooth may produce hypoplasia and hypomaturation of a succedaneous tooth if the inflammatory process occurs at the time of amelogenesis and maturation. Nutritional deficiencies, endocrine disturbances, and other systemic diseases have been suggested as etiologic agents in hypoplastic defects of the enamel. Enamel hypomaturation can be produced by ingestion of an excess of fluorine. Various hereditary defects of the enamel are seen such as amelogenesis imperfecta, hereditary brown teeth, and other hypoplasias of the enamel. Some hereditary enamel defects appear quite similar to those of local or unknown origin.

Enamel hypoplasia may appear as a localized alteration of one or several teeth or involve all the teeth. It may consist of the absence of enamel and dentin or of only the enamel. Its clinical appearance will depend upon the stage of amelogenesis at which the disturbance occurred and the external or environmental factors that have altered the enamel. Frequently enamel hypoplasia of the central incisors will show rather well-defined horizontal lines of pits and grooves (Fig. 140). The levels at which the defects occur represent an expression of the rhythmic or intermittent character of the interference in the development of the tooth structure. A comparison of levels of hypoplasia from one area of the mouth to another serves to point out the chronologic period or stage of development that various teeth were in during the period of disturbance. While the time period for the defect may be established, it is only rarely that a history of systemic disease will correspond to this time period. A recent study by Witkop indicates that many forms of enamel defects loosely classified as amelogenesis imperfecta may be distinct clinical and genetic entities. Thus a history of similar hypoplastic and hypomaturation defects of the enamel and dentin in other members of the patient's family should be determined.

Single or multiple chalky-white opaque spots may be present on the teeth. These spots are most obvious on the central incisors (Fig. 141). With eruption of teeth and recession of the gingiva, they may appear to the patient to be of recent origin; however, the defect actually occurs during the formation of the enamel. Clinically the enamel in an opaque spot may be soft and can be penetrated by an explorer if the surface is worn away; however, if the overlying enamel has

Fig. 141. *Teeth—altered color and texture.* Opaque spots due to hypomaturation of enamel.

remained intact, the surface will be granular but hard, and the explorer will not penetrate into the opaque spot. Not infrequently removal of the surface for restoration purposes reveals for the first time that the underlying enamel is softer than normal. Opaque spots may also be due to faulty matrix apposition which changes the index of refraction.

The greatest difficulty in arriving at a diagnosis of opacity of the enamel appears to be centered around the difference between hypocalcified and decalcified enamel. Clinically both appear white and opaque in character. No difficulty arises if the surface of the opaque spot is glazed and smooth since the defect of decalcification results in a granular, rough, and soft surface that can be penetrated with a sharp explorer. However, if both surfaces have a similar texture, some difficulty may arise. The white opaque areas of decalcification associated with the early phases of dental decay are usually found beneath soft masses of materia alba along the cervical one-third of the crowns of teeth adjacent to the free gingival margin and in areas which are not self-cleansing (Fig. 142). Opaque spots due to hypomaturation, hypoplasia, or altered pigmentation may be found anywhere on the teeth, including self-cleansing areas.

Endemic dental fluorosis (mottled enamel) is an acquired form of enamel hypoplasia resulting from the consumption of water containing an excess of fluorine. Mottled enamel may be mild or severe in character. Unless the concentration of fluorine is high, enamel apposition will proceed normally. The clinical manifestation will consist of cloudy opaque areas or of yellow or brown areas if extrinsic material has pigmented the areas (Fig. 143). Since mottled enamel is only one of the signs by hypomaturation, the unequivocal diagnosis of mottled enamel cannot be made without a positive history of excessive fluoride ingestion.

The differential diagnosis of Hutchinson's teeth, mulberry molars, and hypoplastic defects may be the most difficult. The difficulty involved in making a diagnosis of Hutchinson's incisors and mulberry molars can usually be attributed to an inadequate understanding of the morphologic and histologic characteristics of these manifestations of congenital syphilis. The most common error regarding Hutchinson's incisors occurs when the examiner attributes the notching of the incisor teeth to an underdevelopment of the central developmental lobe rather than to the loss of tooth structure from trauma. It must be remembered that the characteristic shape of a Hutchinson's incisor is due to the underdevelopment of the central developmental lobe with a collapse of the lateral developmental lobes. This causes the incisal edge to be narrower than the cervical portion of the tooth, thus giving it a characteristic screw driver shape (Fig.

Fig. 142. *Teeth—altered texture and color.* Cervical decalcification.

A   B

C   D

Fig. 143. *Teeth—altered texture and color.* Fluorosis.

Fig. 144. *Teeth—altered form.* **A** and **B**, Hutchinson's incisors. **C**, Mulberry molars.

144, *A* and *B*). Therefore, the examiner should not consider notching of the incisal edge of the incisors as evidence of the absence of the middle developmental lobe unless the width of the incisal edge is less than that of the cervical portion of the tooth.

Mulberry molars are also suggestive of congenital syphilis (Fig. 144, *C*). They are characterized by normal buccal and lingual surfaces but have occlusal surfaces analogous to a mulberry. A variation of this type of molar has pinched-in buccal and lingual surfaces and is called a bud molar. Localized defects of the occlusal surface of the molar teeth have at times been incorrectly diagnosed as mulberry molars. These dental stigmas do not occur in all cases of congenital syphilis, and the final diagnosis of congenital syphilis cannot be made purely on the basis of hypoplastic defects which are suggestive of Hutchinson's incisors and mulberry molars. In a few instances, Hutchinson's triad of notched incisors, deafness, and interstitial keratitis may be present.

Another form of enamel dysplasia is amelogenesis imperfecta. This designation has been loosely applied to many disturbances of the enamel involving hypoplasia, dysplasia, hypocalcification, hypomaturation, altered pigmentation, and defects involving hereditary or genetic linkages. Most of these defects are generalized throughout the teeth; however, they also may be localized. The involvement in amelogenesis imperfecta may vary from a complete lack of enamel to an immature enamel matrix. The enamel, where present, is soft, poorly calcified, and easily abraded (Fig. 145). A form of amelogenesis imperfecta in which the enamel is apparently normal in thickness and surface consistency is hereditary brown teeth (Fig. 145, *C*). The enamel is not so hard as normal and tends to chip on the incisal and occlusal surfaces. Extension of the brown color throughout the enamel and involvement of all the teeth are rather characteristic. The absence of enamel, poorly formed enamel, hyperpigmented enamel, and a hereditary background of amelogenesis imperfecta are the points to be remembered in a differential diagnosis.

Defects of the dentin which are distinct genetic and clinical entities include dentinogenesis imperfecta and dentin dysplasia. Dentinogenesis imperfecta is characterized by opalescence, abnormal coloration, absence of pulp canals, poorly calcified dentin, and constricted roots (Fig. 146, *A* to *C*). The enamel tends to chip away from the dentin and leaves a surface which is easily abraded. The clinical and radiographic findings are typical with little alteration in the usual pattern. Once this defect is seen, usually no diagnostic problems occur.

A   **B**

C

Fig. 145. *Teeth—altered color, form, and texture.* **A** and **B**, Amelogenesis imperfecta; note small area of enamel remaining on left maxillary central incisor in **A** and complete absence of enamel of maxillary incisors in **B**. **C**, Hereditary brown teeth.

A   B

C

D

Fig. 146. *Teeth—altered color and form.* **A-C,** Dentinogenesis imperfecta. **D,** Dentin dysplasia.

Dentin dysplasia is clinically manifested by wandering and malposed teeth.
Radiographically the teeth affected show absence of pulp canals, decreased
density of dentin, and short narrow roots. Radiolucent apical areas are also
frequently present (Fig. 146, *D*). Radiographically chevronlike areas may appear in the remaining portion of the pulp chamber.

It is important to determine the number of teeth which are present because
of the significance of supernumerary teeth and the congenital absence of teeth
in diagnosis and treatment planning. The clinical absence of teeth should always be verified by radiographic examination.

The maxillary lateral incisors and the mandibular second bicuspids are congenitally absent more often than any teeth except the third molars. The congenital absence of teeth is usually bilateral. Congenital absence is an important

consideration in orthodontic treatment and space management. Anodontia may be associated with other ectodermal defects such an anhidrosis, asteatosis, hypotrichosis, and defects of the salivary glands. One such defect is anhidrotic ectodermal dysplasia (Fig. 147, A and B). Partial anodontia is seen frequently in this ectodermal defect.

Supernumerary teeth refer to an increase in the normal number of teeth present in the dentition (Fig. 147, C). The presence of extra teeth, whether normal or abnormal in form, is an important factor in disturbances of occlusion. Supernumerary teeth may interfere with normal eruption of the teeth, may erupt outside the normal line of the dental arch, and may occasionally give rise to dentigerous cysts.

Numerous unerupted supernumerary teeth can be seen radiographically in persons with cleidocranial dysostosis, although clincally such patients may not show obvious signs of unerupted teeth. Since this disease is often associated with a failure of permanent dentition to erupt, the kind and number of teeth present may suggest to the examiner simple delayed eruption or partial anodontia. However, radiographs will show the presence of supernumerary teeth. In addition to the dental defect, defective ossification of the clavicles and bones of the

A   B

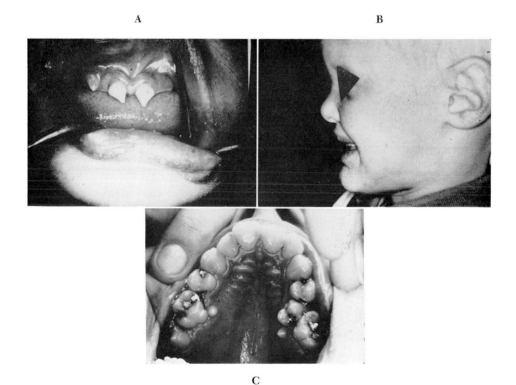

C

Fig. 147. *Teeth—altered number.* **A** and **B,** Anhidrotic ectodermal dysplasia; note congenitally missing teeth, abnormal form of those present, and absence of eyebrows and coarse hair. **C,** Supernumerary teeth.

skull can be noted. It is not uncommon for these persons to completely lack clavicles.

Erosion, Abrasion, and Fractures.—The examiner should note the presence of defects caused by abrasion and erosion and, if possible, the etiologic agent should be determined. Erosion results from a chemical process, and the defects are usually limited to the labial and buccal surfaces of the teeth. These defects vary in shape from saucerlike depressions to deep wedgelike grooves. The base presents a hard, polished surface. The lesions are seen most often on the labio-

Fig. 148. *Teeth—altered form.* **A,** Idiopathic erosion. **B,** Lemon juice erosion. **C,** Abrasion due to thread biting. **D,** Abrasion due to biting pipestem. **E,** Toothbrush abrasion.

cervical portions of the maxillary incisors (Fig. 148). They differ from those caused by decalcification in that their base is hard, smooth, and polished and their cause cannot be determined.

Abrasion may occur anywhere on the enamel surfaces or the cervical area of the root and is related to mechanical wearing of the tooth structure by physical agents such as toothbrushes, abrasive powders, hair pins, nails, clay pipestems, glass, toothpicks, dental tape, sand, thread, etc. (Fig. 148). Abrasion may affect any hard dental structures, whereas erosion is generally limited to the enamel surface. Abrasion of the cementum and dentin in the cervical area is frequently encountered in the presence of gingival recession. The location and character of the lesions produced by abrasion are related to the type of mechanical agent which produces the defect. Exposure of the cementoenamel junction and the cementum by recession of the gingiva may give rise to softening and brown discoloration of the cementum or exposed dentin. The softening is associated with decalcification and/or maceration of the cementum or dentin by the fluids of the mouth. Changes in color are associated with exogenous pigments. Exposure of the cementum and dentin of the cervical area by erosion frequently leads to cervical decay and hypersensitive cervical areas.

Fractures of teeth may involve both the crowns and roots (Fig. 149). Although coronal fractures are obvious, root fractures require radiographic evaluation. Radiographic examination should be a part of any examination involving traumatic fractures of the teeth. Two factors must be determined in the evaluation of a fractured tooth: whether or not the fracture directly involves the pulp and whether or not the pulp has been secondarily involved by injury at the apex. Unfortunately many fractures occur in young individuals when the pulp spaces are large. It must be remembered, however, that the spaces are generally more open than in an adult, and the pulp is more vulnerable to injury. Many times it is possible to observe that the pulp is involved in a fracture; at other times direct involvement may be difficult, if not impossible, to detect. The presence of hemorrhage is good evidence of direct involvement. The final diagnosis

Fig. 149. *Teeth—altered form.* Fracture; no change in color of tooth.

of pulpitis may not be realized in some instances until the pulpal tissues have fully reacted to the injury. It can be said that trauma will always produce, either directly or indirectly, pulp disease; however, the response of the pulp may vary considerably. In general, the pulps of young teeth respond more favorably than those of older teeth. Pulp testing immediately after a fracture has occurred would appear to serve no useful purpose since the full extent of pulpal damage will not have had time to manifest itself. Immediately after fracture, most teeth are hypersensitive to electric stimulation.

Vitality.—All questionable teeth should be examined for vitality. The state of the pulp may be questioned because of the history given by the patient, radiographic signs of disease, discoloration of the teeth, hypersensitivity of the teeth, and the presence of referred pain. Routine testing of all the teeth should be a part of a thorough and complete examination. This is of particular value when the operator is able to compare several evaluations in a program of periodic examinations. Present methods of pulp testing do not allow any great degree of correlation between the diseased state of the pulp and the clinical evidence of pulp disease. However, when the operator understands the principles of pulp testing and uses standardized methods, a certain amount of useful correlative data may be found. Details of pulp testing by thermal and electric means can be found in Chapter 7.

Functional Contours.—The labial, lingual, and buccal curvatures at the cervical and middle thirds of the crowns of the teeth are related to the protection of the periodontal tissues. When the teeth are in normal position and carious lesions have been properly restored, the convexity of the labial, lingual, and buccal surfaces prevents food from being forced into the gingival crevice and at the same time allows the food to pass over the gingiva to provide stimulation and massage of the gingival tissues. If these curvatures are too convex or too flat or are improperly placed in the dental restoration, normal cleansing action may be lost or food may be forced into the gingival crevices. The examiner should give careful attention to these factors since the health of the supporting structures is directly related to the form and function of the teeth. The apparent absence of disease of the supporting structures does not necessarily indicate that poor form of the contact areas, marginal ridges, and deflection curves will not ultimately produce injuries to the tissues.

Carious Lesions.—A periodic examination of the teeth is indicated for all individuals regardless of their age. The interval of time between examinations depends upon many factors such as rate of development of caries, Lactobacillus count, sugar intake, age, and susceptibility to decay. New carious lesions may develop within six months or take as long as one or two years. Extension of the lesion may be rapid in some individuals, while in others it may be exceedingly slow. Rampant decay is seen most frequently in children and in older adults (Fig. 150). It is obvious that the periodic examination of individuals with a high caries rate should be more often than those with a low caries rate. This does not imply that the rate will be constant; it may increase. It may also be reduced by natural or acquired preventive measures. The evaluation of carious activity can be accomplished by caries activity tests (Chapter 7). In many individuals certain areas of the mouth appear to be more susceptible to decay than others. This may be due to unknown factors or to acquired factors such as exposure of the cementum, improper extension of restorations for prevention of decay, or malposed teeth. This does not imply that these affect the basic mechanism of dental decay; it does suggest that faulty developmental grooves, overhanging margins, and rough cementum are much more prone to the deposition and maintenance of bacterial plaques than areas which are naturally more self-cleansing or can be reached by home-care methods. All the factors are important in the initiation of dental caries, especially if the sugar intake and Lactobacillus count is high. Periodic examinations of the teeth should be based on the need of each individual. All individuals should be examined at least once a year or more often not only for carious lesions, but also for all the other abnormalities which may occur in the oral cavity and contiguous structures.

Carious lesions develop frequently in the pits, fissures, and developmental grooves of the occlusal surfaces of the teeth and in the nonself-cleansing areas such as the interproximal surfaces at or near the contact areas. Areas less commonly affected initially are the buccal, labial, and lingual surfaces which are generally considered to be self-cleansing areas. Not infrequently, carious lesions

A   B

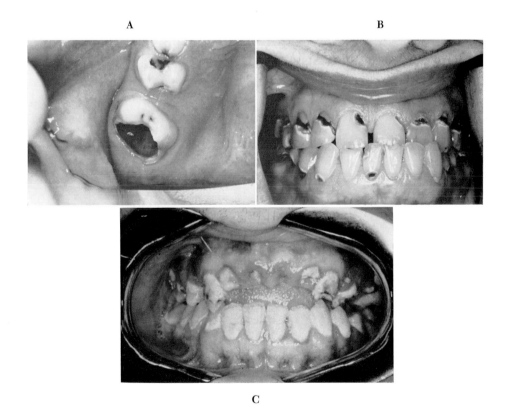

C

Fig. 150. *Teeth—caries.* A, Caries of primary teeth. B, Rampant caries. C, Extensive caries in hemophiliac.

may extend to these areas or be initiated in buccal developmental grooves and in the labiocervical and buccocervical surfaces adjacent to the gingival margins. Occasionally carious lesions may initiate in the lingual cervical surfaces of the molar teeth.

Special attention should be given not only to susceptible regions of dental decay, but also to all the tooth surfaces. Those areas which are considered to be nonself-cleansing and the margins of proximal restorations are difficult to assess without the aid of radiographs. The examiner should carry out his clinical examination and utilize dental radiographs. The radiographs are of special value in locating recurrent decay, occlusal caries, and proximal carious lesions. It must be emphasized that clinical examination of the teeth with a mouth mirror and explorer only or by radiographs alone is never sufficiently accurate.

The examination should be done by combining clinical exploration and radiographs. The use of posterior bite-wing films alone cannot be considered to be more effective than exploration, nor can exploration alone be considered more effective than the use of posterior bite-wings since both methods of examination have inherent weaknesses that the examiner must take into consideration. It is not a question of which method of examination is better or which one may be omitted but a matter of using both to their fullest extent for the most effective demonstration of carious lesions. The diagnosis of recurrent proximal caries by radiograph may be difficult in the presence of restorations which hide carious lesions because of the angulation of the central ray at the time the radiographs are taken or because of the location of the caries within the boundaries of the margins of the restoration. While the posterior bite-wing tends to eliminate much of this error, inaccuracies in positioning of the central ray are frequent. Obviously recurrent caries lying on the buccal or lingual aspect of the restoration may be completely obliterated by the shadow cast by the restoration. There can be no question that combined radiographic and visual inspection and exploration for occlusal decay are superior to the use of radiographic methods of examination alone.

The accuracy of both the clinical and radiographic examinations is limited to some extent by the form and position of the teeth. Those teeth which present large convex approximating surfaces are easier to examine clinically and radiographically than those which present flat approximating surfaces. Broad contact areas in the mandibular bicuspid and maxillary molar regions are especially troublesome at times in the radiographic examination because it is difficult to take radiographs with the central ray exactly parallel to the proximal surfaces of these teeth so that no superimpositioning of the proximal surfaces occurs. The clinical examination may also be complicated because of the difficulty in gaining access to these contact areas with an explorer. The clinical examination may be more effective in these instances especially where separation of the teeth will allow entrance of an explorer tine into the area in question. Thus, the detection of early carious lesions of the contact areas may present difficulties even when both clinical and radiographic examination methods are used.

While a radiographic examination tends to be more effective in detecting initial carious lesions of the proximal contact areas, clinical exploration and separation of the teeth may be necessary to remove any question of doubt regarding the presence of recurrent lesions.

An incipient lesion first appears clinically as an opaque white spot which presents a rough surface to the explorer; it may not be sufficiently advanced to cause the exploring tine to catch or hang. When the convexity of the contact area is great and the central x-ray is parallel to its surface, an initial lesion of the proximal surface may appear radiographically to be slightly roughened or etched. With further advance of the lesion, perforation of the enamel can be seen radiographically; clinically the enamel shows discoloration, and upon pressure the exploring tine hangs in the opening of the lesion. Careful consideration of the interproximal surfaces of the teeth should include not only the contact areas, but also the cervical areas above and below the gingival margin. Not infrequently the initial lesion is on the labiocervical or buccocervical surfaces of the teeth and is manifested as a chalky white area of decalcification that spreads from this area to the proximal and subgingival surfaces of the teeth. Careful attention should be given to this type of carious lesion, especially around the distal, buccal, and proximal surfaces of the teeth.

All restorations should be carefully inspected for secondary or recurrent carious lesions by clinical and radiographic examination. Open margins, overhanging margins, and broken restorations that are found on clinical examination should alert the examiner to the presence of caries which may not be found on clinical examination alone. The radiographs should be studied in detail, and when necessary new radiographs using a different angulation should be taken. The principles of radiographic interpretation of dental caries is given in Chapter 6.

The examination for carious lesions may require the use of different explorers to adequately examine all the surfaces of a tooth. Those shown in Fig. 151 may be used; however, other types may be more desirable for some exam-

Fig. 151. *Explorers* for examination of teeth.

iners. The main requirements are that the explorer be sharp and be suited to the area to be examined.

The examination should be systematic and include both clinical and radio-graphic methods. It should begin at a specific location and proceed systematically tooth by tooth throughout the whole mouth and should be made with the aid of a mouth mirror and a fine sharp explorer (Fig. 152). The field of observation should be dry and well illuminated. Special attention should be given to variations in shade or color of the enamel and changes in its texture and hardness; these are significantly changed in the presence of dental decay. The initial lesion of dental decay is generally seen as an opaque or white spot. This area may later become pigmented or stained.

Unless the explorer is fine and sharp, many areas of occlusal decay may be

Fig. 152. *Examination of teeth.* **A** and **B,** Use of mirror and explorer. **C-F,** Exploration for interproximal caries.

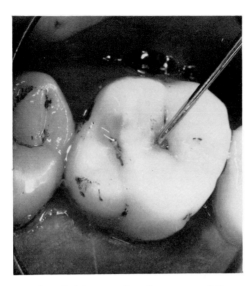

Fig. 153. *Examination of teeth.* Mirror and explorer; pit and fissure caries; explorer caught in the carious lesion.

overlooked. Use of posterior bite-wing radiographs will enhance the yield of carious lesions. Manipulation of the explorer and sufficient pressure to push the exploring tine into soft decayed tooth structure will result in a "hang" or "catch" (Fig. 153).

The examination should begin with a specific tooth and proceed systematically throughout the arches. All surfaces of a tooth should be examined completely before proceeding to the next tooth. The examination may begin at the occlusal surfaces, proceed to the proximal surfaces, and then proceed to the labial and lingual surfaces.

No examination of the teeth can be considered to be thorough without a complete examination of all the pits, grooves, and fissures that are vulnerable to decay. This is especially true in children, since a significant percentage of the first permanent molars are lost six months after eruption and an even greater percentage may be lost before the age of 12 years. Even in the adult a large percentage are lost before the age of 25 years. In effect, the chance of decay occurring in pits, grooves, and fissures is significantly probable. It must be remembered that teeth in fluoride areas will show a significant number of defects in the occlusal developmental grooves. These should not be mistaken for carious lesions. Special attention should be given to mesial and distal occlusal pits and grooves and to the lingual groove of the maxillary permanent molars; their depth, overhanging edges, and inaccessibility to toothbrushing make them ideal places for the initiation of decay. Similar defects may be present in the occlusal buccal grooves of the mandibular permanent molars as well as in the bicuspids. Careful consideration should also be given the lingual pits in the cingulum area of the maxillary central and lateral incisors. Frequently very deep pits occur on the lateral incisors in this area and can be fully evaluated only with radiographs. The frequency of occurrence of deep pits on the maxillary lateral incisors and cuspids and their relationship to dens in dente are well known.

Gross occlusal decay may be present without obvious clinical signs; therefore, use of radiographs is necessary for an evaluation of the extent of decay.

The proximal surfaces should be examined next. Since initial decay here may be difficult to detect with only an explorer, use of radiographs should be made also. The determination of recurrent decay around the margins of restorations requires the use of both explorer and radiographs. The margins of restorations should be explored with a No. 3 or No. 17 explorer to determine the presence of open margins, soft tooth structure, and overhanging margins. The extent of the carious lesion can most generally be determined from the radiographs. In many instances, however, exploration is the only method possible. The removal of calculus and debris is essential before an adequate diagnosis can be made. In some instances gingival packs may be necessary before the evaluation can be made successfully. In rare instances a separation may be required to adequately probe the gingival margins of a restoration. This is true when access is limited and the radiographs do not give conclusive evidence of an open margin. Hypersensitive cervical areas are not in themselves evidence of dental decay. Rarely resorption of the tooth occurs externally or in conjunction with internal resorption. These areas appear to be dental decay radiographically; however, exploration will reveal their true nature. These areas are filled with soft tissue, and the margins are generally firm and hard. This is in contradistinction to carious lesions whose margins and centers are soft.

Examination of the labial, buccal, and lingual-cervical surfaces is best accomplished with a No. 3 explorer. It is imperative that the examiner be able to determine the location of the cementoenamel junction. Changes in the texture and hardness of the cementum as compared to the enamel are sometimes confusing to the dental student. This is especially true where recession of the free gingival margin has exposed the cementum to fluids and stains. Cementum so exposed tends to become macerated, soft, and darkly stained. It is not infrequent that this condition is mistaken for dental caries. When decay involves both the cementum and the enamel and the cementum is soft from exposure to the fluids of the oral cavity, the extent of the decay may be difficult to determine without careful attention to the difference between texture and softness of decay and cementum. Smoothing of the surface with periodontal files may serve to facilitate delineation of the lesion. Opaque and white areas of decalcification on the cervical areas of the molar teeth are frequently mistaken for calculus by dental students. These areas generally follow the line of the free gingival margin and may extend around to distal and mesial surfaces of the teeth involved. The ability to penetrate this area with an explorer generally serves to differentiate decalcification from calculus. In addition, repeated scaling has little effect on removing it, and the curvature of the tooth indicates that the opaque area is a part of the tooth structure.

Contact Relationship.—Dental floss should be used to determine the tight-

A   B

Fig. 154. *Examination of contact relationship* by use of dental floss.

ness of contact areas throughout the mouth. It should be unwaxed and fine enough to pass between the proximal contact without undue pressure (Fig. 154). Thick, flat, and waxed dental tape which is suitable for interproximal cleaning is not suitable for this test since it does not slide easily and its thickness does not permit an adequate evaluation of the proper contact relationship. Thin round unwaxed nylon has the optimum characteristics for delicate manipulation of the floss between the contact areas. Dental floss should pass through the contact area without being torn or shredded. Tearing or shredding of the tape or obstruction of its passage is usually indicative of dental caries or overhanging dental restorations. Using radiographs as a guide, overhanging cervical margins of dental restorations should be examined with the tine of a sharp explorer. Careful examination of this area will aid in determining whether these margins can be recontoured or whether the whole restoration must be replaced. Both clinical examination and radiographic examination of the cervical areas of restorations may be necessary for complete evaluation of overhanging margins of restorations.

An improper contact relation is indicated when the floss can be pulled easily through the contact areas. Also, the gingival tissues will show evidence of food impaction—detachment, enlargement, and alteration of normal color. They will also show evidence of disease if contact areas are incorrectly placed, if marginal ridges are faulty, and if a restoration encroaches upon the interproximal spaces. Normally, the form and position of the mesial and distal marginal ridges and the interproximal contact areas of the teeth prevent food from being driven between the teeth. When the marginal ridges and the contact areas are lost from decay or are improperly placed in restoration, food impactions usually occur. Unfavorable alterations of the interproximal space by dental restoration, abnormal tooth positions, and disease are common causes of gingival disturbances.

The examiner should inspect the contact area from the occlusal and incisal surfaces of the teeth and at the same time observe the gingival tissue. Observation of the interdental papillae from the occlusal and incisal views will aid considerably in assessing the health of these tissues in relation to the contact area, marginal ridges, and lingual, labial, and buccal curvatures of the teeth.

Charting.—Charting of teeth may be accomplished by the use of a printed form (Fig. 155). This form has been prepared to be used both for periodontal and dental findings. Charting is a useful procedure since any part of the derived data can be readily seen in relation to the whole picture. The form presented here is only one of the many that might be used. However, most other charting forms do not include provisions for both periodontal and dental findings. Combining the results of the examination into a single form greatly enhances the correlation between the teeth and the supporting structures.

SYMBOLS FOR CHARTING

1. Missing	5. Open Contact	9. Bridge
2. Cavity	6. Mobility	10. Periapical Area
3. Decalcified Area	7. Bifurcation Exposed	11. Hypoplasia
4. Food Impaction	8. Drifted, Extrusion	12. Overhang
		13. Extract

Fig. 155. *Examination of teeth.* Typical chart showing periodontal disease and dental caries. (See also Fig. 157 for work sheet.)

Fig. 156. *Examination and charting of teeth.* **A-F,** Clinical examination of the teeth in one quadrant of the mouth. **G** and **H,** Corresponding radiographic examination of the same quadrant. **I,** Completed dental chart of the corresponding quadrant showing clinical and radiographic findings.

The charting of carious lesions, decalcification, and recurrent decay may be accomplished first by clinical examination with the aid of a mouth mirror and explorer. An example of the examination and charting procedure is given in Fig. 156. The results of the clinical examination may be indicated on the chart first. The radiographs should also be examined and the charting completed (Fig. 156). The periodontal examination in the example has already been completed. For clarity, carious lesions, decalcified areas, and areas of recurrent decay are first outlined only; those findings derived from the radiographic examination are indicated by blocked-out areas. In the completed chart all initial and recurrent carious lesions are indicated by blocked-out areas.

In addition to the chart, a work sheet may be utilized for the listing of carious lesions and the preparation of a tentative treatment plan (Fig. 157). One system of indicating a particular tooth is to number the permanent teeth from

WORK SHEET

RADIOGRAPHIC FINDINGS		ORAL FINDINGS	SUMMATION	TREATMENT PLAN
PBW	FM			

(Work sheet chart, rows 1–32)

PERIODONTICS

OPERATIVE
10 E (ENDO.)
151-5 A
153 A
154 A
156 A
142-6 A
143 A
144 A
91 S
92 S
101-4 G (D)
281-5 G (D)
286 F
29

SURGERY
EXTRACT
3,7,31,32

PROSTHETICS
BRIDGE
2-4, 6-8
PART. DENT.
CLASS II

Oral findings / summation entries:
5 — 45
1-4 — 71 74
2 — 82
1-2 — 91 92
1-4 — 101 104
3-4-6 — 142-6 143 144
3-4-5-6 — 151-5 153 154 156
5-6 — 281-5 286.
5-4 — 31 1-5-4

Fig. 157. *Examination of teeth.* Treatment plan work sheet. **PBW,** Posterior bite-wings; **FM,** full mouth radiographs. (See also Fig. 155 for charting.)

1 to 32. Starting with the maxillary right third molar as 1, the teeth are numbered consecutively around the arch to the maxillary left third molar, which is numbered 16. Then dropping down to the mandibular left third molar, which is numbered 17, the teeth are given consecutive numbers to the mandibular right third molar, which is numbered 32. The primary teeth are numbered in the same manner using 1d through 20d. Another system for symbolic designation of teeth is recommended by the Committee on Nomenclature of the American Dental Association. This plan divides the arches into four quadrants. Each arch is divided into halves by a median plane, and each arch is separated from the other by a horizontal plane. In the permanent dentition, numbering starts with the central incisor on each side of the midline and proceeds with the sequence of 1 through 8. The teeth of the primary dentition are designated by the letters A through E. Thus the symbol |6 would indicate the mandibular left sixth-year molar and 6| would indicate the maxillary right sixth-year molar. The symbol |C would indicate the primary mandibular left cuspid and C| the primary maxillary right cuspid. Both this plan and the preceding plan for the symbolic designation of teeth have advantages and disadvantages.

Numbering the teeth from 1 through 32 eliminates the necessity of using brackets and can be used to indicate various surfaces of the teeth involved in dental decay. The surfaces are numbered from 1 through 6; these numbers are added as superscripts to the number of the tooth; e.g., carious lesions involving all the surfaces of the maxillary right third molar would be indicated by the symbol

$32^{1\text{-}2\text{-}3\text{-}4\text{-}5\text{-}6}$. The surfaces are numbered as follows: 1, mesial; 2, distal; 3, labial or buccal; 4, lingual; 5, occlusal; and 6, distal fossae and pits of the mandibular first bicuspids and the maxillary molars. Thus a carious lesion of the mesial surfaces of the maxillary right central incisor would be indicated by 8^{1}. Lesions present on the mesial, distal, and occlusal surfaces of the mandibular right second permanent molar would be indicated by $31^{1\text{-}2\text{-}5}$. A lesion involving only the buccal surface of the mandibular left cuspid would be indicated by 22^{3}.

A temporary work sheet may be used to facilitate the clinical examination and charting procedure. It should not take the place of charting but should be used for summation and treatment planning while the patient is present. It can then be utilized for a more elaborate write-up and treatment plan when the patient is not present. The work sheet shown in Fig. 157 is arranged in five columns. The number of the tooth is given at the extreme left. Under radiographic findings and oral findings, only the surfaces involved by carious lesions are listed. In the summation column the number of the tooth is repeated and the surfaces involved are given. The treatment plan column is merely an outline of the treatment to be rendered and the type of restorative material to be used. Letter abbreviations to indicate the restorative material are used as follows: S, silicate; A, amalgam; G, gold; G (D), gold, direct; G (I), gold, indirect; F, gold foil; E, emergency treatment.

Occlusion

With the growth of dental specialties such as pedodontics, orthodontics, and periodontics, the general practitioner has come to regard the recognition of malocclusion and periodontal disease as being in the private domain of these specialties. However, in order for a general practitioner to fulfill his responsibility in the field of preventive dentistry, it is necessary that he recognize those changes which may be predisposing factors in diseases of the mouth of the adult; he must also be able to recognize the initiation of disease in the child or adolescent in order that effective preventive measures may be applied. This is not only true in operative dentistry and periodontics, but also in the field of orthodontics. The prevention of dental disease should begin at an early age. Preventive dentistry as it relates to malocclusion and periodontal disease is based upon the recognition and diagnosis of deviations from the normal pattern of growth and the recognition of factors which may predispose to disease at a later time.

Many times a dentist will tolerate an undisciplined child in his practice merely to retain the mother or father as a patient. With this attitude it is impossible for him to provide adequate service to the child. In such instances, and occasionally in the offices of those who specialize in dentistry for children, examination of the child consists only of a search for cavities or the treatment of an aching tooth.

Whether he is a specialist in the field of dentistry for children or a general practitioner, the dentist should be thoroughly familiar with the examination and diagnostic procedures necessary for interception of dental disease in patients of any age. In view of the prevalence of malocclusion and periodontal disease in the adolescent and adult, it is necessary that the dentist be aware of the many abnormalities that may have their inception in young children. The initiation of periodontal disease occurs at a much earlier age than was previously thought; malocclusion frequently is an initiating cause. Thus, a careful examination of a child will not only serve to provide an adequate diagnosis of abnormalities already present but will also enable the examiner to recognize factors in the mouth which predispose to disease at a later time.

The examination suggested here is of a screening nature and should not be construed as a complete orthodontic examination since this field of endeavor is outside the objective of this text. The development of occlusion is presented in order to provide the student and the general practitioner with certain basic landmarks and examination procedures for the early detection of occlusal disturbances. The orthodontic literature is replete with the basic principles of examination for the interception of malocclusion and for efficient and rational referral to an orthodontist. Although this type of examination is primarily screening in nature and is not intended to be a complete coverage of all the necessary diagnostic procedures necessary for complete evaluation, it is hoped that it will alert the general practitioner and student to their responsibilities in the field of preventive dentistry, e.g., the prevention and interception of disturbances of the developing occlusion.

The principles for the recognition of incipient malocclusion are based on a knowledge of the normal growth and development of the teeth, jaws, and face and of those etiologic factors which may produce malocclusion. The factors which influence the development of occlusion are genetic and/or environmental in nature. The latter may be local or systemic in origin. Inasmuch as the development of occlusion is based on genetic, dental, and muscle factors, it may be related to abnormalities in any or all of these. Thus, malocclusion may be skeletal, dental, or functional in origin, and the examination of the young patient should consist of an evaluation of these factors. The examination should begin with a complete history and an evaluation of the patient's past and present health. It has been well established that constitutional factors and systemic disease have an important effect upon general health and upon those tissues which are responsible for the development and establishment of occlusion. It goes without saying that the general health of the patient must be appraised before an examination can be considered complete. No practitioner of dentistry should become so engrossed in his particular specialty or field of interest that the rest of the mouth and body is completely overlooked.

In addition to the information considered in Chapter 4 on the skull and facies, the examiner must also consider the form of the face as it relates to the occlusion. There is a close relationship between the development of occlusion and the development of the face. This is well known to the orthodontist, but the general practitioner has at times failed to fully appreciate this fact. This situation is not without foundation; the pattern of facial growth is complex and the determination of facial disharmony is not generally considered in the usual examination procedures used by the general practitioner.

The development of occlusion does not originate solely from processes in the mouth; it is also derived from the skeletal parts responsible for the development of the face. When a facial disharmony is present, it does not necessarily follow that there will be a disturbance in the development of the occlusion. However, there are certain alterations in the proportions of the face which are considered to be outside the range of normal; these alterations are quite likely to be associated with a disturbance in the development of the occlusion. Thus, when evaluating the occlusion, it is necessary to consider the facial form as well as the alveolar processes and the jaws.

Facial Form Analysis.—An analysis of facial form will serve to appraise the harmony of growth and development of the facial skeleton as it relates to the support of the dentition. The examination should show the presence or absence of abnormal anteroposterior relationships and asymmetries of the dentofacial parts. It will also indicate to the examiner the possibility of a difference in the absolute size of the parts of the dentofacial complex and will point out the variations in dental and occlusal relationships which have resulted from the combination of parts of abnormal size and form. It must be pointed out again that the facial form is not entirely dependent upon the facial skeleton; it is also dependent upon the teeth.

One of the difficulties that the general practitioner must face in his examination of a growing child is the fact that the facial form is an ever-changing pattern and that no clearly defined or static standard of dentofacial relationship exists. Thus, the concept of normality or the range of normal is difficult to visualize and even more difficult for the general practitioner to measure without the equipment and training necessary to utilize comprehensive gnathometric and cephalometric indexes of so-called normal relationships between the occlusion, face, and skull. However, it is possible for him to evaluate gross skeletal variations by direct observation of the facial form. He can learn much about the position of the teeth by observing the facial profile and the facial musculature. While this type of examination fails to give the exact and precise results of a complete facial form analysis, it does keep the examiner from having to evaluate an occlusion on a purely intraoral basis without due regard for other dependent relationships.

The examiner should not base his entire evaluation of malocclusion on the relationship of the first permanent molars and/or the relationship of opposing arches since the remainder of the face and muscles are often intimately related to malocclusion. From a practical standpoint, the occlusion and dentofacial structures should be related to established planes of the face and skull; this relationship then can be used to grossly evaluate obvious variations from the normal. The planes which are used relate to the facial profile and to a division of the face into two equal parts. Abnormalities of the profile are related to the profile plane; abnormalities of asymmetry are related to the midsagittal plane.

An appraisal of the profile may be made by use of the Frankfort horizontal (eye-ear) plane and a plane perpendicular to the Frankfort plane which passes through the nasion, called the anterior facial plane (Fig. 158, *A*). An appraisal of facial symmetry may be made by using the midsagittal plane; this plane is perpendicular to a plane through the orbitale and vertically divides the face and head into two equal parts (Fig. 158, *B*).

By using these reference planes the examiner can determine the antero-

A   B

C

Fig. 158. *Facial form analysis.* A, Frankfort horizontal and anterior facial planes. B, Mid-sagittal plan. C, Displacement reference points; found by palpation. From top to bottom—sub-spinale, prostheon, infradentale, and pogonion.

posterior relationships between the dentofacial parts and also the presence of asymmetries of the dentofacial parts. This procedure serves to estimate the difference in size of one facial part as compared with another, to indicate angle variations between the maxillary occlusal and Frankfort planes, and to provide a plane of reference for the evaluation of inclinations of the anterior maxillary and mandibular teeth. Thus, the information may reveal whether the abnormality is symmetrical or asymmetrical, bilateral or unilateral, anterior or posterior; whether or not the condition extends beyond the boundaries of the maxilla and mandible or both; or whether a deviation in the anteroposterior relationship involves the upper or lower teeth or both groups of teeth or other parts of the dentofacial structure.

Four points of reference may be used to evaluate changes in the anteroposterior relationship of the parts making up the facial profile. These can only be approximated in the living; however, their determination serves a useful purpose. The points of reference are skeletal areas whose placement provides the basis for the facial profile, and they must be visualized on soft tissues. They are the subspinale for the midfacial region—where the ala of the nose meets the cheek, the prostheon for the maxillary alveolar region, the infradentale for the mandibular alveolar region—deepest point of the mentolabial sulcus, and the pogonion for the chin point (Fig. 158, C). Relating these points to the facial profile serves to point out abnormal anteroposterior displacements of the midfacial region, the maxillary and mandibular alveolar denture bases, and the chin. In general, these points lie harmoniously along the facial profile plane; any different relationship should alert the examiner to abnormalities of facial form. Any of the parts of the face represented by the four reference points may be deviated or displaced in an anteroposterior direction relative to the profile plane. The area of deviation may indicate to the examiner where the disharmony of dentofacial form exists; e.g., a positive posterior displacement of the chin point is suggestive of retrognathism; an anterior displacement suggests prognathism. It must be borne in mind that the displacement of the mandible may be skeletal, dental, or functional in origin. Thus, the points of reference should be observed when the mandible is at rest position, when the mandible is in centric relation, and when the teeth are in complete occlusion.

The relative size or mass of the maxilla and the mandible should be noted. This can be visualized as prominent, moderate, or reduced. The vertical proportions of the face should also be considered. Visual inspection of the space occupied by the nose, upper lip, lower lip, and chin while the lips are brought together lightly usually indicates that nasal height constitutes about 43 per cent of the vertical height while the region below constitutes 57 per cent (Dempster). Proportionate lengths of the body and ramus of the mandible also should be evaluated.

An estimate of the angles of the mandible, the angle between the maxillary occlusal and Frankfort planes, and the angle of inclination of the maxillary and mandibular teeth should be made. In children 8 to 12 years of age, the angle made by the base of the mandible and the ascending ramus should be an obtuse angle of about 140 degrees (McCoy). This is not a fixed value and only represents the average. Actual angular measurements need not be made; a general appraisal of the angle at the gonion is all that is necessary. Extreme variations are not difficult to observe. The inclination of the mandibular and maxillary anterior teeth should be approximately parallel with the median and facial profile planes. The angulation of the maxillary occlusal plane with reference to the Frankfort horizontal plane should be noted. While this angle is generally in the region of 12 degrees, observations need only indicate that the angle is reduced, normal, or increased.

Asymmetries of the frontal facial form are best considered relative to the midsagittal plane. While features tend to be associated with common patterns, the general proportions of the facial mass are symmetrical. A systematic comparison of definite areas should be carried out, e.g., frontal bones, orbital regions, malar regions, maxillary region, and mandibular region.

Some generalities of dentofacial form may alert the examiner to analyze the facial form. For instance, some facial features appear to be associated very frequently with certain types of malocclusion, e.g., the adenoid facies associated with habitual mouth breathing. The typical adenoid facies is characterized by a thin face, pinced nose, high arched palate, and often retrognathia. The typical mouth breather shows a short upper lip and a lower lip which rests between the maxillary and the mandibular incisors. The maxillary incisors are frequently in labioversion and the mandibular incisors in linguoversion. In other instances, where the maxillary incisor teeth are in linguoversion to the mandibular incisors, the lower lip may be unusually prominent and the upper lip underdeveloped. The position and form of the lips are greatly influenced by the teeth and by breathing. It is also true that lip habits can produce changes in the position of the teeth and that abnormalities of occlusion can affect the position of the lips. It must be remembered that the position of the lips is directly related to the musculature and directly or indirectly related to the position of the teeth. In some instances the examiner may be alerted to the possibility of retrognathism by the presence of a rather pronounced mentolabial sulcus; this finding is not uncommon in this type of malocclusion. The presence of unusual facial forms generally referred to as hatchet face, flat face, mouse face, and dish face are obvious indications for an analysis of the facial form.

It is not necessary to take cephalograms or photographs to generally appraise the form of the facial skeletal structures. The structures can be visualized in relation to the profile and midsagittal plane by holding up a piece of cardboard or other suitable material to the patient's face in approximate alignment with the reference landmarks (Fig. 159). The examiner should inspect the approximate placement of the chin point, the mandibular alveolar point, the maxillary alveolar point, and the midfacial region individually. Palpation of these bony landmarks may be necessary while the examiner holds the reference plane up to the face in order to determine their location. This is especially true if the lips, nose, and soft tissues are large in relation to the skeletal structures. In general, these reference landmarks lie along the facial profile plane in the average face. The degree of anterior or posterior displacement of each area (midfacial, maxillary alveolar, mandibular alveolar, and the chin) should be noted. Generally, the examiner expresses his findings of a variation in facial relationships by a reference to the facial angle and to the angle of convexity (Fig. 160). The facial angle is an expression of anteroposterior displacement of the chin. It is determined by a gross appraisal of the angle made by the Frankfort and facial planes. A facial angle of less than 90 degrees is suggestive of a retrognathic or Class II type of face; a right angle, an orthognathic or Class I type of face; an angle slightly greater than 90 degrees, a mesognathic face; and a marked obtuse angle, a prognathic or Class III type of face (Downs). The angle of convexity is formed by the intersection of a line drawn from the nasion to the nasospinale and a line drawn from the pogonion to the nasospinale. The angle formed by these two intersecting lines is a measure of the anteroposterior displacement of the maxillary part of the face to the total profile. As indicated in Fig. 160, the angle made

A   B

Fig. 159. *Facial form analysis.* **A,** Clinical method of determining the facial angle and alignment of the reference landmarks of the anterior facial plane. **B,** Checking symmetry by use of midsagittal plane.

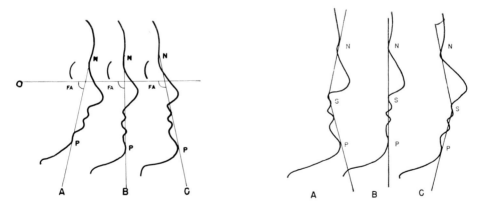

Fig. 160. *Facial form analysis.* Left: variations in facial relationships by reference to the facial angle (**FA**). **A,** Retrognathic type of face. **B,** Straight or orthognathic face. **C,** Prognathic face. Right: variations in facial relationships by reference to angle of convexity (**S**). **A,** Dish or concave face. **B,** Straight face. **C,** Hatchet or convex face. (After Downs.)

by these intersecting lines may be concave (dish face), straight, or convex (hatchet face).

The angular relationship of the occlusal and Frankfort planes is generally related to the facial angle. The cant of the occlusal plane is relatively steep in retrognathism and approaches parallelism in severe prognathism.

The inspection of the facial form for skeletal asymmetry may be accomplished by observing both sides of the face when the piece of cardboard is placed in the midsagittal plane (Fig. 159). Palpation of the skeletal structures may be necessary to differentiate between soft tissue, muscle, and skeletal asymmetry. As prevoiusly mentioned, asymmetry may be muscular, soft tissue, or skeletal in nature and these may be genetic, developmental, or pathologic in origin. The degree of asymmetry should be indicated in the same terms used previously— small, moderate, and marked. The examination of the facial form in the midsagittal planes should be made while the patient is closing his teeth together and when the teeth are in occlusion. A deviation from the midline of the maxillary incisors may indicate a skeletal asymmetry or a malposition of the teeth in the arch. Asymmetry of the midline of the mandibular central incisors may indicate malposition of the incisors, asymmetry of the mandibular arch, or functional displacement of the mandible. It must also be remembered that an abnormal anteroposterior relationship of the mandible may be on a functional basis; i.e., the mandible may be prevented from closing in the normal anteroposterior relationship because of premature contacts or occlusal interference. It is not uncommon to find what appears to be mandibular prognathism when the teeth are together yet find that the anteroposterior relationship is normal when the jaws are separated in centric relation.

Standardization of the relationships between facial structures cannot be dogmatized even with comprehensive methods of analysis. The evaluation of the findings of the type of facial form analysis presented here is based on the examiner's visual judgment and a sense of facial harmony. Thus, in most instances, the general practitioner is well equipped to detect moderate to severe abnormalities of the facial skeleton and relate them to malocclusion.

After the examiner has completed his analysis of the facial form, he will have some idea of the presence or absence of unfavorable or disharmonious bone growth and how they may relate to the development of the occlusion. In general his findings of disharmony will be those of skeletal displacement or asymmetry of the face. (Skeletal displacement is a term used to mean the malposition or maldevelopment of the arches.) Insufficient bony support for the size of the teeth may also be noted. It was previously stated that the development of malocclusion is related not only to skeletal development, but also to dental development. Therefore, in order to understand all the factors which may cause abnormal development of occlusion, it is necessary that the examiner know something about the normal development of occlusion.

The development of occlusion is related to the harmonious development of the facial skeleton and to the functional harmony of the teeth, jaws, and musculature. Thus, while the development is in process, the examination of the patient for disturbances in this process must be related to the signs of disharmony or abnormality in all of the areas responsible for the development of the occlusion. The following presentation of the development of the occlusion is related to the position of the teeth in a more or less "ideal" arrangement for certain arbitrary set stages of occlusal development. These stages are related to the completion of the primary dentition, the mixed dentition, the occlusion of the permanent teeth in young adults, and a fourth stage which takes into consideration the changes in occlusion which result from wear. The descriptions of so-called ideal or normal occlusions for any particular stage cannot be considered absolute. This arbitrary categorization is only of value when the examiner is able to visualize what variations of occlusion may exist and still be within the range of normal. Thus, the clinician should strive to use his knowledge of the development of occlusion and his knowledge of those factors which may alter the normal development of occlusion rather than to base his evaluation of occlusion on an ideal arrangement of the teeth.

Primary Dentition Analysis.—The development of the primary occlusion is usually completed between the third and fifth year of life; it is generally considered to be more stable and to show fewer anomalies than either the mixed or permanent dentitions. It does, however, show a wide range of normal variation. Apparently there are no essential changes in the occlusion once an interdigitation of the primary teeth has occurred. Growth in the height of the alveolar process and sagittal growth distal to the dentition continues to occur. Most primary dentitions show a generalized spacing of the anterior teeth, and there may be wide spaces mesial to the maxillary cuspids and distal to the mandibular cuspids. Spacing is normal and does not change, i.e., spaces do not close. An absence of spacing is normal, and spaces do not occur with advancing age.

The shape of the arch is usually ovoid. The length of the arch, from the distal surface of the second primary molar around to the distal surface of the opposite second primary molar, decreases following the eruption of the second primary molars. This decrease continues until the completion of the primary dentition and is due to the mesial migration of the maxillary and mandibular second primary molars. The termination of the occlusion at the posterior surfaces of the second primary molars usually forms a straight terminal plane—vertical line tangent to the distal surfaces of second primary molars. Deformity of the facial skeleton, premature interproximal cavities, and sucking habits may cause the premature development of a terminal plane with a distal step. In other instances the anteroposterior occlusal relationship may be normal as manifested by a symmetrical midline and a satisfactory maxillary and mandibular cuspid position. However, a straight terminal plane is a more favorable condition for the establishment of the occlusal relationship of the first permanent molars. Occlusal irregularities of the primary dentition may result from severe sucking habits and from space closure associated with the premature loss of primary teeth.

In general, the primary dentition is characterized by a straight axial inclination of the incisors with an almost end-to-end relationship of these teeth. The mandibular teeth occlude one cusp anteriorly to the corresponding tooth in the maxilla. Deviations from this pattern are suggestive of malocclusion. In addition to an evaluation of the characteristics of the normal primary dentition, the examiner should search for all the local causes capable of bringing about irregularities of occlusion.

Due consideration should be given the prevention of malocclusion arising from neglect of the primary teeth and their early loss, from prolonged retention of the primary teeth, and from the presence of severe sucking and other oral habits. The premature loss of primary teeth from dental neglect and interproximal decay is quite likely to cause a loss of arch length with a consequent tendency for crowding of the permanent teeth. Retention of the primary teeth beyond their normal period of exfoliation may cause their permanent successors to erupt in an abnormal position. If a child persists in thumb sucking, an anterior open-bite usually results. In the presence of an abnormal anteroposterior relationship of the occlusion, severe malocclusion of the permanent dentition may result; however, where the anteroposterior relationship is normal, an open-bite of this type may be self-correcting provided the child ceases his severe sucking habit by the age of 4 years.

Mixed Dentition Analysis.—The first permanent molars erupt at 6 to 7 years of age and represent the beginning of mixed dentition. The mandibular incisors usually follow the sixth-year molars and are frequently noted to be in a crowded and rotated position. At this age such crowding is not considered to be abnormal but may be abnormal in those instances where tooth eruption has preceded the growth of the jaw (dental age exceeds skeletal age). The crowding may be self-correcting because vertical growth of the alveolar processes up to the age of 9 or 10 years will usually allow for their proper positioning.

The first permanent molars may frequently erupt in a cusp-to-cusp relationship when there is no spacing in the primary arches and the terminal plane is straight. This molar relationship is of no significance provided the mandibular second primary molar is shed prior to the maxillary second primary molar so that a mesial shift (late mesial shift) of the lower permanent molar may take place (Baume). In the presence of generalized spacing of the primary arches the mandibular first permanent molar should erupt before the maxillary first molar to prevent the formation of an unfavorable distal step in the terminal plane. If the maxillary first permanent molar erupts first, a distal step is established, and the mandibular first permanent molar may become locked in distal occlusion.

It has been shown by Lo and Moyers that a certain sequence of eruption is most favorable to the development of a normal occlusion. This sequence in the maxilla and mandible is shown in Fig. 161. In the maxillary arch the first molar (6) is the first to erupt, the central incisor (1) is second, the lateral incisor (2) is third, the first bicuspid (4) is fourth, the second bicuspid (5) is fifth, the cuspid (3) is sixth, and the second molar (7) is seventh. In the mandibular arch the first molar (6) is first to erupt, the central incisor (1) is second, the lateral incisor (2) is third, the cuspid (3) is fourth, the first bicuspid (4) is fifth, the second bicuspid (5) is sixth, and the second molar (7) is seventh to erupt.

Certain other sequences of eruption have been found to be associated with an unfavorable development of the occlusion. In the maxilla the early eruption of the premolars or cuspid often results in Class II molar relationships. The most

Fig. 161. *Mixed dentition analysis.* Most favorable sequence of eruption. Numbers indicate numerical order of sequence of eruption. (After Lo and Moyers.)

unfavorable sequence in the mandible is associated with the late eruption of the cuspid or the early eruption of the second molar. There appears to be a significant tendency for a Class II molar relationship to result when the maxillary molars erupt before the mandibular molars. Any clinical examination of the primary dentition cannot be considered complete without a radiographic study of the sequence of eruption. A study of radiographs will be of considerable aid in studying the sequence of eruption and anticipating the development of malocclusion. It should be noted, however, that a prediction of malocclusion based on the sequence of eruption without a consideration of such factors as endocrine disturbances, familial tendencies, density of bone, scar tissue, and keratinization of the epithelium may lead to an incorrect anticipation of occlusal irregularities.

Between the ages of 6 and 8, the incisors in the anterior segments of the mouth begin to erupt into occlusion. The lower central incisors erupt first and then the lower lateral. In the absence of retained primary incisors, these teeth move labially from the lingual aspect of the jaw. The primary incisors should be shed before the eruption of the permanent incisors so that the latter do not erupt lingual to the deciduous incisors. In general where there is no spacing in the primary dentition, the permanent mandibular lateral incisors tend to become crowded. While there is some lateral displacement of the deciduous cuspids to compensate for simple crowding, there will be no displacement when the mandibular lateral incisors erupt lingually and are rotated. Excessive crowding of the lower central incisors can produce abnormal lateral displacement of the primary cuspids and cause them to be lost prematurely or produce a functional retraction of the mandible with distal occlusion of the arches to utilize the increased intercanine width in the lower arch.

Careful attention should be given at this time to the premature loss of primary cuspids since their loss may prevent the normal rate of growth and development of the anterior segment of the jaw. The eruption of the maxillary central incisors occurs just after eruption of the mandibular central incisors. The permanent maxillary incisors erupt in a more labial inclination than the almost vertically positioned primary teeth. This inclination accompanied by spacing of the teeth is often considered to be a sign of serious malocclusion by anxious parents. However, this appearance is within the range of normal, and, if significant space is available, the teeth will erupt in their normal positions provided no abnormal oral habits are present.

Not infrequently a diastema is seen between the maxillary central incisors, and the incisors will exhibit some distal inclination. This should not be considered abnormal unless the opening is extreme and interferes with the normal eruption of the lateral incisors. Closure of this space usually occurs in conjunction with the eruption of the permanent cuspids about the twelfth year. The maxillary lateral incisors may show some tendency for labioversion because of the close approximation of the roots of the lateral incisors with the crowns of the erupting cuspids. However, as the cuspids erupt, their relationship with the lateral incisors changes and allows the latter to assume a more favorable position.

The development of the lateral segments of the mouth occurs between the ages of 9 and 12 years. At this time the sequence of eruption, the size of the teeth, and a normal retention of the primary cuspids and second molars are of

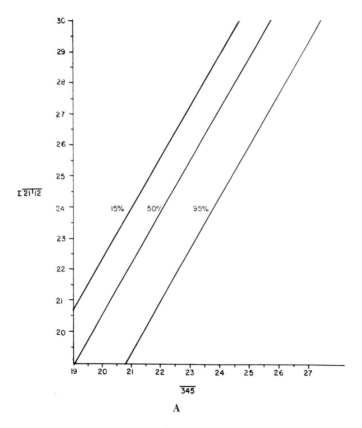

A

Fig. 162. *Mixed dentition analysis.* Per cent probability of predicted tooth size of cuspids and premolars based on the sum of the widths of the mandibular incisors. If the sum of the widths in millimeters of the mandibular incisors is known (vertical axis), the sum of the widths of the cuspids and premolars can be predicted (horizontal axis) at the indicated probability (15%, 50%, 95%). **A,** Maxilla. **B,** Mandible. (From Moyers, R. E.: Handbook of Orthodontics, Chicago, 1958, Year Book Publishers, Inc.)

considerable importance. As indicated previously, the most favorable sequence of eruption in the lateral segment of the mandible is cuspid, first bicuspid, second bicuspid, and then the second molar (provided the sixth-year molars and the lateral and central incisors have already erupted). The eruption of the man-dibular cuspids first tends to maintain a normal arch length and prevent a deep overbite which is usually associated with the lingual collapse of the anterior seg-ments. If the mandibular first bicuspid erupts before the cuspid, there is a tend-ency for the bicuspid to be tipped mesially, thereby preventing the cuspid from erupting normally. This occurs not infrequently when the primary cuspid is lost prematurely. If the mandibular second permanent molar erupts before the second bicuspid, there tends to be a loss of arch length and a mesial drift of the first molar which blocks the second bicuspid out of its normal eruption position. This may also occur with the premature loss of the mandibular second primary molar although a certain amount of mesial drift is to be expected because of a favorable leeway space that usually exists due to the difference in tooth size be-tween primary dentition and permanent dentition in this area. However, it is important that excessive mesial migration of the first permanent molar be pre-vented and sufficient space maintained to allow for the permanent successors.

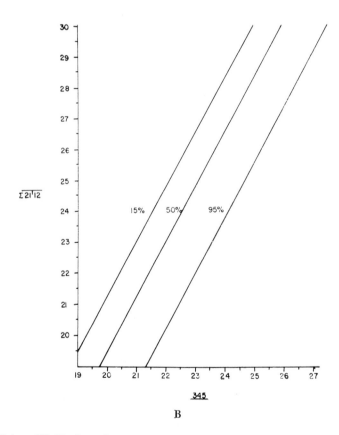

B

Fig. 162 (cont'd). For legend see opposite page.

Thus, there must be sufficient leeway space available for the size of the teeth that are to erupt; otherwise crowding and malocclusion will result.

Fortunately the examiner can predict the sum of the width of the cuspid, bicuspid, and second bicuspid within certain limits of probability by measuring the widths of the lower incisors. Thus, the sum of the widths of the four incisors is related to the sum of the widths of the teeth which are to erupt in the lateral segments of the jaw. This can be predicted with a certain level of confidence as indicated in Fig. 162 (Moyers). This chart may be used to predict, within certain limits of probability, the tooth size of the permanent cuspid and the first and second premolars if the sum of the widths of the incisors is known. A prediction of the arch space available for these permanent teeth by such a probability chart is not clinically useful in all cases. However, a negative predicted value may be used as a basis for a referral to an orthodontist for consultation.

For example, in an 8-year-old child an end-to-end relationship of the first permanent molars and a predicted tooth size of 23.1 mm. for the mandibular cuspids and premolars suggest that the optimum space needed as measured from the distal aspect of the lateral incisor to the mesial aspect of the first permanent molar should be 24.8 mm. Crowding of the lower anterior teeth may be present, and the degree of crowding measured in millimeters has to be considered. In this example if 2 mm. of crowding exists in the four mandibular incisors, 1 mm. has to be added to the optimum space needed in each lateral segment of the arches. The figure 24.8 is derived by adding the mean increment of 1.7 mm. for the late mesial shift of the sixth-year molar to the predicted tooth size of the mandibular cuspids and premolars. A negative predicted value should alert the examiner to the probability of malocclusion because of a lack of arch space.

Many factors can influence tooth-to-tooth relationship, e.g., shape of the dental arch, inclination of the teeth, loss of teeth, sequence of eruption, and environmental factors. From a practical standpoint the general practitioner may use this method of prediction of arch space reliably in a percentage of his cases. In fact, if the measurements are precise, there is a 95 per cent probability that the predicted arch space will be correct within 2.5 mm. (Moyers). It is to be expected that a more precise evaluation will be undertaken by the orthodontist whenever a general practitioner has referred such cases because of a predicted negative mixed dentition value for the arch space.

The most favorable sequence of eruption of the teeth in the lateral segments of the maxilla is first bicuspid, second bicuspid, cuspid, and then second molar. Variations in this sequence in the first bicuspid and cuspid area are not so significant as those in the mandible. Mesial migration of the maxillary first permanent molar from a premature loss of the primary second molar tends to allow a mesial drift of the first molar and the first and second bicuspids and often blocks out the normal eruption of the maxillary permanent cuspids. In some instances the second bicuspid is also crowded out of position. In general, the leeway space in the maxilla is less than that in the mandible, and therefore less mesial migration of the first permanent molar can be tolerated. It can be seen that the most favorable sequence in the lateral segment of the arch occurs when the eruption of the mandibular teeth precedes the eruption of the maxillary teeth. Thus, the most favorable relationship between the upper and lower lateral segments of the arches is in large part dependent upon a favorable sequence of eruption of the teeth in this area.

Many of the problems which arise in the development of the occlusion arise from local factors which occur during the primary and mixed dentitions. Thus, the examiner should direct his attention not only to those factors affecting general facial and craniofacial development and imbalance of oral and facial musculature, but also to etiologic factors which can contribute to a loss of space. The premature loss of primary teeth, retention of primary teeth, congenital absence of teeth, dental anomalies, ectopic eruptions, and abnormal diastemas should be considered as important factors in the initiation and contribution to the development of an abnormal occlusion.

Functional as well as skeletal and dental factors are important for the development of a normal occlusion. Not only is the proper functioning of jaws and musculature important to the position of the teeth in the jaws, but also it is significant in its influence upon dentofacial growth. The importance of a harmonious balance between the oral and facial musculature and the teeth must not be minimized. Abnormal shifting of the mandible associated with occlusal interferences contributes to facial asymmetry, temporomandibular joint disturbances, and disturbances in the teeth and supporting structures. Malposed teeth, cross-bite, faulty restorations, and other occlusal interferences that produce unfavorable shifting of the mandible or of the teeth may affect the normal process of growth and development so that a more severe type of malocclusion results, e.g., maxillary protrusion may be seen in association with hypotonicity of the upper lip, mouth breathing, or excessive lingual forces from abnormal tongue thrusting. A functional prognathic position of the mandible may be due to muscle reflexes that are elicited to avoid occlusal interferences such as malposed teeth, faulty restorations, or occlusal anomalies. In these instances the lower jaw is habitually protruded to a point where the teeth can come together without interference. Lateral and other abnormal shifts of the mandible may be observed by the examiner when the patient is requested to occlude the teeth from the tonus or rest position of the mandible. Abnormal patterns of closure should be evaluated for the presence of malposed teeth, occlusal interferences, temporomandibular joint disturbances, and abnormal tonicity of the muscles.

•   •   •

In summary, the examination of the development of occlusion should consist of an adequate history, an analysis of the facial form, an analysis of the sequence of eruption and the problems of space management, and an analysis of the function of the masticatory system.

Although judging malocclusion from a purely intraoral standpoint without regard for other dependent relationships has many shortcomings, a description or classification of the various types and forms of occluding teeth is a useful adjunct to occlusal deviations and terminology. However, two important considerations must be pointed out: a classification of malocclusion, per se, is never a diagnosis, and the determination of malocclusion simply on the basis of a description or classification of occlusal relationships is misleading and only a part of the total picture of malocclusion.

Angle introduced a system of classifying occlusal relationships into orthodontics in 1887. This classification was based on the assumption that the maxillary first permanent molar is always in the same position in the maxilla in relation to the base of the skull. He divided occlusal relationships into three classes according to the relationship of the maxillary and mandibular first permanent molars.

Class I comprises those arches which show a normal relationship of the maxillary and mandibular first permanent molars (mesiobuccal cusp of the maxillary molar fitting into the buccal groove of the mandibular first molar). This class also includes individual or groups of malposed teeth in which there is a normal molar relationship. Class II is comprised of those cases of malocclusion in which the mandibular first permanent molar is in distal relationship to the maxillary first permanent molar. This class is divided in two divisions. Division 1 includes protruding maxillary incisors and distoclusion of the lower molars and premolars in their relationship to the maxillary teeth. Mouth breathing, abnormal muscle pressure, and narrow maxillary arch are included. This division is subdivided to include unilateral distal molar relationships. Division 2 includes bilateral distal molar relationships with retruding maxillary incisors; the maxillary arch is of normal width, and there is no mouth breathing or abnormal muscle pressure. This division is also subdivided to include unilateral cases. Class III includes all the cases of malocclusion in which there is mesial occlusion of both sides of the mandibular arch. The mesial occlusion must be one-half the width of the molar. Thus, the mesiobuccal cusp fits into the embrasure between the first and second mandibular molars. This classification of malocclusion based on molar relationship can be utilized even after extractions if the teeth are envisaged as replaced.

Although Angle's classification is simple and creates a framework for classifying malocclusion, it has many obvious shortcomings. The position of the maxillary first permanent molar is not constant in relation to the base of the skull; many factors may influence its position. For example, the signs of Class II, Division 1 or 2, may merely represent an exacerbation of a Class I and not the primary or essential changes underlying a true distal occlusion. Thus, a Class I occlusion may have the symptoms of a Class II, Division 1, malocclusion. Or the early loss of sixth-year molars may result in the mesial migration and tipping of the twelfth-year molars into a position that would simulate a Class I molar relationship when in reality there is a Class II relationship present.

Adult Occlusion.—An examination of the occlusion in the adult is necessarily concerned with those changes which occur with physiologic and pathologic processes. An occlusion that is considered normal at the age of 18 years cannot be considered normal for the same individual at the age of 40 or 50 years. Even though the occlusion at 18 years of age may meet the criteria for ideal alignment and contact relation of the teeth, drifting, eruption, abrasion, extractions, loss of bone support, and prosthetic reconstructions continually alter the occlusion. These factors are of primary consideration in the continually changing pattern of occlusion and are difficult to separate from those changes which may be considered to be physiologic in nature. Therefore, it is difficult to state unequiv-ocally what might be a normal occlusion for the adult. If it were possible to study the changes of occlusion over the years from adolescence to old age with-out the presence of pathologic disturbances, it might be considerably easier to establish a range of normal occlusion for an adult at any given age. The ar-rangement of the teeth and the occlusion of an adult are the results of changes which occur throughout life.

The occlusion of an adult at the time of examination cannot be assumed to have been constant over a long period of time. Other than extractions and re-placement of teeth, attrition, extrusion, tipping, and migration appear to be the most obvious signs of occlusal changes in adult dentition. Attrition is a wear-ing away of the tooth surface from chewing foods which have a rough and gritty consistency. The condition progresses with advancing age. The pattern and degree of attrition are determined by the hardness of the teeth, the shape of the teeth, the amount of grit in the food, the age of the individual, the amount of force exerted on the teeth during the whole process of mastication, and the individual pattern of biting movements of the mandible. Attrition begins as soon as the teeth come into occlusal function. This is readily apparent in newly erupted incisors where the mamelons are soon worn down by incisal wear. Ab-normal patterns of wear may be seen in localized areas where premature occlu-sion occurs or where abnormal occlusal surfaces are present. After second molars have erupted, there is little change in the width of the alveolar arches, but there is a slight increase in the length of the dental arches during the time that the third molars are erupting. It is impossible to tell exactly what the initial adult occlusion will be until all the permanent teeth have erupted.

In this country the development of an edge-to-edge bite is not seen frequently either in the molar area of the primary dentition or in the incisor region of the adult dentition. As mentioned previously, characteristics of a normal primary dentition are the straight terminal plane and the almost end-to-end relationship of the maxillary and mandibular incisors. It is possible, however, for a step to develop in the terminal plane due to a forward shifting of the mandible associated with occlusal wear or because of a wide primary maxillary second molar. The edge-to-edge bite does not occur frequently in this country because of our diet of soft and refined foods. In persons who eat a gritty diet, such as the Eskimos and aborigines, an edge-to-edge bite is common in the anterior teeth. Appar-ently the edge-to-edge bite is not manifest during the eruption of the perma-nent teeth and only occurs as a result of eating coarse and gritty foods. (Fig. 163.) Though there is a tendency for mesial shifting of the mandible in the primary dentition and the permanent dentition associated with attrition of the teeth, sufficient wearing of the teeth does not occur frequently enough for evalua-tion of the full manifestations of this type of occlusion.

Overjet and overbite relationship is related to the development of the oc-clusion and to function. Thus, a certain amount of overjet and overbite must be considered normal. The degree of overbite must be related to the functional movements of the mandible, the presence or absence of extrusion of the max-illary and mandibular incisors, and the presence or absence of abnormal facial

Fig. 163. *Occlusion.* Marked occlusal attrition sometimes associated with bruxism; note end-to-end relationship of anterior teeth and gemination of lower central incisor.

proportions. Abnormal overjet may be due to maxillary protrusion, mandibular retrusion, labioversion of the maxillary incisors, or linguoversion of the mandibular incisors. Generally the maxillary incisors overhang the lower incisors about one-third the length of their crowns. The degree of overbite in the primary dentition is related to the amount of overbite in the mixed dentition; the overbite in the permanent dentition is influenced by the sequence of eruption of the permanent canines and premolars. A normal overbite usually results when the sequence of eruption is cuspid, first premolar, and second premolar in the mandibular arch and first premolar, cuspid, and second bicuspid in the maxillary arch.

From a practical standpoint the evaluation of the degree of overbite in the adult dentition should be related to the presence of impaired occlusal function, loss of vertical dimension in the posterior part of the mouth from extractions and loss of centric stops, extrusion of the maxillary and mandibular incisors associated with lack of centric stops, and impingement of the supporting structures by the maxillary and mandibular anterior teeth. Thus, a deep overbite in itself cannot be considered pathologic without evidence of contributory signs of disease.

The form and localization of the occlusal changes associated with attrition apparently develop in accordance with the individual pattern of gliding movements. Thus, occlusal wear or attrition is related to the function of the masticatory system. Another important factor in the changes in occlusion in the adult dentition is a forward movement of the teeth by interproximal attrition. It is known that considerable interproximal wear of the teeth occurs and that a loss of up to 1 cm. from the length of the arch may be manifested in the older adult.

The significance of occlusal wear is directly related to the health of the supporting structures. Thus, in evaluating the relationship of attrition and the presence or absence of unfavorable stresses upon the supporting structure, it is necessary to consider the direction of the stresses transmitted to the supporting structures. In general, excessive attrition tends to produce oblique planes of wear which imply an increase in the horizontal stress on the teeth during mastication. If there is a general diminishing of cusp height and overbite, the teeth will receive a more favorable axially directed occlusal stress. Also, the smooth gliding movements of the mandible induced by this type of occlusal wear are more favorable to these supporting structures.

Another type of occlusal wear that has an unfavorable influence on the supporting structures can be observed when the incline planes of the cusps become steeper than usual and form plunger cusps. This pattern of wear seems to be seen most often when bilateral movements of the mandible predominate during mastication (Beyron). Other patterns of wear can be observed in association with restricted lateral movements of the mandible and when a patient chews only by moving the jaws up and down.

For some individuals protrusive movements seem to be most comfortable, and the occlusal changes brought on by these movements are primarily in the anterior teeth; these teeth frequently show marked attrition, labial tipping of the maxillary incisors, and development of secondary spaces. In these instances there is a decrease in the incisor inclination and an increase in the cuspal inclination of the bicuspids and molars. The occlusal changes associated with unilateral and unilateral-diagonal movements during mastication and related to irregularities of the dentition, including so-called unilateral cross-bite, are characterized by marked attrition on the side used for mastication and a tendency for opening of the contacts of the anterior teeth (Beyron). Where unilateral movements predominate, the pattern of wear appears to be related to a combined lateral and up-and-down movement of the mandible. In unilateral-diagonal movements the patient is able to produce diagonal protrusive movements as well as lateral movements to one side, and the pattern of wear is related to these movements. Thus, more incisal wear may be observed in the unilateral-diagonal gliding movement than in the straight unilateral type of movements (Beyron). Extrusion and tipping of the most distal mandibular molars may result in a unilateral-diagonal restricted type of movement in which there is attrition of the bicuspids on a side of the extruded molar and extrusion of the maxillary anterior teeth diagonally opposite the extruded molar (Thielemann) (Fig. 164). Disturbances in the supporting structures in these types of movements appear to be related more to the lack of function than to the teeth which show the effects of attrition.

Functional Analysis.—The masticatory system has been described as a functional unit comprised of the teeth and their supporting structures, the jaws, the temporomandibular joints, the muscles attached to the mandible, the lips and tongue, and the vascular and nerve supply to these tissues. Thus, the so-called masticatory system constitutes groups of integrated parts capable of acting as a unit not only for the purpose of mastication, but also for the purpose of sucking, speaking, and any other function that reflects the behavior of the individual. It is impossible to adequately examine any one of the components of this system without consideration of the correlation that exists between the component parts.

Each component of the masticatory system may be examined individually,

A

B   C

Fig. 164. *Occlusion.* A, Extruded upper right second molar in premature centric contact.
B and C, Example of Thielemann's law.

but the findings should be correlated by a functional analysis of the whole system. Thus, an analysis of the temporomandibular joint will not be adequate
without an evaluation of the neuromuscular system which makes the functional
activities of the masticatory system possible. Furthermore, it is necessary to
evaluate the physiologic adaptation of the masticatory system to functional
wear and tear by compensatory eruption of the teeth, mesial drift, and changes
in occlusal pattern. A practical approach to the analysis of disturbances of any
of the components of the masticatory system demands that a clinical examination be made for the signs and symptoms of organic disease and that the findings be related to the functional or dysfunctional activities of each of the components and to the functional activities of the whole system. This means that
each component part must be analyzed for organic disease, functional incapacitation, and production of disturbances in the rest of the system.

A functional analysis is a systematic examination of the anatomy and function of the masticatory system with special consideration given to functional
disturbances and pathologic changes in the periodontium, teeth, joints, and
muscles of mastication. The analysis should consist of (1) a complete case
history, including a review of the masticatory system for symptoms of dysfunc-

tion of the joints and muscles, psychic factors, fatigue, anxiety, and pain, (2) a clinical examination of the masticatory system, supplemented with (3) a radiographic examination of the teeth and periodontal structures and, where indicated, radiographs of the temporomandibular joint, and (4) an analysis of the occlusion with an articulator.

Temporomandibular Joint.—Though the joints are considered briefly in a general examination (Chapter 5), a more detailed consideration of this area may be necessary during examination of the occlusion. The examination of the temporomandibular joint should begin by inspection and palpation of the tissues contiguous with the joint while it is at rest and during functional movements. Inspection for visible signs of swelling and ecchymosis, palpation for localized tenderness, and inquiry about pain on motion should be carried out in the region of the joint. Subjective complaints as described by the patient during the clinical history should serve to orient the examiner to a correlation of the symptoms of local manifestations of disease. Elevation of temperature, texture and induration of the overlying tissue, presence or absence of tenderness or fluctuation, and the characteristics of any enlargement are determined by palpation. Friction fremitus or joint crepitus can be detected as the joint is moved.

The muscles of mastication should be sufficiently relaxed to permit the patient to move the mandible comfortably through all functional movements. Movements may be restricted because of pain, joint disease, neuromuscular disease, or lack of muscle coordination. The range and freedom of active movements made by the patient should be evaluated in all excursions of the mandible, and, if indicated the patient should be requested to bite on a piece of rubber or orangewood stick. Biting force, per se, probably has little significance to the natural dentition; however, biting down on something hard may produce symptoms that are not otherwise evident.

The temporomandibular joints are subject to luxation, subluxation, traumatic arthritis, acute suppurative arthritis, rheumatoid arthritis, and osteoarthritis associated with generalized degenerative joint disease involving all joints in the body. Traumatic tempromandibular joint arthritis is due to incomplete or complete dislocation of the joint and to traumatic injury of the head of the condyle, the glenoid fossa, and the meniscus. If subluxation or traumatic injury is severe, the signs and symptoms are usually of an acute nature. Movements of the mandible are usually restricted by pain, and pain may be produced when the joints are palpated. On opening, the mandible may be deviated to one side because of unilateral pain involvement or because of immobilization of one side. Occasionally there is radiographic evidence of an increased joint space.

When traumatic injury to the joint is not sudden or severe but is of a low degree, chronic, or of a repeated nature, the history of onset will be vague and insidious. In these instances a disturbance in the other components of the masticatory system, such as occlusal disharmony, may be the factor responsible for trauma to the joints. The etiologic factors causing chronic traumatic arthritis may be present also in those patients exhibiting acute traumatic arthritis; they are not usually the cause of acute signs and symptoms unless they rather suddenly exceed the physiologic limits of the joint. The latter occurs not infrequently with occlusal disharmony. Dental procedures that require the mouth to be open for extended periods, high restorations, blows to the mandible, and extractions can be causes of traumatic injury to the joint. The signs and symptoms of such injury may be severe and of sudden onset or the symptoms may be of a minor nature at first, only to give rise to severe symptoms later, either spontaneously or in association with another traumatic incident even of a minor nature.

The signs and symptoms of chronic temporomandibular arthritis include clicking and snapping noises in the joint when it is being moved, restricted patterns of mandibular movements, pain in the joint when certain movements are attempted, neuralgic pain referred to the ear and surrounding structures, and occasional pain in the muscles of mastication in certain areas. Palpation of the joint area will rarely uncover swelling or pain; however, jerky movements of the head of the condyle may be felt. Visual inspection will only rarely show signs of obvious deformity, but radiographic examination may show evidence of bone resorption or irregularity of the head of the condyle or anterior slope of the glenoid fossa.

An acute suppurative arthritis of the temporomandibular joint is usually a complication of gonorrheal urethritis or of other acute pyogenic joint involvement. Local manifestations consist of spasms of the masseter muscles, difficulty in opening the mouth, and the presence of the cardinal signs of inflammation in and around the affected temporomandibular joint. The systemic reaction consists of an elevation in temperature, leukocytosis, and general malaise. Radiographic examination of the joint will not reveal any change until rather extensive damage has taken place. Thus, it is necessary that early diagnosis and antibiotic treatment be instituted for the maintenance of a functional joint. The diagnosis of gonococcal arthritis can be confirmed by examination of fluid aspirated from the joint. The acute nature of the local and systemic signs and symptoms of disease should direct the examiner's attention to the possibility of an infective arthritis.

Etiologic factors responsible for disharmony of the masticatory system as well as for traumatic temporomandibular joint arthritis are discrepancy between centric relation and centric occlusion, abnormal tonicity of the masticatory muscles, local irritation associated with periodontal disease or dental caries, occlusal interference, psychic tension, loss of vertical dimension, neurologic disorders, abnormal habits of mastication and nonfunctional jaw positions, loss of teeth without replacement and faulty dental therapy, and bruxism.

Examination for Slide in Centric Occlusion.—The examination of the masticatory system should include a search for a discrepancy between centric relation and centric occlusion. Centric relation is the most retruded position of the mandible from which lateral jaw movements can be made comfortably. Centric relation refers to a jaw-to-jaw relationship. The term centric occlusion refers to the position of the teeth when the jaws are closed and the teeth are at a maximum intercuspation with the mandible in centric relation. This is a tooth-to-tooth relationship.

When the mandible is closed in centric relation and there is no occlusal interference, the teeth should be in a position of maximum intercuspation without a sliding movement of the mandible. When there is a forward slide of the mandible and an anterior displacement of the heads of the condyle, the acquired relationship of the teeth is then one of convenience or habitual occlusion. The sliding change from "true" centric to a convenience centric occlusion is called a slide in centric occlusion. There should be no slide in closing in centric relation; however, when premature contacts exist, the shift in the mandible will occur. The initial contact in centric relation that causes the slide is referred to as a premature contact or a centric interference. Thus, the mandible may be deflected during centric relation closure from true centric relation by a premature contact, thereby producing a habitual or convenience occlusion of the teeth. This habitual or convenience occlusion represents a potential source of tissue injury and is a significant etiologic factor in temporomandibular joint arthritis and bruxism.

The success in determining the presence of a slide in centric occlusion is determined by the ability of the examiner to manipulate the mandible about its hinge axis. This maneuver may be complicated by temporomandibular joint dysfunction and by abnormal tonus of the muscles of mastication. The initial objective of the examiner should be to get the patient to assume a relaxed, unstrained retruded position of the mandible without exerting unnecessary pressure. When there is hypertonicity of the muscles, the patient may require considerable training in relaxation of these muscles. The use of relaxant drugs such as Flexin may be of assistance in such cases. The chin should be held between the index finger and thumb (Fig. 165), and the mandible should be moved up and down in small arcs. Initially it may be necessary to ask the patient to assist in making these movements. As the jaw is manipulated, the mandible should be directed passively posteriorly and upward to decrease the inner occlusal distance. When the muscles are completely relaxed and the mandible is in the retruded position and the teeth are in close approximation, the examiner should have a sense of rotary or hinge axis movement. Further slight closure will serve to establish the first occlusal contact. If premature contacts are present, the mandible will be displaced anteriorly on closure. Where no slide in centric occlusion is present, a maximum number of teeth will contact simultaneously. During the hinge axis closure, the examiner may palpate for the tooth exhibiting the first premature contact, for percussion vibrations, and for movements of the teeth.

The areas of premature contact may be marked with articulating paper or 28-gauge wax (Fig. 166). The process should be repeated until the patient is aware of what is being done and until the muscles are completely relaxed. It may take some time to train the patient in centric relation closure. This may require considerable patience on the part of the examiner as well as the patient. The determination of centric relation should be carried out several times in order that the examiner may feel sure that the hinge axis movement is being made without benefit of the patient's muscle effort. In general, the examiner will find that the most retruded position of the mandible becomes more apparent after several manipulations of the mandible. The patient may be requested to

Fig. 165. *Occlusion.* **A,** Examination for premature centric contact. **B,** Centric relation. **C,** Centric occlusion. **D** and **E,** Carbon marks indicating points of premature contact; note marks on mesial aspects of the lingual cusps of the maxillary first bicuspid; this is a common location of premature contacts.

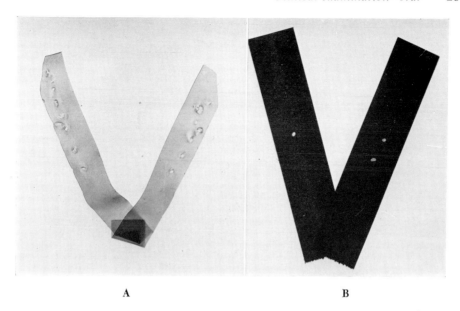

A   B

Fig. 166. *Occlusion.* A, Premature contacts identified by perforations in 28-gauge Kerr green wax. B, Premature contacts identified by perforation in carbon paper; this method also marks the teeth.

stop his centric closure just as he first comes into occlusal contact; at this point visual inspection of the teeth may reveal the position of the premature contact. After this is noted, the patient should be requested to press his teeth together and the path of closure is noted. In some instances it may be difficult to determine the exact position of a premature contact. Various methods are used to determine a position of the premature contacts, depending upon the ability and success of their use by the operator. The examiner should always question the patient regarding his location of a tooth contact, for in many individuals the sense of location is very highly developed; in others misleading information will be given. The sound of the teeth coming together may indicate where the premature contact is located; however, it is only of limited value to most operators. The presence of worn facets on the teeth is suggestive of premature contacts. Polished gold restorations present some difficulty in marking with articulating paper. In these instances especially, the use of 28-gauge green wax may be helpful. In some instances where there is hypermobility of the teeth, the initial occlusal interference will tend to move a tooth in a lateral direction. This movement can be easily felt by the examiner.

Mandibular Movements.—The relation of the teeth to mandibular movements should be observed in working, balancing, and protrusive positions (Fig. 167). In working position the buccal cusps of the mandibular teeth should contact the lingual inclines of the buccal cusps of the maxillary teeth. The position of the cuspid may prevent this from occurring in the posterior teeth except for limited lateral movements. The examiner should determine whether or not se-

A   B

C

Fig. 167. *Occlusion.* **A,** Working position. **B,** Balancing position. **C,** Protrusive position.

lective grinding will allow more contacts to be made over the full extent of tooth contact in lateral working excursions. The extent of improvement will depend to a large degree upon the relationship of the anterior teeth and the amount of grinding that can be accomplished without removing an excessive amount of tooth structure from the cuspids. The degree of overjet and overbite will usually determine the amount of functional improvement that can be accomplished.

Balancing occlusion should be examined when the teeth are together and when lateral excursions are being made. A balancing bite occurs when the buccal cusps of the mandibular teeth occlude with the buccal inclines of the lingual cusps of the maxillary teeth. Balancing occlusion is not necessary in the natural dentition. It should be examined when observing the working bite. Abnormal, jerky, and restricted movements may be due to interferences on the balancing side.

Such movements which result from balancing interferences prevent maximum efficiency on the working side, tend to place undue lateral stress on the teeth on the balancing side, and predispose to temporomandibular joint arthritis.

Protrusive movements should be observed for abnormal patterns of movements. The teeth should be in occlusion when the excursions are performed so that jerky, eccentric, and deviated protrusive movements can be observed. Quite frequently cuspal interferences will prevent the mandible from performing smooth gliding protrusive movements.

The mandibular movements should be repeated while the teeth are out of contact (Fig. 168). In many instances the patient will be able to perform these excursions better than when the teeth are in contact because of the occlusal interferences present which restrict excursions of the mandible when the teeth are in contact. In other instances the patient will not be able to perform the movements adequately because of forced inactivity of some of the usual patterns of muscle activity due to restricted movements resulting from occlusal interferences. Less frequently, muscle spasms, tenderness, or paralysis will prevent certain of the mandibular movements.

Fig. 168. *Mandibular movements.* Observation of mandibular movements. **A,** Centric occlusion. **B,** Protrusive movement without occlusal contact. **C,** Protrusive movement with occlusal contact. **D** and **E,** Lateral excursions without occlusal contact.

A   B

C   D

Fig. 169. *Mandibular positions.* Functional Class III relationship of mandible due to mal-posed maxillary incisors. **A** and **B**, Mandible in centric relation. **C**, Teeth in acquired centric occlusion producing prognathism. **D**, True centric occlusion following labial movement of incisors.

Cases of prognathism should be observed for the possibility of an occlusal interference preventing the closure of the mandible in centric relation.   This functional type of prognathism can be determined easily by having the patient close in centric relation and then in his convenience centric relation. In centric relation a functional prognathism will disappear (Fig. 169).

Tonus or Rest Position of the Mandible.—The involuntary maintenance of the position of the mandible in an individual who is awake and in an upright position is determined by the tonus of the masticatory and functionally related muscles. The reflex contraction of the muscles which results from a pull such as gravity is called the stretch or myotatic reflex. A steady reflex contraction as seen in the muscles which are concerned with posture and gravity is called tonus. Factors such as learning, pain, fear, fatigue, mental relaxation, and the positions of the patient will affect tonus. Occlusal irregularities and periodontal disease may also alter normal tonus position of the mandible.

The tonus or rest position is of clinical importance because of its relationship to the interocclusal space (freeway space) which is usually present between the occlusal surfaces of the maxillary and mandibular teeth. The width of this space varies considerably but most generally is from 2 to 5 mm. in the anterior portion of the mouth. The exact amount of freeway space should be determined independently in each individual.

In order to obtain a dependable recording of the rest position, it is necessary to eliminate factors which can disturb the tonus. Relaxing procedures, such as repeated swallowing, the use of phonetics or word sounds to be repeated by the patient such as "m" or "o" or word syllables such as O-hi-o or Miss-i-ssipp-i, and training in muscle relaxation are of help in obtaining a dependable rest position of the mandible. Such maneuvers will give fairly good results provided there are no disturbing factors such as occlusal interference, periodontal disease, tongue and lip habits, fear, apprehension, and pain. A radiographic registration is probably more accurate than other methods for registration of the rest position of the mandible; however, this method does not lend itself readily to most clinical procedures. Under normal conditions the rest position is considered to be constant except for minor changes with age.

Vertical dimension is the vertical height of the face as determined by muscle relationships and the rest position of the mandible. Its determination is of importance when the examiner seeks to evaluate the possibility of an increase in the freeway space (so-called closed-bite) (Fig. 170).

Inasmuch as vertical dimension is related to the position of rest of the mandible and this rest position is stable, changes in the interocclusal space (freeway space) can be related to the vertical dimension of the face. An increase in the space results occasionally from excessive attrition of the teeth without compensatory eruption. Encroachment on the space may result from extrusion of teeth; this is usually limited to localized areas of the arches where teeth or centric stops have been lost. Not infrequently, encroachment on the freeway space will result from misguided bite-raising procedures. When there has been

Fig. 170. *Functional occlusion.* Attrition of anterior teeth due to deep overbite and loss of posterior teeth; note presence of bite-raising appliance in the mandibular arch.

encroachment upon the space by some bite-raising procedure, there will be a constant undue stimulus to the stretch reflex of the muscles of mastication that will promote undue muscle contractions and produce pathologic sequelae. An increase in the freeway space is not of direct significance for muscle tonus and rest position, but it may directly influence the tonus and other functional relations of the masticatory system by associated abnormal or strained occlusal relations.

The diagnosis of an abnormally wide freeway space or loss of vertical dimension should not be made simply on the basis of altered facial expression, for many factors can produce changes in facial expression. Wrinkles caused by age and the disappearance of fat pads with a loss of tissue contour cannot be considered as signs of loss of vertical dimension. A deep overbite in itself is not a sign of lost vertical dimension. Excessive attrition of the teeth is not necessarily an indication that the patient has a loss of vertical dimension or an abnormally wide freeway space, since a loss of tooth structure may be compensated for by eruption of the teeth and increase in the height of the alveolar process. Where an older individual has what appears to be a closed-bite and an abnormally wide freeway space but does not have untoward signs or symptoms of this condition, the clinician should be very cautious about attempting to greatly reduce the freeway space without an effort to determine the actual status of the vertical dimension and freeway space.

Not infrequently an attempt to restore vertical dimension will result in failure because the appearance of the freeway space was not related to the actual status of the vertical dimension. When extensive reconstruction is planned, it is necessary that the clinician give due consideration to the measurement of vertical dimension. While the vertical dimension may be determined by its relationship to the rest position of the mandible, it has been pointed out that the procedure for obtaining the exact location of the rest position is not precise. A temporary splint may be used as a diagnostic aid for the evaluation of a vertical dimension which is considered to be the right one for the patient. If the patient tolerates the appliance well, the derived freeway space is probably correct. In general, it is better to underdiagnose cases of a loss of vertical dimension than to overdiagnose them. All too frequently a diagnosis is made of a loss and treatment for the loss results in an encroachment upon the freeway space.

When a patient with a deep overbite complains of soreness of the palatal tissue around the incisive papilla, the clinician should not necessarily consider this evidence of a close-bite or loss of vertical dimension unless additional facts justify the diagnosis. Many individuals have a deep overbite that is within the range of normal for them. However, if a patient complains of an incisive papilla being painful because of traumatization from the lower incisors, the clinician should determine whether or not there is a loss of centric stop on these teeth, whether or not there is extrusion of these teeth, or whether or not there is hyperplasia of the gingival tissues and incisive papilla.

Quite frequently the inclination and the anatomy of the maxillary central incisors do not present adequate centric stop for the lower incisor teeth. This may be accompanied by an extrusion of the lower incisors with impingement upon the incisive papilla, causing an inflammatory reaction. Although this may be considered an anterior closed-bite or an encroachment upon the freeway space, it is not satisfactory evidence of a generalized change in the vertical dimension. In the great majority of these cases there is no change in the posterior vertical dimension. Unfortunately many of these cases are diagnosed as having loss of vertical dimension, and attempts are made to intrude the anterior teeth and cause eruption of the posterior teeth. Such a diagnosis and treatment plan are based on lack of understanding of the rest position of the mandible and the freeway space. The difference in the occlusal plane between the anterior portion of the mouth and the posterior teeth in such cases does not represent a lack of development of the alveolar process and eruption of the posterior teeth but reflects the lack of centric stops on the maxillary teeth by an extrusion of the mandibular and/or maxillary central incisors. Thus, the treatment should not be based upon a loss of vertical dimension but upon a correction of the factors responsible for it. In this particular instance a diagnosis is directed toward the extrusion of teeth in the absence of adequate centric stops. Therefore, the treatment plan should be based upon the establishment of centric stops either by orthodontic movements of the teeth and/or restoration to provide centric stops for the lower incisors. In either event, some occlusal adjustment will be necessary for the correction of the height of the lower incisors and in some instances for the correction of the length of the maxillary incisors. A more detailed study of the occlusion may be necessary, and the examiner may desire to mount the models of the patient's teeth on an articulator. This is accomplished by a face-bow registration, a centric relation wax bite, and a protrusive relation wax bite. Casts of the teeth to be studied may be mounted on an adjustable articulator. Articulation of the models is an important aid in the functional analysis of occlusal relations and is of significant value many times in diagnosis and treatment planning (see Chapter 7).

Edentulous Mouth

The examination of the edentulous patient should include all the components of a complete and thorough examination except for those parts concerned with the evaluation of the natural dentition. The examination of the patient in preparation for the construction of dentures differs only slightly from that of the patient already wearing dentures. The main difference lies in analysis. The analysis of the areas to receive dentures relates to effective impressions for adequate construction of denture bases, whereas the analysis of denture-bearing areas relates to dentures already in use.

Periodic examination of denture-bearing areas and artificial dentures is as important as the periodic examination of the natural dentition. It should serve to outline the denture-bearing areas, to determine structures or areas that may require relief, to ascertain what anatomic features can be found in the impression, to evaluate the hard and soft structures which are used for the denture base, and to evaluate dentures already being worn.

The preparation of the mouth for dentures may require the removal of bony spines, unerupted teeth, retained roots, hyperplastic tissue, tori, and pro-

tuberant localized areas of the alveolar ridges that would prevent proper placement of dentures because of lack of intermaxillary space. Occasionally it may
be necessary to push back the frenula and deepen the mucobuccal fold. These
factors should be taken into consideration before denture construction is started.
Although dentists are quite adept at compensating for many defects of the denture-bearing areas, alveolectomies and other surgical procedures many times
provide a more favorable denture base than can be obtained by compensatory
procedures.

The anatomic features which should be considered prior to taking an impression are those hard and soft tissue landmarks which must be identified in
the impression and those tissues which may, because of their consistency and
contour, interfere with the taking of an impression. It is very necessary that
the examiner determine what soft tissue displacements must be considered before
taking the impression. Inspection and palpation of the structures of the denture-

Fig. 171. *Examination of edentulous patient.* **A,** Tongue position. **B,** Position of labial
frenulum. **C,** Position of lingual attachment of soft tissue. **D,** Retromolar pad and lateral
throat form.

A   B

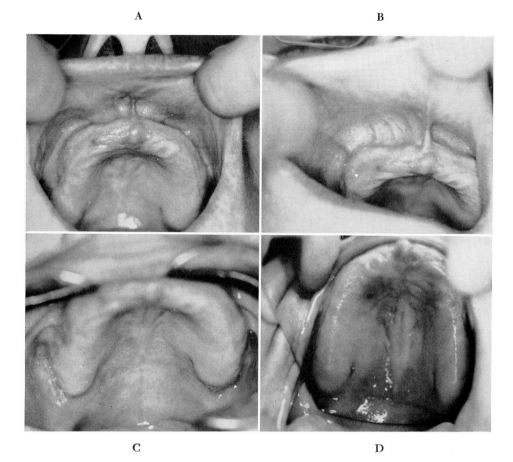

C   D

Fig. 172. *Examination of edentulous patient.* **A,** Labial frenulum. **B,** Buccal frenulum. **C,** Vibrating line (junction of hard and soft palates). **D,** Tuberosity and midsagittal suture; note relationship of pterygomandibular raphe to palate.

bearing areas and periphery will enable the clinician to interpret these structures in the impression. It will also enable him to determine what areas are to bear the dentures and what areas must be relieved to prevent interference with function, movement, retention, and placement of the dentures.

Inspection and palpation of the edentulous areas should be systematic and should follow a routine procedure so that no feature will be overlooked (Figs. 171 and 172). The following characteristics of the ridges should be noted: roughness, sharpness, flatness, height, and relation to the opposing arches; relation to the anterior nasal spine, zygomatic process of the maxilla, hamulus, mental foramen, mental trigone, buccal shelf, retromolar trigone, genial tubercles, and mylohyoid line; and relation to position of the tongue and the floor of the mouth.

Inspection and palpation of the maxillary arch can begin at the midline. The prominence of the anterior nasal spine and its relationship to the alveolar ridges can be noted by pressing a finger lightly over the midline above the attached gingiva. By palpating laterally, the examiner can feel the slight con-cavity of the canine fossa just anterior to the canine eminence. The alveolar ridge should be palpated in these areas for evidence of sharp bony spicules. Then, by palpating posteriorly, the examiner can feel the maxillary buttress of the zygomatic arch and should note its relation to the alveolar ridge. Its oblique-ness and prominence should be related to the position of the periphery of the denture. The position and prominence of labial and buccal frenula should be noted; when the attachment is high on the ridge, special consideration may be necessary. The superior buccal fornix should be considered in relation to its depth and position of the buccal flange of the denture. The maxillary tuberosity should be inspected and palpated for hyperplastic tissue and nearness to the opposing alveolar ridge. Occasionally the tuberosity extends to the mandibular ridge and makes recontouring necessary.

The relation of the pterygoid hamulus to the hamular notch should be noted. The position of the posterior palatal seal must be accurately determined to avoid interference with the action of the tensor veli palatini muscle. The lo-cation of the distal posterior palatal seal must be visualized at the junction of the hard and soft palates (vibrating line). The junction can be seen clearly when the patient says "aah." The tissue over the greater palatine foramen should be palpated for texture and softness. Not infrequently these tissues are soft, fluctuant, and easily compressed by impression materials. The tissues of the palate and alveolar ridges should be palpated and the compressibility of these areas compared. This comparison should extend from the midline to the alve-olar ridges and from the junction of the hard and soft palates to the incisive papilla. Obviously, the degree of compressibility is of considerable importance in recording an accurate impression. The presence of a palatine torus can present denture problems (Fig. 6, A). The incisive papilla may lie on a level with the alveolar ridge, and, if it is soft and hyperplastic, relief of this area may be necessary. This is especially true if on palpation the patient complains of tenderness.

The position of the palatine foveas is often used as a landmark for the es-tablishment of the posterior border of the upper denture (Fig. 172). However, because of considerable variation and difficulty in seeing these depressions, these foveas cannot be relied upon as landmarks for the peripheral posterior border of the denture.

The mandibular buccal fornix and the buccal shelf should be palpated in the molar region to determine the direction of the slant of the surface of the shelf and the relationship to the attachment of the buccinator muscle fibers. It is necessary to determine these anatomic landmarks since the buccal flange or periphery of the lower denture is related to the usable surface presented here. Palpation will also facilitate the determination of the periphery of the impres-sion tray. The buccal fornix is also frequently involved in overextension of the buccal flange of dentures and should be inspected for signs and symptoms of this condition.

The anterior border of the ramus of the mandible should be palpated at rest and during movements of the mandible. The relationship between the alveolar ridge, retromolar pad, pterygomandibular raphe, and buccinator muscle should be evaluated. The pterygomandibular ligament passes by the lateral posterior palatal seal area and frequently impinges on the junction of the alveolar ridge and the palate (Fig. 172, *D*). The attachment of the pterygomandibular ligament must not impinge upon the periphery of the denture. Dislodgement of the denture may result when the mouth is opened wide if this area of attachment is not considered.

The anteroposterior ridge relationship is of considerable importance in the placement and arrangement of the teeth. The mandibular alveolar ridge may be in distal or mesial relation to the maxillary ridge and occasionally presents difficulties in the placement of teeth and the retention of the dentures. The lateral ridge relationship is also of similar importance to the stability of the dentures.

Vertical dimension should be established during the initial phases of the examination and more accurately during the construction of the denture. Some change in the rest position of the mandible may occur with older age. This fact must be considered when evaluating vertical dimension. The external features of the face should be noted from frontal and profile aspects (Fig. 173). Loss of tissue tone does not in itself indicate a loss of vertical dimension.

The tissues which are to bear the dentures should be evaluated for their

A   B

C   D

Fig. 173. *Examination of edentulous patient.* **A,** With denture. **B,** Without denture; note depth of labial folds and loss of support for cheeks. **C** and **D,** Examination of profile with and without dentures.

ability to support dentures. Thin, atrophic, and spongy tissues are easily traumatized, and special consideration may be necessary to prepare them for dentures. Older patients, especially women past the menopause, may require massage of the tissues, small posterior teeth, and a special soft lining over the surfaces of knifelike alveolar ridges. It may also be necessary for these patients to alternately leave out one of their dentures at night.

The periphery of the buccal posterior border of the lower denture can be estimated by palpation during functional movements of the mandible and later can be fully evaluated by a functional impression. The lingual tubercle (the mandibular eminence below and medial to the most distal lower molar) and the postmylohyoid fossa of the mandible should be palpated to determine the undercut that this eminence and fossa present in order that some idea of the extent of the lingual flange of the lower denture can be made. It is important in the selection of an impression tray since an overextended flange of an impression tray can injure the bony tissue and also prevent an adequate impression. The position of the attachment of the lingual frenulum is of significance in establishing the periphery of the denture. If the alveolar ridge height is minimal and the attachment high, there may be difficulty in establishing a proper lingual flange in this region. This area is also of significance in the placement of lingual bars of partial dentures.

The alveololingual sulcus should be palpated since the floor of the mouth and the prominent structures that lie in it may be raised during the impression taking and may obliterate a portion of the ridge in the impression. This is especially true if there are prominent glands in the floor of the mouth together with extensive resorption of the molar area of the mandibular alveolar ridge. When this arrangement of structures is known, the examiner can prevent them from affecting the impression by modifying the impression tray.

The examiner should observe and palpate the lingual aspects of the mandible in the region of the bicuspids for the presence of mandibular tori since these structures occasionally prevent the proper placing of dentures and of necessity have to be removed surgically. The location of the mylohyoid ridge should be determined by palpation, especially in cases of extreme absorption of the alveolar ridge; the effect that the position of the mylohyoid ridge will have on the periphery of the lingual flange of the lower denture should be visualized.

The examination of the patient with dentures should consist of an evaluation of the response of the tissues to the dentures, the patient's adjustment to the dentures, and an analysis of the function of the dentures. The response of the tissues may be that of physiologic adaptation or pathologic regression. While most patients adjust esthetically, functionally, and emotionally to the dentures, some patients refuse to wear dentures because of a lack of adjustment in any one or all of these areas. A patient may be completely satisfied with his dentures, yet an analysis of their function may reveal many shortcomings which prevent their maximum efficiency. It is not uncommon in such instances for pathologic factors to be present which the patient has unknowingly tolerated. Some patients with a high degree of tolerance believe that soreness, looseness, and poor chewing ability are inherent qualities of all dentures. At the other extreme are those who refuse to adjust to any denture regardless of its perfection. The emotional aspects of complete denture service and the adjustment of the patient make it imperative that the examination of dentures and denture-bearing areas for determination of proper function and the presence of disease be thorough and complete.

The diagnosis of complaints regarding complete dentures may present serious difficulty (Fig. 174). The separation of complaints of organic origin from those due to lack of adjustment often taxes the skill and patience of the examiner. A well-taken history is often of significant value in making the differentiation. Proper preparation of the mouth and proper psychologic preparation of the patient are important considerations in the avoidance of denture problems.

The patient's complaints are usually directed toward soreness of the tissues following insertion of the dentures. Another common complaint during the adjustment period is lack of stability of the dentures. It must be pointed out that patients must learn to wear dentures, and the importance of this fact is sometimes completely overlooked by the patient. From the dentist's standpoint, many complaints may arise from a lack of adjustment of the patient to the dentures.

A complaint of soreness should be evaluated in terms of an overextension or overpressure of the denture, faulty occlusion, excessive vertical dimension, and a lack of patient adjustment. Localized areas of soreness may be manifested by a break in the mucosa or by areas of tenderness that can be determined by palpation. Ulceration of the tissues may arise because of overpressure from the denture or because of bony spicules beneath the mucosa. The exact location of the area of overpressure may be localized on the denture by using soft wax. This is painted on the mucosal surface of the denture in the general location of the offending area. Replacement of the dentures and functional movements of the mandible will displace the wax if overpressure or extension is present.

Fig. 174. *Examination of edentulous patient.* Lesion detected in patient who has worn same denture for thirty-five years. There is palatal papillomatosis and large fungating carcinoma with central necrosis involving left tuberosity. This lesion almost hidden by the denture was undetected through three periods of hospitalization for cataract removal.

Generalized soreness of the alveolar crest may be related to excessive vertical dimension, encroachment on the freeway space, locked occlusion, lack of accommodation for Bennett's movement, or the presence of tissues which are not capable of denture support (Kingery). Denture-sore mouth is commonly caused by lack of denture stability, rarely by a sensitivity to the denture material itself. The stability of the dentures is related to occlusal balance, peripheral seal, vertical dimension, and the freeway space. Constant rocking and displacement result in chronic irritation of the underlying soft tissues.

Soreness at the periphery of the denture in the mucobuccal fold is usually due to an overextension or overpressure of the buccal or lingual flange. The soreness is related to abrasion or ulceration of the mucosa. Soreness in the anterior part of the mouth can result from an overextension of the lingual flange, excessive pressure due to a slide in centric occlusion, or overextension of the buccal flange in the molar region. Soreness on the lingual aspect of the denture flange may be caused by overextension on the labial or buccal side, occlusal interference on the same or opposite side, or warpage of the denture (Kingery). Soreness in the posterior part of the mouth may result from occlusal interference or overextension of the labial flange in the anterior part of the mouth.

Looseness of dentures is another complaint which the examiner may encounter either shortly after the denture has been delivered to the patient or after it has been worn for a considerable length of time. The patient may complain of the maxillary denture dropping each time the mouth is opened or only occasionally. The causes may be multiple, and the occlusion, posterior seal, and overextension of the denture should be evaluated. Not infrequently a patient will complain that the upper denture drops when he talks or sings; this may be due to overextension of the periphery of the denture or overactivity of the soft palate.

If the denture becomes loose on one side while the patient chews on the other side, the occlusion should be checked for teeth set too wide on the denture, inadequate overjet, and entrapment of food because of the inclination of the buccal cusps. Cheek chewing may result from inadequate overjet of the maxillary molars both buccally and distally. A denture may come loose after being worn for only a few hours; this is frequently caused by accumulation of thick mucinous saliva under it. Having the patient wash the denture off occasionally will usually indicate whether or not this is the cause.

The stability of the lower denture is related, among other things, to the position of the bicuspids and the thickness of the periphery of the denture. The buccal aspect of the first bicuspid should not be more prominent bucally than the buccal flange of the denture. The peripheral flange should be thin in the region of frenula, lips, and molar region.

Partially Edentulous Mouth

Examination of the partially edentulous mouth includes a thorough examination of the whole mouth, the remaining teeth, and the denture-bearing areas (Fig. 175). The examination may be given for the purpose of considering the mouth preparatory to partial dentures, for evaluating dentures which are al-

A   B

C

Fig. 175. *Examination of partially edentulous mouth.* **A,** Relation of maxillary molars to edentulous area. **B,** Position of sublingual tissue to edentulous area. **C,** Clinical survey regarding planes of insertion of an appliance.

ready in use, or for appraising the response of the tissues to the dentures. Whatever the reason for the examination, the mouth should be completely examined for the presence of disease or potentially harmful conditions.

It goes without saying that a complete examination of the mouth is necessary prior to the preparation for partial dentures. The prerequisite of a complete examination has been discussed previously. The condition of the teeth and their supporting structures must be known prior to the construction of partial dentures. It is only after these structures have been evaluated that the dentist can know what elements of the partial denture prosthesis have to be considered. Whether or not a tooth and its supporting structure is a suitable abutment can be determined only by an examination of these structures. Thus, periodontal disease, carious lesions, devital teeth, poor root form, malposed teeth, teeth with abnormal anatomic crowns, unerupted teeth, root fragments, soft tissue lesions, and systemic disease are factors which have an important bearing on the placement of partial dentures; each must be evaluated by history and examination.

It is not the purpose of this book to dwell on the indications and contraindications for partial dentures or to justify the use of fixed or removable appliances. Both forms of appliances have common aims: to increase the function of mastication; to prevent extrusion, drifting, and hyperfunction of the remaining teeth; and to improve esthetic and phonetic qualities of the mouth.

The examination of the partially edentulous mouth should consider the following items: (1) vitality of the teeth, caries, attrition, (2) condition of the supporting tissues of the teeth, (3) status of the edentulous areas, (4) arrangement and position of the remaining teeth, (5) occlusal relationships, (6) intermaxillary space and vertical dimension, (7) oral hygiene, (8) form of roots and crowns of the teeth to be used as abutments, (9) relationship of the alveolar ridge to frenula, soft tissues, and bony eminences, (10) relationship of free gingival margin to placement of the appliance, (11) anteroposterior and lateral relationship of opposing arches, and (12) ability of the tissues of the edentulous areas to act as a denture-bearing area. These are the basic principles of the examination necessary for the restoration of any edentulous space, whether it be with a fixed or removable appliance.

The examination of the appliance already placed should consider all of the preceding factors plus an evaluation of the adjustment of both the tissues and the patient to the appliance. These factors should be brought out and elaborated upon in the history and examination of the patient. A periodic examination of appliances as well as the structures of the masticatory system should be a part of an efficient dental practice.

The consideration and selection of abutment teeth for a fixed or removable appliance must follow the needs and dictates of each case, and consideration must be given to the status of the pulp, the form and length of the root, the stability of the tooth, and the condition of the supporting tissues. Irrespective of the type of appliance, the ability of the tooth to be used and retained as an abutment must receive due consideration. Thus, the first step in an examination of the teeth and arches for a prosthetic appliance should be the determination of the status of the teeth and supporting structures.

The vitality of any tooth to be used or that has been used as an abutment should be routinely tested. Retrograde pulp changes may not be obvious to the patient or to the examiner until the extra load on an abutment tooth causes a rapid deterioration of the pulp. While pulp testing may not completely appraise minor pulp abnormalities, a sufficient number of abnormal teeth may be discovered by routine testing to make the effort well worth while. The location and extent of carious lesions should be determined. Such a determination may require removal of all the decay before a final evaluation can be made.

The condition of the supporting structures of the teeth also has to be evaluated before proceeding with the construction of an appliance. If periodontal disease is present, extensive treatment may be required to prepare the mouth for an appliance. In many instances teeth which appear to be good abutments superficially have to be extracted because of bifurcation and trifurcation involvement.

Edentulous areas should be examined clinically and radiographically for the presence of lesions, unerupted teeth, retained root tips, and foreign objects such as amalgam.

The arrangement and position of the teeth are directly related to the design of an appliance. Malposed teeth present problems in the final placement of fixed appliances, preparation of the teeth for retainers, and interocclusal harmony. They also present problems in the design of clasps, line of insertion, and line of draw for removable appliances. These factors can best be evaluated by the use of a surveyor.

The location of edentulous areas is of importance in determining whether or not an appliance is to be fixed or removable. The use of a classification system to describe the type of partial edentulism present facilitates the discussion of a case without resorting to the cumbersome task of naming all the teeth present in the arch. Such a classification as advocated by Kennedy is an aid to the terminology used in oral diagnosis and has practical application in partial denture design. It must be remembered that such a classification is never a diagnosis. The designation Class I is given to those cases in which bilateral edentulous areas are located posterior to the remaining teeth; Class II, to those cases in which a unilateral edentulous area is located posterior to the remaining teeth; Class III, to those cases in which there is a unilateral edentulous space with teeth remaining posterior and anterior to it; and Class IV, to those cases in which a unilateral edentulous space is present involving the midline.

Occlusal relationships are important to the stability, retention, and maintenance of appliances as well as to trauma of the remaining teeth when occlusal disharmony exists. Extruded and drifted teeth should be analyzed in their functional relations and in relation to the appliance which is to be placed (Fig. 176). Equilibration of the natural dentition may be necessary for the preparation of

A   B

Fig. 176. *Examination of partially edentulous mouth.* **A,** Cast showing relationship of teeth to edentulous area. **B,** Root form unfavorable for an abutment tooth.

the mouth. This must be considered before construction of the appliance begins. Working, balancing, and protrusive relationships should be evaluated. An alteration of the form of the remaining teeth should be considered in relation to improving the function of the occlusion. Not infrequently an appliance is constructed without first considering what modification of the teeth can be accomplished to improve the number of harmonious contacts in lateral excursion. Unfortunately in many such instances the working bite will consist of only one or two teeth being in contact in lateral movements of the jaw. In a large number of instances judicious grinding will result in bringing more of the remaining teeth into contact in the working bite. It will also allow the replacement of the missing teeth in the appliance in a functional position for lateral movements.

The intermaxillary space should be evaluated since in many instances little space may be present for the placement of teeth or the ideal placement of the metal framework, connectors, and occlusal rests (Fig. 170). Frequently a patient will have lost all the lower molars with the result that the upper molars have drifted and encroached upon the denture area of the lower arch (Fig. 176). This is a significant finding and has an important bearing on the preparation of the mouth for an appliance and on the design of the appliance.

Oral hygiene is an important factor in the maintenance of any appliance. Establishing good oral hygiene and teaching the patient to maintain it are important factors in the health of the supporting structures. This phase of treatment should be considered prior to the placement of an appliance. Any type of appliance requires that the patient take additional care of the mouth to prevent the accumulation of debris in abutment areas. Poor oral hygiene in itself may be a strong contraindication for many or all appliances.

The form of the roots of teeth that are to be used as support for an appliance is of considerable importance. Short conical roots may preclude the use of a tooth for an abutment (Fig. 176, *B*). The form of the crown is important to the type of retainer which may be used and to the placement of clasps if the appliance is of the removable type. The presence and location of undercuts in the anatomic crown of an abutment tooth are directly related to the position and design of the retaining parts of the appliance. In some instances the crown of a tooth may have to be completely altered either by grinding or by full crown restorations in order to have a line of draw or retention areas for clasps.

The relationship of the alveolar crest to frenula, soft tissues, and bony eminences should be determined (Fig. 177). Lingual bars of lower partial dentures may encroach upon the lingual frenulum when its attachment is high or when the alveolar process has been resorbed. When this occurs, frenula attachments may have to be altered, or the design of the partial denture may have to be altered to the point that the lingual bar does not rest on soft tissue but on the teeth. The presence of undercuts in the alveolar ridge and adjacent tissues may of necessity require that the line of draw be altered or the undercut removed. Such conditions should be evaluated during the examination of the mouth; in some instances such an evaluation may determine what type of appliance, if any, can be constructed for the patient. The use of casts and a surveyor will be of significant benefit in evaluation of the undercut areas. The

Fig. 177. *Examination of partially edentulous mouth.* Relationship of remaining teeth to edentulous arch.

presence of large bony eminences like palatine and mandibular tori directly affects the design and position of palatal and lingual bars if not removed. These protuberances should be noted in the examination and considered in the treatment plan.

The location of the gingival margin should be considered in relation to the design and placement of the framework of partial dentures. Also of importance is the relationship of the gingival margin to the placement of the gingival margin of a retainer. In some instances its position may also affect the placement of clasps. Hyperplastic papillae on the mesial or distal aspects of an abutment tooth are a potential source of trouble and can also interfere with the design of an appliance. This tissue with its relationship to the appliance and abutment predisposes to the development of deep crevices or even periodontal pockets. Removal of the tissue should be considered in the examination and related to the preparation of the mouth for the appliance. Lingual bars and connectors of partial dentures have to be designed in order to avoid encroachment on the free gingival margin.

The anteroposterior and lateral relationships of the opposing arches should be noted and evaluated. As in the construction of full dentures, the proper relationship of the teeth to the arches is an important consideration. The anteroposterior relationship of the maxillary and mandibular arches should be determined in centric relation as well as in centric occlusion. Premature contacts may result in a false anterior displacement of the mandible.

The state of the soft and hard tissues which are to bear the prosthetic appliance is an important factor in the successful wearing of the appliance. Thin, atrophic, or soft and hyperplastic tissue is not a good base for partial dentures; the examiner should evaluate all such areas which are to be used for supporting the denture. Older patients may frequently have thin and atrophic tissue which cannot stand the trauma of an appliance. Patients with Plummer-Vinson syndrome frequently complain of the inability to wear any type of tissue-borne appliance. When the examination reveals that tissue is soft and atrophic in those areas to be used as a denture base, careful consideration must be given to the design of the appliance and the possibility of toughening the tissue by massage.

Complaints relative to partial dentures already being worn are similar to those relative to full dentures. In addition, complaints concerning sore teeth may be found. Sore teeth may result from occlusal trauma, especially associated with occlusal rests being "high," from constant displacement of the teeth by excessively tight clasps, and from displacement of the teeth during the insertion of the appliance. Complaints concerning fixed appliances are usually related to occlusal trauma, balancing interferences, and heavy loading of an abutment tooth not accustomed to its increased function.

REFERENCES

Anderson, G. M.: Practical Orthodontics, St. Louis, 1948, The C. V. Mosby Co.

Baume, L. J.: Physiological Tooth Migration and Its Significance for the Development of Occlusion: I. Biogenetic Course of Deciduous Dentition, J. D. Res. **29**:123-132, 1950; II. Biogenesis of Accessional Dentition, J. D. Res. **29**:331-337, 1950; III. Biogenesis of the Successional Dentition, J. D. Res. **29**:338-348, 1950; IV. The Biogenesis of Overbite, J. D. Res. **29**:440-447, 1950.

Beyron, H.: Occlusal Changes in the Adult Dentition, Sv. Tandl.-Tskr. **45**:119-169, 1952.

Committee on Nomenclature: Committee Adopts Official Method for the Symbolic Designation of Teeth, J.A.D.A. **34**:647, 1947.

Dempster, W. T.: Selected Dissections of the Facial Regions for Advanced Dental Students, Ann Arbor, 1956, The Overbeck Co.

Downs, W. B.: Variations in Facial Relationships: Their Significance in Treatment and Prognoses, Am. J. Orthodontics **34**:812-840, 1948.

Friel, S.: The Development of Ideal Occlusion of the Gum Pads and Teeth, Am. J. Orthodontics **40**:196-227, 1954.

Hals, Einar, and Olow, Märta: Turner Teeth, Odont. Tskr. **66**:199-212, 1958.

Kingery, R. H.: Lectures on Complete Dentures, Ann Arbor, 1958, University of Michigan, School of Dentistry.

Lo, R. T., and Moyers, R. E.: Studies in the Etiology and Prevention of Malocclusion, Am. J. Orthodontics **39**:460-467, 1953.

McCoy, J. D.: Applied Orthodontics, Philadelphia, 1941, Lea & Febiger.

Moyers, R. E.: Handbook of Orthodontics, Chicago, 1958, Year Book Publishers, Inc.

Thielemann, K.: Biomechanik der paradentose, Leipzig, 1938, Herman Meusser.

Witkop, C. J.: Hereditary Defects in Enamel and Dentin, Acta genet. (Basel) **7**:236-9, 1957.

Wright, C. R., and others: A Study of the Tongue and Its Relation to Denture Stability, J.A.D.A. **39**:269, 1949.

Radiographic examination

Dental radiographs, when correlated with the case history and clinical examination, are among the most important diagnostic supplements in oral diagnosis. Well-taken radiographs examined under the proper conditions may reveal evidence of disease which cannot be discovered by any other method. There are numerous pathologic situations which cannot be detected clinically until a large amount of normal tissue is involved; yet, a radiograph may reveal such a situation while it is still incipient. This can be said of such entities as odontogenic cysts and tumors, neoplasms of bone, reaction of bone to devital teeth, and many others. If the dentist neglects to use an adequate number of radiographs at regular intervals, he ignores an extremely valuable diagnostic procedure. Misuse of radiographs by using them only for the detection of dental caries encourages neglect of other major dental problems.

There has been much discussion among dental radiologists relative to the most desirable method or technic for obtaining radiographs. Regardless of the preference for a particular technic, the final product is, of course, of the utmost importance. The technic used should be mastered so that all of the features which a diagnostician desires in a radiograph are present. The requirements of any good radiograph, regardless of technic, are (1) a clear sharp image of the anatomic area involved, (2) inclusion of a sufficient normal area surrounding the pathologic area being examined, (3) proper contrast between tissues of varying densities, and (4) minimal distortion.

It is important that radiographs be examined under proper lighting conditions. Properly exposed radiographs will show varying amounts of detail, depending upon the intensity of the light used to view them. Quite frequently detail is not seen in a radiograph because the lighting is too dim, and, in many instances, a bright light will bring out detail which is not seen under ordinary lighting conditions.

The most common mistake made in radiographic examinations is that of omission. It is not an uncommon practice in dentistry to include posterior bite-wing radiographs and periapical radiographs of the anterior teeth only in the initial radiographic examination and then to repeat only the posterior bite-wing

A

B

Fig. 178. *Radiographic examination.* **A,** Posterior bite-wing radiographs. **B,** Periapical radiographs. **B** shows that posterior bite-wing radiographs are inadequate to demonstrate findings other than those associated with the crowns of the teeth; note that dentigerous cyst and impacted molar are not seen in posterior bite-wing radiographs.

radiographs in subsequent examinations at six-month or yearly intervals. In instance after instance it can be shown that posterior bite-wing radiographs without periapical radiographs of the complete mouth are far from sufficient (Fig. 178). Too frequently, pathologic areas involving the apices and radicular portions of teeth are missed because an insufficient number of radiographs are taken. The minimum to be taken in the initial examination of any patient, dentulous or edentulous, should include radiographs of the complete mouth as well as posterior bite-wing radiographs if the posterior teeth are present.

It is a common practice to charge a separate fee for radiographs. This makes it seem as though the dentist is offering a product for that fee. It is far more desirable to charge one fee for the service of conducting a thorough and efficient examination, including interpretation of the radiographs. The radiographs in themselves are of no value to the patient—it is the ability of the dentist to interpret those radiographs accurately for which the patient pays the fee.

INTERPRETATION OF NORMAL RADIOGRAPHS

The basic prerequisite for radiographic interpretation is an understanding of what constitutes normal. The normal architecture of the hard tissues as seen radiographically, as well as the normal landmarks, must be recognized by the examiner and distinguished from pathologic conditions. It must be remembered that the radiographic image seen on the x-ray film is a "shadow" of hard tissues which do not permit the complete passage of x-rays through them. The varying degrees of density or calcification of bone and teeth permit varying amounts of x-rays to reach the x-ray film. The areas occupied by the denser structures such as teeth and bone appear lighter (radiopaque) on x-ray film, since a large portion of the x-rays is stopped and therefore not permitted to reach and expose the x-ray film. Areas occupied by the soft tissues or by air allow the passage of almost all of the x-rays and appear black (radiolucent) on film. What one actually sees when he examines a radiograph is a two-dimensional shadow of the structure radiographed. The fact that the radiograph is only two dimensional permits superimposition of one structure upon another in the radiograph. When the diagnostician examines a radiograph, he must always keep in mind that what he sees is merely variations in density of hard tissues and that he also sees a shadow of all of the tissue which occupied the space between the x-ray film and the source of the x-rays.

Normal Landmarks—Periapical Radiographs

There are several normal anatomic landmarks which can be recognized on radiographs taken in different parts of the mouth. These landmarks vary in position, size, and clarity from one individual to another, and they correspond to normal anatomic structures which are seen by every dental student in anatomy dissections.

The Maxilla (Fig. 179).—The following landmarks are recognizable in radiographs of the maxilla.

Incisive Foramen.—The incisive foramen is visible in the anterior midline of the maxilla between the roots of the maxillary incisor teeth. The foramen usually appears as an oval-shaped, somewhat radiolucent area surrounded by a relatively dense layer of bone.

Nasal Septum.—The nasal septum is visible as a vertical radiopaque band well above the apices of the central incisors and is centrally located in the radiograph.

Incisive Fossa.—Between the roots of the cuspid and central incisor teeth and over the apex of the lateral incisor tooth is an area which appears to be less dense than the surrounding tissue. This corresponds to the incisive fossa and is in fact an anatomic area which contains less thickness of bone than the areas lateral to it.

Maxillary Sinus.—The maxillary sinus produces a large radiolucent area usually extending from the bicuspid area posteriorly to the second molar region. Sinus septa can be seen as radiopaque lines running through the maxillary sinus, and an important landmark, the so-called antral Y, marks the separation of the anterior portion of the maxillary sinus from the nasal cavity. The antral Y is seen in the radiograph of the cuspid region. In young persons the maxillary sinus is confined to an area near the apices of the teeth, while in older persons this sinus extends well down toward the alveolar crest, and it may appear as though the roots of the maxillary bicuspid and molar teeth actually project into the maxillary sinus.

A   B   C

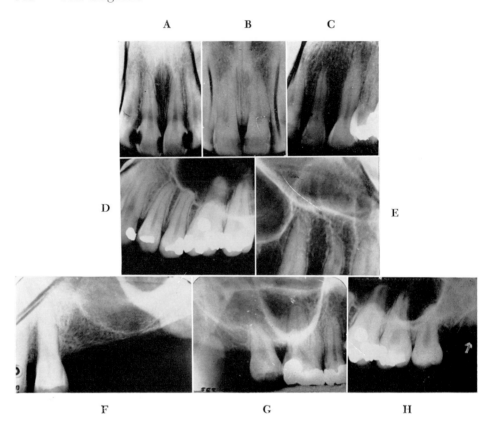

D

E

F   G   H

Fig. 179. *Radiographic examination—landmarks.* **A,** Incisive canal. **B,** Nasal septum. **C,** Incisive fossa. **D,** Maxillary sinus. **E,** Antral Y. **F,** Molar bone. **G,** Coronoid process. **H,** Hamular process.

Malar Bone.—This appears radiographically as a U-shaped radiopaque band at the maxillary first molar area and is frequently superimposed on the roots of the maxillary first molar.

Coronoid Process.—Quite frequently when the second molar region is radiographed, a fingerlike projection can be seen in the inferior and posterior corner of the film. This bony structure represents the coronoid process of the mandible.

Hamulus.—A small projection of bone may be seen just posterior to the maxillary tuberosity in many radiographs of the second molar region. This represents the hamular process of the medial pterygoid plate.

•   •   •

The maxillary radiographic landmarks which are likely to cause confusion are the maxillary sinus, which is often confused with a cystic area by the inexperienced examiner; the incisive fossa, which may give the impression of a rarefied area about the lateral incisor root apex; and the incisive foramen, which, when rather large, may suggest the presence of an incisive canal cyst or an area

A   B

Fig. 180. *Radiographic examination—landmarks.* Incisive foramen superimposed on apex of central incisor.

of bone rarefaction over the central incisor if superimposed on the apex of the central incisor (Fig. 180).

The Mandible (Fig. 181).—The following landmarks are recognizable in radiographs of the mandible.

Lingual Foramen.—In the anterior midline of the mandible inferior to the apices of the central incisor teeth is the lingual foramen. This is not seen on all mandibular incisor radiographs. However, when visualized, it is a circumscribed radiopaque area with a center which is radiolucent and about 0.5 mm. in diameter.

Genial Tubercles.—The genial tubercles can be seen only when the base of the mandible is visible in the mandibular central incisor radiograph. They appear as sharp radiopaque projections from the lingual cortical plate of bone.

Mental Foramen.—The mental foramen is located near the apices of the bicuspid teeth in the mandible. In the greatest percentage of human jaws the mental foramen is seen radiographically between the two bicuspid teeth. However, its position may vary from a position anterior to the first bicuspid to one which is posterior to the second bicuspid. Multiple mental foramens do occur.

Mental Ridge.—Due to the heavy cortical plate of bone in certain areas of the mandible, there are definite linear structures which produce normal radiographic landmarks. The mental ridge is one of these structures. It appears as an inverted V-shaped radiopaque structure and may be superimposed on the incisor roots.

Submaxillary Fossa.—Another normal radiographic finding on the mandible is that of the depression beneath the mandibular molar roots which is occupied by the submaxillary salivary gland. This area of the mandible is somewhat thinner than the surrounding bone and therefore may lack trabecular pattern and may appear comparatively radiolucent.

Mandibular Canal.—In the area beneath the first, second, and third molar roots the mandibular canal appears as a horizontal linear radiolucent band bordered by two radiopaque lines.

Fig. 181. *Radiographic examination—landmarks.* **A,** Lingual foramen. **B,** Genial tubercle. **C** and **D,** Mental foramen. **E,** Mental ridge. **F,** Submaxillary fossa. **G,** Mandibular canal, mylohyoid and external oblique line moving from inferior to superior. **H,** Projection of impacted third molar roots into inferior alveolar canal.

External Oblique Line.—Immediately superior to the mandibular canal is another radiopaque linear structure which represents the external oblique line.

• • •

The areas in the mandible which produce confusion in interpretation of radiographs for the inexperienced examiner are the mental foramen, particularly when it is superimposed over the apex of one of the bicuspid teeth, and the submaxillary gland fossa which sometimes appears as an area of bone rarefaction.

General Landmarks (Fig. 182).—The general landmarks recognizable in radiographs include the alveolar process, alveolar bone, and periodontal space.

Alveolar Process.—The alveolar process is that bone which is trabecular in pattern and surrounds the roots of the teeth. The bony architecture of the alveolar process varies from one area to another, particularly in the size of the trabeculae and the size of the marrow spaces. Patterns of trabeculae also vary from one person to another. One particularly characteristic variation in pattern is that of the so-called "stepladder" trabecular arrangement which is frequently seen between the roots of the mandibular incisor teeth.

Alveolar Bone.—The alveolar bone is the cortical bone which immediately surrounds the teeth and therefore lines the alveolus of the tooth. It is often referred to as the lamina dura radiographically and under normal circumstances is a radiopaque line of relatively uniform thickness which is continuous around the entire root of the tooth. The term lamina dura also includes the cortical bone which extends over the alveolar crest and gives the impression that the lamina dura is a continuous line from one alveolus to another. The most coronal portion of the alveolar process, as well as the lamina dura which occupies the space between two adjacent teeth, is referred to as the alveolar crest. The crest is normally within 1 to 1.5 mm. of the cementoenamel junction of the adjacent tooth.

Periodontal Space.—The radiolucent line between the root of the tooth and the alveolar bone represents the space occupied by the periodontal membrane. Normally the periodontal space is of nearly uniform width around the entire root of the tooth.

Fig. 182. *Radiographic examination—landmarks.* Alveolar process and alveolar bone.

METHOD OF RADIOGRAPHIC EXAMINATION

As previously stated, the minimum dental radiographic examination should include radiographs of the complete mouth (14 periapical films) and posterior bite-wing radiographs (No. 1 and No. 2 size films to allow two views with different horizontal angulations in order to reduce overlap areas) if enough posterior teeth are present to warrant them. Auxiliary radiographs may be used wherever indicated and will be discussed later.

Well-organized, methodic examination of the radiograph is imperative if the dentist is to make complete use of this valuable diagnostic aid. Whenever possible, correlation between clinical and radiographic findings is extremely important to minimize the interpretation of an artifact in the radiograph as a disease process. The organization of the radiograph viewing procedure minimizes the possibility of overlooking important details. A methodic approach to radiographic viewing develops the habit of examining all radiographs in the same sequence, thereby increasing the accuracy of the viewing procedure.

OUTLINE OF THE SEQUENCE FOR VIEWING RADIOGRAPHS

Complete Mouth Radiographs

1. Lamina dura associated with teeth and the cortical bone associated with denture-bearing areas—continuity and thickness
2. Periodontal spaces—variations in width
3. Level of the alveolar crest in relation to cementoenamel junction
4. Periapical radiolucency
5. Pathologic conditions of the teeth
6. Pathologic conditions of the jaws—osseous radiolucencies and osseous radiopacities
7. Other dental findings

Posterior Bite-wing Radiographs

1. Lamina dura continuity at the alveolar crest
2. Alveolar crest level in relation to the cementoenamel junction
3. Tooth crown shape and formative defects of the tooth crown
4. Pulp size and degree of pulpal calcification
5. Existing restorations
6. Location of calculus
7. Location of carious lesions

RADIOGRAPHS OF THE COMPLETE MOUTH
Lamina Dura—Continuity and Thickness

The lamina dura normally forms a continuous line around the roots of the teeth and over the alveolar crest between the teeth. It should be examined in the same numerical sequence as the teeth are examined to preclude the possibility of missing any area. Periapical films provide the means for examining the lamina dura in most areas, although the bite-wing films are often helpful in determining its continuity over the alveolar crest in the posterior part of the dental arch.

A lack of continuity of alveolar crest lamina dura is indicative of active periodontal disease (Fig. 183). This very important finding, if overlooked, can cause the examiner to miss the diagnosis of incipient periodontal disease, since resorption of the alveolar crest lamina dura is the initial bone loss which occurs

Fig. 183. *Absence of lamina dura* at alveolar crest and lateral surface of root.

Fig. 184. *Absence of lamina dura* at apex of mesial root of first molar due to devital pulp.

in periodontitis. The success of periodontal treatment can be evaluated radiographically in many cases since the lamina dura will reappear when the gingival inflammatory process is eliminated.

A break in continuity of lamina dura at the apical area of the tooth occurs as the result of inflammatory reaction of the periapical tissue to a devital pulp (Fig. 184). The break will occur in either an acute or chronic periapical inflammation and the extent of the lack of continuity is dependent on the extent of the inflammatory process. An acute periapical inflammatory process can always be correlated with the clinical findings of a tooth which is painful to percussion or biting pressures and the presence of swelling or abscess formation, depending on how marked the inflammatory response is and how far it has progressed. A chronic inflammatory process will show varying degress of involvement of the lamina dura and usually will be asymptomatic.

Interruption of the lamina dura associated with the lateral aspect of the root of a tooth is usually due to the extension of periodontal disease. In acute periodontal abscess the resorption of the lamina dura occurs very rapidly and is accompanied by clinical signs and symptoms of abscess formation (Fig. 185). A periodontal pocket which is progressing rapidly also shows interruption of the lamina dura and can be demonstrated clinically, although it may be asymptomatic. When no periodontal pocket or abscess formation can be demonstrated clinically in relation to the disappearance of the lamina dura from the lateral root surface, then the possibilities of trauma, lateral root cyst formation, or neoplasm should be considered. Other radiographic evidence of lateral root cyst or neoplasm usually accompanies the disappearance of lamina dura.

Fig. 185. *Absence of lamina dura* from lateral root surface associated with periodontal abscess. Note probe in the area of abscess.

Fig. 186. *Absence of lamina dura* in bifurcation area of mandibular second molar.

In radiographs which show considerable periodontal disease, examination for continuity of the lamina dura in the trifurcation area of maxillary molars and the bifurcation area of mandibular molars is very important (Fig. 186). A disappearance of lamina dura in these areas indicates that the periodontal destruction has advanced to the area of root division and the degree of destruction becomes very important in the consideration of retention of teeth so involved.

The cortical bone is continuous in edentulous arches under normal conditions. It should appear as a regular unbroken line at the crest of the well-healed edentulous ridge (Fig. 187). The cortical bone in edentulous areas is susceptible to the same resorptive changes as the lamina dura about functioning teeth. Pressure and inflammation are capable of disrupting the cortical bone at the crest of the edentulous ridge. By far the most common resorptive change in cortical bone over the edentulous ridge occurs in the situation in which a maxillary denture is worn opposing natural mandibular anterior teeth and without posterior support. When a mandibular partial denture which needs rebasing is worn and does not support the posterior part of the maxillary complete denture, anterior resorption will occur in the maxilla. Radiographically this type of resorption is

A

B

Fig. 187. *Continuity of cortical layer of bone* in edentulous arch. **A,** Lack of continuity in left cuspid region. **B,** Lack of continuity in right and left cuspid regions.

Fig. 188. *Increased width of lamina dura* and *widened periodontal space* due to occlusal trauma.

evident from bicuspid to bicuspid region of the anterior portion of the edentulous maxillary arch. The resorption can be correlated with the clinical finding of a flabby ridge and in many instances with an accompanying inflammatory reaction in the overlying tissue. The patient in such instances complains of looseness of the maxillary denture or uses denture adhesive constantly to provide denture stability.

The thickness of the lamina dura about the roots of teeth is, in general, uniform. There are minor degrees of variation from one area of the mouth to another, but the radiographic interpreter should be alerted by variations of thickness of lamina dura on the same tooth. The changes which occur in traumatic occlusion are evidenced by a compensatory widening of lamina dura associated with the portion of the tooth where tension is applied to the periodontal membrane as the tooth is traumatized (Fig. 188). A clinical appraisal of occlusal function will usually substantiate the radiographic findings.

Periodontal Spaces—Variations in Width

Uniformity of the width of the periodontal space is evident about teeth which are functioning normally. The space averages from 0.18 to 0.25 mm. in width (Kronfeld). The minor variations in width depend on the level of the periodontal membrane under consideration. Physiologic movement of a tooth results in slightly wider periodontal membrane at the apical and cervical regions due to movement about a fulcrum point near the midpoint of the root of the tooth. Nonfunctional teeth show narrowing of the periodontal space. A tooth in traumatic occlusion shows characteristic excessive widening of the periodontal space near the alveolar crest (Fig. 189). Excessive widening of the periodontal space is often visible near the apical portion of the root on the contralateral side of the traumatized tooth. The horizontal angulation of the radiograph sometimes masks one or both of these changes because the variation of breadth of periodontal space that is parallel to the x-ray at different horizontal angulations and because the involved surface of the tooth may be buccal or lingual and therefore not visualized. Widening of the periodontal space in the bifurcation and trifurcation areas of molars may be suggestive of either advance of periodontal disease to these areas or traumatic occlusion (Fig. 186). Widened periodontal spaces may be confirmed by clinical examination of the traumatized tooth

Fig. 189. *Widened periodontal space, calculus on distal aspect of second bicuspid, and loss of alveolar bone.*

which frequently shows increased mobility and produces a dull percussion note.

Initial periapical reactions to devital pulps are manifest radiographically as widened periodontal spaces at the apices of involved teeth. Recognition of this incipient finding may prevent extensive periapical involvement or severe pain and possibly severe infection. Confusion in diagnosis may arise when the periapical periodontal membrane is widened as a result of vertical occlusal trauma to the affected tooth. The suspicion of a devital tooth in the course of the radiographic examination should always be confirmed by the appropriate pulp tests.

Level of the Alveolar Crest in Relation to the Cementoenamel Junction

The normal level of the alveolar crest is from 1 to 1.5 mm. apical to the cementoenamel junction (Fig. 190). Reduction of the level is indicative of the extent of periodontal disease but not always indicative of active periodontal disease; however, when the alveolar crest is seen at a reduced level without the lamina dura intact over it, the examiner can assume that the periodontal disease is active.

There may be confusion in judging the level of the alveolar crest in the maxillary molar region due to the vertical angulation at which this area is radiographed and the buccolingual width of the crest. The vertical angulation

Fig. 190. *Normal complete mouth radiograph.*

results in a projection of the buccal portion of the alveolar crest coronally (Fig. 191). The "long cone" technic is capable of producing a truer radiographic reproduction of this area.

The level of the alveolar crest is a very important consideration in the selection of teeth to be retained in periodontal treatment and in the selection of abutment teeth for prosthetic appliances. No rule of thumb will hold true for the acceptable level of the alveolar crest due to the variation in root form and root size. However, when a tooth has less than half its original periodontal support, it is usually not able to withstand the additional load of a prosthesis.

The terms horizontal and vertical bone loss have been applied loosely to the two different patterns of reduction in height of the alveolar crest. The term horizontal bone loss applies to a more or less uniform reduction of the alveolar crest which is associated with periodontal disease on the basis of a uniform inflammatory process (Fig. 192). The inflammatory process is mainly due to calculus and poorly adapted cervical margins of restorations. Vertical bone loss, on the other hand, refers to localized reduction in height of the alveolar crest, in which case one or several teeth will show supporting bone destruction while adjacent teeth show little or none (Fig. 193). Vertical bone loss is usually at-

Fig. 191. *Demonstration of buccal and lingual bone levels.* Note trifurcation involvement of first molar and deep caries on mesial aspect of second biscuspid and distal aspect of second molar.

Fig. 192. *Horizontal loss of alveolar bone and alveolar process.* Note bifurcation involvement on first and second molars.

Fig. 193. *Vertical loss of alveolar bone.* **A,** Lingual aspect of lateral incisor. **B,** Distal and lingual aspect of second molar. **C,** Single area of involvement on mesial aspect of maxillary right central incisor.

tributed to traumatic factors such as traumatic occlusion, food impaction, and periodontal abscess formation.

Examination of the level of the alveolar crest is particularly important in relation to molar teeth when the level of the crest is lowered to the bifurcation or trifurcation area. Due to the angulation of maxillary molar radiographs, the involvement of root trifurcations is difficult to determine. The difficulty arises because, as stated before, the buccal level of alveolar crest is projected more to the occlusal than to the lingual level. Careful examination in the maxillary molar region will reveal the lingual level of the alveolar crest as an indistinct line apical to the buccal level. The lingual level is a more accurate level since it is the anatomic portion of the jaw in that area which is closest to the film and, therefore, less subject to distortions of angulation. It is not always possible, on clinical examination, to determine the involvement of trifurcation areas in periodontal disease, but a radiographic finding suggestive of trifurcation involvement should prompt specific clinical examination procedures for confirmation.

Periapical Radiolucency

Periapical radiolucency usually indicates a devital tooth. The exceptions to this are frequent enough, however, to warrant clinical confirmation by pulp test of any tooth suspected of being devital on the basis of radiographic findings (Fig. 194).

Periapical radiolucencies may be due to a variety of causes such as chronic periapical granuloma, radicular cyst, periapical abscess, and neoplasms. The most common causes are periapical granuloma and periapical abscess. Neoplasms are infrequently responsible for periapical rarefaction of bone, but when neoplasia is the cause this finding may be of grave importance. The odontogenic neoplasm, cementoma, in its osteolytic stage may be the cause of periapical radiolucency.

Acute periapical abscess in its initial stages may produce very little periapical change in radiodensity of bone, but as it becomes recurrent or long standing, the area of apical bone destruction becomes obvious. Usually there is sufficient clinical evidence of acute periapical inflammation to confirm early bone rarefaction at the apex of the tooth.

Fig. 194. *Periapical radiolucency* of first molar roots due to devital pulp.

Fig. 195. *Periapical radiolucency.* Radicular cyst on devital central incisor. Cuspid and lateral incisor are vital.

Chronic periapical granuloma is a chronic inflammatory process which represents reaction to a devital pulp. The area of bone involved varies considerably, depending on the period of time the tooth has been devital and on the individual human defense mechanism. There is a variation in relative radiolucency of granulomas which makes one easily discernible and another difficult to detect radiographically. There is seldom any clinical symptom to indicate that a tooth has a chronic periapical radiolucency.

Radicular cysts are always associated with devital teeth (Fig. 195). In their initial stages they cannot be distinguished with any accuracy from chronic periapical granuloma. When large, they have the characteristics of any bony cyst. A large radicular cyst is a radiolucent area surrounded by a thin layer of compact bone appearing radiographically similar to lamina dura. Radicular cysts are products of proliferation of the epithelial rests of Malassez in a chronic periapical granuloma. Such cysts are not accompanied by clinical symptoms unless secondarily infected, but, if they are large enough, they may produce local swelling and looseness of teeth.

Multiple cementoma is an odontogenic tumor which, at different stages of its development, produces both periapical radiolucency and radiopacity. The most common area of involvement is the mandibular anterior region. The initial stage is the osteolytic stage in which one or more teeth are involved, and this stage presents a radiographic picture identical to that of chronic periapical granuloma. Pulp testing will show the involved teeth to be vital.

Traumatic devitalization of teeth occurs readily in the mandibular anterior region. Teeth devitalized by trauma are often free of caries; therefore, a radiolucent zone at the apex of a mandibular anterior tooth which is free of caries may lead to confusion between periapical granuloma and cementoma. Vitality tests by reliable means provide the diagnosis.

Pathologic Conditions of the Teeth

Calcification of the Pulp.—Complete calcification of the pulp occurs for the most part in the incisor and cuspid teeth. In most cases of complete calcification,

Fig 196. *Secondary dentin formation* associated with deep restoration on distal aspect of first molar.

Fig. 197. *Pulp stones.*

a history of trauma to the involved tooth can be obtained. While complete calcification does occur following trauma it is not unusual for only part of the pulp to become calcified. Quite frequently the entire coronal portion of the pulp calcifies in a relatively short period of time following acute trauma to the tooth. In most instances teeth which show a marked degree of calcification of the pulp are vital and clinically they will show changes in color when compared to the adjacent teeth.

Minor degrees of calcification are seen in the dental pulp shortly after the tooth has reached occlusal contact and has received a functional load. Secondary dentin is laid down at a rate which varies with many factors such as occlusal attrition, dental caries, and the size of restorations and their proximity to the pulp (Fig. 196). Calcification of the pulp is a continuous process which is seen to a minor degree in the teeth of young persons and to a greater extent in older individuals.

Pulp stones are frequently seen in various places in the pulp. They occur in the chamber and in the canals. Radiographically they appear as radiopaque, regular, round areas of calcification and may be isolated in the center of the pulp chamber or apparently attached to one of the walls of the chamber (Fig.

197). Pulp stones, as well as the amount of secondary dentin which can be seen radiographically in the pulp canals, are of particular importance when a tooth is being evaluated for root canal therapy.

Caries.—Dental caries is by far the commonest pathologic change that will be seen radiographically in the teeth (Fig. 198). It is necessary that radiographs have proper contrast in order to show dental caries in all of the areas of the tooth in which decay occurs. Radiographs should be examined for caries in the same sequence each time. The carious lesions should be listed in numerical order as they are discovered on the radiograph. The list may be supplemented during the clinical examination, and, at the same time, lesions found radiographically can be verified clinically.

Initially, the carious process will appear as a V-shaped radiolucent zone in the enamel, with the apex of the V toward the dentoenamel junction when it occurs at the contact point of the tooth. When an initial carious area is in an

A

B   C

Fig. 198. *Dental caries.* **A**, Early interproximal dental caries on mandibular first and second molars; recurrent caries beneath and distal to occlusal restoration of second molar. **B**, Occlusal caries. **C**, Interproximal caries in mandibular anterior teeth.

occlusal developmental fissure, the process involving enamel is not easily detected, so that occlusal caries involves dentin before it is discovered radiographically. As the carious process involves the dentin, a wider radiolucent zone can be seen extending well beyond the apex of the lesion in the enamel along the junction between the enamel and dentin. In advanced dental caries the radiolucency will appear as a large dished-out area. When dental caries is advanced, it is quite simple to interpret radiographically. However, initial incipient caries involving occlusal fissures requires close examination of the radiographic film. It is important to confirm clinically the radiographic findings of dental caries whenever possible. Clinical confirmation of caries is particularly important in the anterior part of the mouth where silicate restorations are placed, since silicate restorations are radiolucent and may resemble caries radiographically. Silicate or plastic restorations are sometimes placed in bicuspid teeth in an attempt to preserve esthetics, and these also appear radiolucent and may be mistaken for carious lesions radiographically.

One of the most difficult of carious lesions to interpret on the dental radiograph is that of recurrent caries at the margins of existing restorations. Recurrent caries is particularly difficult to interpret in radiographs where steep vertical angulations have been used. Recurrent caries is virtually impossible to detect radiographically when it occurs beneath a buccal or lingual restoration. The commonest picture of recurrent marginal caries is that of a radiolucent zone extending inward from the cervical margin of interproximal restorations. Another location in which recurrent dental caries is somewhat difficult to detect radiographically is under existing silicate fillings in the anterior part of the mouth. A loss of the sharp outline of the cavity preparation may be the only radiographic evidence of recurrent caries under a silicate restoration.

Attrition.—Occlusal attrition is an obvious clinical finding which may be confused radiographically with extensive occlusal caries. Of course, clinical confirmation of attrition is readily made; even so, attrition and dental caries are occasionally coexistent.

Calculus.—Certain types of calculus can be seen radiographically on careful inspection of the x-ray film (Fig. 199). Calculus may appear as a spurlike projection near the proximocervical aspect of the tooth or as a linear radiopaque

Fig. 199. *Calculus.* Spurs of calculus and linear pattern of calculus; note also the cemental caries on the distal aspect of the second molar associated with periodontal disease.

Fig. 200. *Overhanging restorations.* Massive overhang on distocervical margin of first molar; note impaction of third molar associated with lack of bone support on distal root of second molar.

line running from mesial to distal aspects of the tooth, representing calculus on the buccal or lingual aspect of the tooth. Calculus which has been altered in contour with a scaler but incompletely removed will lose its angular appearance radiographically and will appear as a somewhat rounded elevation along the root surface of the tooth. The fine flat type of calculus which is tenaciously adherent to the root surface of the tooth is virtually impossible to detect radiographically, and therefore clinical examination is always important in spite of a lack of radiographic evidence of calculus.

Conditions Due to Overhanging Restorations.—Overhanging restorations at the proximocervical margin are rather easy to detect when the filling material is radiopaque in nature (Fig. 200). Overhanging margins of restorations on the buccal and lingual aspects of interproximal restorations or on buccal or lingual restorations are difficult to detect radiographically. However, careful clinical examination of the buccal and lingual areas will reveal any existing overhanging margins and the gingival inflammation which they produce.

Resorption.—Root resorption is not an uncommon radiographic finding and may be described as external and internal (Fig. 201). External root resorption may occur anywhere along the root of the tooth. Areas of root resorption give a radiographic picture of a noticeable irregularity in the contour of the root surface of the tooth. When resorption has occurred to a somewhat advanced degree at the apex, it may give the impression that the apical portion of the tooth has been cut off. Root resorption which occurs in an area where the periodontal membrane is intact is almost without exception due to trauma of some type. Types of trauma to be considered are traumatic occlusion, orthodontic movement, and prosthetic abutment overload. When external root resorption occurs opposite a radiolucent zone and the lamina dura and periodontal space are not intact, it should be a matter for serious consideration since neoplasms occurring about the roots of teeth have the ability to erode through the lamina dura and produce resorption of the root.

Internal resorption is a less frequent finding than external resorption and always occurs somewhere along the pulp canal or adjacent to the pulp chamber.

Fig. 201. *Root resorption.* **A,** External resorption associated with occlusal trauma. **B,** Internal resorption.

Fig. 202. *Hypercementosis* of first molar roots.

Radiographically it will appear as an indistinct and irregular zone of radio-lucency and may be confused with dental caries when the coronal pulp is involved. Where there has been extensive buccal recession of the gingiva, allowing the occurrence of carious lesions on the buccal or lingual root surface of the tooth, the carious lesion may give a radiographic impression of internal resorption.

Hypercementosis.—Hypercementosis, or excessive cementum deposition on the roots of the teeth, varies in degree from a situation which is barely discernible to one in which a rather massive amount of cementum has been laid down. The radiographic picture of hypercementosis shows an increase in the bulk of the root, and usually the portion of the root involved is easily detected radio-graphically since there is some change from expected contour of the root surface (Fig. 202).

A   B

Fig. 203. *Dilaceration.* A, Cuspid root; periapical granuloma on lateral incisor. B, Second bicuspid.

Dilaceration.—Dilaceration, or marked angular curvature of the root, is readily detected on periapical radiographs (Fig. 203). It occurs in varying degrees and may involve the root at any level. A very common area in which minimal dilaceration is seen is at the apical one-third of the maxillary lateral incisors. Dilaceration is an important consideration in the diagnosis of teeth which require endodontic treatment or extraction, since there is a limit to the root curvature which will permit passage of a root canal file and which will permit simple extraction without fracture of the root. Occasionally dilaceration is a factor in the selection of abutment teeth for bridges and partial dentures.

Abnormalities of Root Form.—Root form and length, the number of roots on teeth, and the portion of root supported by bone are important considerations in the selection of abutment teeth for dental prosthesis and are readily discernible on properly taken periapical x-ray films. It is especially important to minimize distortion of root length in obtaining periapical radiographs of possible abutments.

The degree of calcification of the radicular (root) portion of the pulp canal, the degree of curvature of the pulp canals, and the number of pulp canals present are important considerations in endodontic treatment. No arbitrary limits on the degree of curvature which can be negotiated by a root canal instrument are in existence, so the radiograph and the amount of root curvature will be regarded differently, depending on the ability of the individual dentist.

Formative Defects.—Formative defects (see Chapter 5) of enamel may be localized or generalized. Radiographically, localized areas of hypoplastic enamel appear similar to dental caries. Localized areas of hyperplasia are frequently multiple, round radiolucent zones. It is not unusual to see hypoplastic pits with associated underlying carious areas.

There are several different types of generalized defects of enamel, all of which have a hereditary etiology. Radiographically the findings in all the types are similar because of the tendency for the enamel to be thin and to abrade or fracture easily. The teeth tend to appear small radiographically due to the thinness of enamel. Attrition varies in degree with the age of the affected individual. Absence of pieces of enamel may be seen radiographically if fractures have occurred.

Turner's teeth show a deformity of the crown of the tooth which may involve only the incisal or occlusal portion of the enamel. Hutchinson's incisors have a screw driver shape radiographically, with the cervical width of the tooth being greater than the incisal width. They may also show a notched incisal edge. Mulberry molars have the radiographic appearance of a constricted occlusal surface without the normal cuspal pattern.

Defects of dentin are hereditary in etiology. Two important hereditary entities are dentinogenesis imperfecta and dentin dysplasia. Dentinogenesis imperfecta, or hereditary opalescent dentin, produces a radiographic picture of attrition, absence or near absence of root canals and pulps, and inconstant periapical radiolucency. Dentin dysplasia is characterized radiographically by absent or poorly developed roots, absence of root canals and pulp chambers, and presence of periapical radiolucencies on all teeth.

Other minor formative defects of teeth such as dens en dente, gemination, fusion, and concrescence are well described in oral pathology textbooks.

Pathologic Conditions of the Jaws

At this point in the radiographic examination the parts of the radiograph which have not received specific attention are inspected. There are numerous pathologic processes which might be cited under each of the subheadings; however, it is not the purpose of this book to present specific pathologic entities other than as examples to illustrate general principles.

Due to the wide variety of pathologic conditions which could be included, it is necessary to organize the possible findings into large general groups which have some common characteristics. Characteristics listed in the accompanying outline can serve as a guide to the examiner and lead him to a tentative diagnosis.

OUTLINE OF RADIOGRAPHIC CHARACTERISTICS OF OSSEOUS LESIONS

I. Osseous radiolucencies
   A. Osteolytic lesions
      1. Cysts (other than radicular)
      2. Neoplasms
         a. Benign
            (1) Odontogenic
            (2) Nonodontogenic
         b. Malignant
            (1) Primary
            (2) Secondary
      3. Endocrinopathic bone dysplasia
   B. Systemic disease
   C. Osteomyelitis
   D. Residual postoperative osseous defect

II. Osseous radiopacities
  A. Tumors
    1. Odontogenic
    2. Nonodontogenic
  B. Foreign bodies
  C. Bone dysplasias
III. Combination of osseous radiolucency and radiopacity
  A. Neoplasms
    1. Benign
      a. Odontogenic
      b. Nonodontogenic
    2. Malignant—primary
  B. Bone dysplasias
  C. Osteomyelitis
  D. Foreign bodies
IV. Other dental findings—impacted teeth, supernumerary teeth, root canal fillings

Osseous Radiolucencies

When a radiolucent area is discovered in radiographs of the complete mouth, the examiner should evaluate the lesion in a specific way. There is no justification for an examiner merely "feeling" a diagnosis; a diagnosis should be based on sound principles. Because of the great variation possible in each type of radiolucent lesion, in examining a pathologic area specific attention must be given to certain details and characteristics of the lesion. In evaluating radiolucent areas, the following should be considered: (1) location and extent of the radiolucency in reference to teeth, normal landmarks, and anatomic region, (2) relative degree of radiolucency, (3) presence or absence of any radiopaque areas or lines in the substance of the lesion, (4) nature of the borders of the lesion, (5) apparent effect of the process which is producing the radiolucency on the teeth and anatomic landmarks, and (6) possible origin of the lesion.

The location and extent of the radiolucency in reference to teeth, normal landmarks, and anatomic region reveal important information about the degree of involvement and the nature of a lesion of the bone. It is important to note whether a radiolucent zone is associated with an area from which teeth have been extracted or are congenitally absent. Certain pathologic conditions of the jaws have a tendency to occur in a certain area of either jaw or in one jaw in particular. In many pathologic conditions, location does not aid in the diagnosis. The amount of involvement is extremely variable in different radiolucent lesions; nevertheless, more extensive involvement may be expected of certain diseases. The extension and location are extremely important in considering the type of treatment and the prognosis.

The relative degree of radiolucency of different lesions is quite variable, depending on the nature of the pathologic process. Some processes produce tissue which is less radiolucent than that produced by other pathologic entities. A cystic process is generally more radiolucent than a process which is producing soft tissue. The amount of normal bone superimposed on a radiolucent area will alter the degree of radiolucency.

The presence or absence of radiopaque areas in the substance of a radiolucent lesion will reveal evidence of ossification centers or sequestra in the lesion. Radiopaque lines may show a tendency toward formation of compartments within a zone of osseous destruction. While loculation is not characteristic of a specific pathologic process, it is a radiographic feature which characterizes certain processes.

The nature of the borders of a radiolucency relates to some degree the growth characteristics of certain lesions of the jaws. Infiltrative, invasive lesions are not well demarcated by a sharp line of contrast between the normal and the radiolucent area. Lesions which grow rather slowly and are not invasive tend to be well outlined, and in many instances slow-growing lesions are surrounded by a definite layer of compact bone. Certain pathologic processes tend to invade surrounding bone in a locular or budding pattern and therefore present a rather characteristic border between the lesion and normal tissue.

The apparent effect of the pathologic process which is producing the radiolucency on the teeth and anatomic landmarks may help the examiner further characterize a radiolucent zone. There are a number of pathologic processes which produce resorption of the roots of the teeth adjacent to, or involved in, the process. Root resorption is by no means diagnostic of a particular lesion, but it should call several possible causes to the examiner's mind. Root resorption associated with a radiolucent zone should always be regarded seriously since it is seen in association with infiltrative neoplasms. Effects on landmarks such as obliteration of normal detail or expansion of normal boundaries of the jaws must also be considered as evidence of a pathologic process of an extensive and serious nature.

Possible origin of the lesion may be derived from its location and general characteristics. If the other considerations for examining radiolucent zones are carefully evaluated, the examiner should have at least one or several possible diagnoses in mind. He should consider the possibility of origin from tissues normally present in the jaws, from direct extension from outside the jaws such as from the maxillary sinus or oral mucosa, or from some distant tissue by indirect extension or metastasis.

The summary of the six general considerations for radiolucent zones should channel the possible diagnoses into the general areas listed previously.

Osteolytic Lesions.—Osteolytic lesions visible as radiolucent lesions include cysts, benign and malignant neoplasms, and endocrinopathic bone dysplasia.

Cysts.—Cysts are osteolytic in that they destroy bone by expansion. Because of their lack of clinical symptoms (unless very large or secondarily infected), they are usually discovered radiographically. They vary considerably in size, depending on the length of time they have been actively enlarging. Cysts adjacent to the maxillary sinus have been known to increase in size until the sinus is replaced by cystic structure.

In general, cysts are very radiolucent. Due to their expansion in all directions and to the limited buccolingual spaces in the jaws, there is usually little or no normal trabecular pattern superimposed on the cyst. The central portion may show signs of septal separation of locules or compartments. The borders are usually distinct due to a tendency for a thin cortical layer of bone to be main-

A   B   C

Fig. 204. *Osseous radiolucencies.* A, Nasopalatine cyst. B, Residual cyst. C, Dentigerous cyst.

tained at the walls of the cyst. The borders appear similar to lamina dura. The presence of a radiopaque cyst wall is not a constant criterion for radiographic diagnosis, since it does not always occur and because other lesions may form a similar boundary pattern.

The effects on structures surrounding a cyst are mainly the result of pressure from expansion of the cyst. Spreading of teeth, expansion of the normal buccal or lingual plate of the maxilla or mandible, and obliteration of normal radiographic landmarks are radiographic changes which may be caused by a cyst (Fig. 204).

Cysts, other than radicular, may arise from residual epithelium in lines of fusion of the jaws and are known as fissural cysts. Cysts may arise from primordial or residual odontogenic tissue in the jaws from the development of the dentition or from periodontal epithelial debris residual after the extraction of the teeth. The location of a cyst is suggestive of the origin of the lesion. Fissural cysts are seen in the midline of the maxilla or between the maxillary cuspid and lateral incisors or rarely at the symphysis of the mandible. Fissural cysts, particularly the globulomaxillary (arising between the maxillary cuspid and lateral incisor), may extend to involve the apices of adjacent teeth. When this occurs, it is difficult to differentiate between a fissural and a radicular cyst radiographically. When the apices of teeth are involved, the vitality of the teeth must be established to rule out radicular cyst. This distinction is important since the treatment of a fissural cyst differs from treatment of a radicular cyst.

Benign Neoplasms.—Benign neoplasms visible as radiolucent zones may be divided into odontogenic and nonodontogenic.

Odontogenic neoplasms: Neoplasms arising from odontogenic tissue which produce radiolucent areas in the radiograph are those which do not have the ability to form calcified structures. Since this group of odontogenic neoplasms includes ameloblastomas, there is a marked variation in the extent of involvement of the jaws in this group of lesions. In general, "soft" or radiolucent odontogenic neoplasms may arise in any area where there is or has been odontogenic tissue. In particular, ameloblastomas show a marked tendency to arise in the mandibular third molar area, and, depending upon the time at which they are discovered, may involve small to very large areas of the jaw.

The relative degree of radiolucency varies according to the type of neoplasm.

The ameloblastoma shows a great deal of variation from one type to another, since it may be solid or cystic. Cystic ameloblastomas may be a single cystic mass or multilocular in character. The single cystic mass shows the marked degree of radiolucency that characterizes most cysts, while the bony septa of the multilocular cystic ameloblastoma results in less penetration of x-rays; therefore, the cyst is less radiolucent. Other soft odontogenic neoplasms, such as soft mixed odontogenic tumors and odontogenic myxomas, show a relative radiolucency similar to that of any soft tissue in an area of bone destruction.

Radiopaque lines and areas are frequently seen in soft odontogenic neoplasms. A multilocular cystic ameloblastoma shows multiple trabeculae which represent the thin bony walls of the multiple compartments of the cyst. The mixed odontogenic neoplasm which has some potential for forming enamel, cementum, or dentin may show small areas of radiopacity within the substance of the radiolucent mass.

The borders of odontogenic neoplasms in general are not clearly defined. Even the cystic ameloblastoma tends to grow in a budding, invasive pattern, thereby producing an indistinct boundary compared to the relatively distinct border of cysts which are increasing in size by expansion only. Solid ameloblastomas also are invasive in growth character and offer no distinct radiographic boundary. Other soft odontogenic tumors are less invasive in character and therefore show more distinct radiographic delimitation.

Teeth and anatomic structure approximating a soft odontogenic neoplasm may show minimal to marked change radiographically as the result of pressure or expansion of the neoplastic mass. Disappearance of the lamina dura about the roots of teeth encroached upon by the mass is a common finding. Ameloblastomas are well known for their ability to produce external resorption of the roots which they involve. When large enough, any of the soft odontogenic tumors may produce expansion of the cortical plate.

The origin of soft odontogenic tumors is, of course, from the dental anlage. The degree of differentiation, when the tissue becomes neoplastic, and the tissue involved determine the type of tumor. None of the tumors can be classified positively by radiographic means alone.

Nonodontogenic neoplasms: Benign neoplasms of the jaws are difficult to characterize due to the variety of radiographic patterns which they may produce and due to their rarity. Their general characteristics may be similar to those attributed to a multilocular cystic lesion or a soft odontogenic tumor. The variation in pattern should impress the examiner with the need for establishing a diagnosis by means of biopsy.

Benign neoplasms may arise from any connective tissue element present in the jaws; therefore, they include myxomas, fibromas, chondromas, neurofibromas, or salivary gland adenomas.

Malignant Neoplasms.—Malignant neoplasms visible as radiolucent zones may be either primary or secondary.

Primary malignant neoplasms: Different types of malignant neoplasms will show different patterns of radiolucency depending upon the origin of the neoplastic cells. These neoplasms are characterized by their rapid growth and their

Fig. 205. *Osseous radiolucency.* Neurogenic sarcoma involving mental foramen and extending along the inferior alveolar canal to the retromolar area; note innocent appearance of this lesion on routine radiographic examination.

ability to invade surrounding tissue and become widespread in their involvement. If discovered on routine radiographic examination, they are likely to be small, but in many instances they rapidly involve a large area (Fig. 205).

The primary malignant neoplasms of the jaws arise from connective tissue. Only on rare occasions is a primary intraosseous malignant neoplasm of epithelial origin. Epithelial neoplasms usually involve the jaws secondarily by local invasion or by metastasis. The primary radiolucent lesions include fibrosarcoma and multiple myeloma for the most part.

Fibrosarcoma gives a radiographic picture of widespread, diffuse involvement, while multiple myeloma tends to produce round radiolucent zones which are often referred to as "punched out" in character. In multiple myeloma, complete skeletal radiographs usually reveal involvement of other bones. Fibrosarcoma has no distinct radiolucent character nor characteristic border; rather, it is the aggressive nature of the process which impresses the examiner. The tentative radiographic diagnosis of any malignant intraosseous neoplasm requires prompt action in obtaining the positive diagnosis by means of biopsy so that therapeutic measures can be undertaken as soon as possible.

Secondary malignant neoplasms: Malignant neoplasms may involve the jaws secondarily by local invasion or by metastasis. For the most part these lesions are epithelial in origin. Squamous cell carcinoma of the alveolar ridge and other areas of the mouth adjacent to bone may invade the underlying osseous structures. Radiographic findings are supported by clinical evidence or history of carcinoma. On rare occasions the first evidence of a carcinoma originating in the oral mucosa may be that of diffuse radiolucency beneath the mucosal origin of the lesion. Osseous involvement by a carcinoma is more likely to occur in the endophytic type rather than in the exophytic type of carcinoma.

Metastatic involvement of the jaws by carcinoma is relatively rare. Certain types of carcinoma, namely, thyroid, breast, and prostatic, and hypernephroma have a marked tendency to metastasize to bone. No distinct radiographic characteristic can be stated for metastatic lesions in the jaws. They appear as nonspecific areas of radiolucency in any location. By the time there is radiographic evidence of metastasis to the jaws, the primary lesion usually has been discovered.

Endocrinopathic Bone Dysplasia.—Radiolucency seen in endocrine dysfunction is the result of hyperparathyroidism. The involvement may be more extensive, but otherwise the process is indistinguishable from central giant cell tumor. The histologic findings must be supported by proper blood studies to establish the diagnosis (see Chapter 7).

Systemic Disease.—Systemic diseases producing an osseous radiolucency include such entities as eosinophilic granuloma and Hand-Schüller-Christian disease. Both of these diseases may produce destruction of the alveolar process in a somewhat generalized pattern. Eosinophilic granuloma may produce solitary or multiple lesions. The radiolucency produced is distinct, and the borders of the lesions are not well defined. The radiolucent zone is not trabeculated and may show some angularity of outline in eosinophilic granuloma. Often the teeth are involved and appear radiographically to have lost all of their bony support. Hand-Schüller-Christian disease may involve developing teeth, resulting in destruction of the follicle or malformation.

A   B

Fig. 206. *Osseous radiolucencies.* **A,** Postoperative defect following removal of third molar. **B,** Oro-antral fistula.

Osteomyelitis.—Osteomyelitis, a suppurative inflammatory process, is accompanied by radiographic changes of radiolucency in its earlier stages while bone is being destroyed. The bone appears to be "moth-eaten," and zones of radiolucency surround islands of necrotic bone or sequestra.

The margins of the radiolucency are ill defined. Later stages of the process show new bone formation with areas of destruction. Clinical manifestations of osteomyelitis should be correlated with radiographic findings.

Residual Postoperative Defects.—Postoperative defects are seen following extraction of mandibular third molars (Fig. 206, *A*). Incomplete repair of an osseous defect in the maxilla usually results in a round radiolucent area which is well defined and surrounded by normal bone. Occasionally a cyst may be suspected, but the history of a surgical procedure will aid considerably in establishing a diagnosis. An oro-antral fistula may be detected as a radiolucent zone between the floor of the sinus and the alveolar crest (Fig. 206, *B*).

Osseous Radiopacities

Radiopacities in general do not have the grave significance that radiolucencies sometimes have. Nevertheless, in evaluating radiopacities a diagnosis must be made because of the potential destructive processes associated with some of them. The following should be considered in evaluating radiopacities: (1) location and extent, (2) relative degree of radiopacity, (3) variations in radiopacity within the radiopaque lesion, (4) nature of the area immediately surrounding the radiopacity, and (5) possible origin of the lesion.

The location and extent often suggest a specific process. For example, torus mandibularis will usually appear as a radiopacity superimposed on the roots of the mandibular bicuspids. The extent of radiopacities, whether they are generalized or localized, offers much information toward a diagnosis. The extent of localized radiopacities may be an important consideration in the surgical attack of such a lesion.

The relative degree of radiopacity is helpful in determining whether the lesion is made up of bone, tooth tissue, or a metallic foreign object. Bone is generally less radiopaque than tooth structure, and both bone and tooth allow passage of more x-rays than metallic objects and are less radiopaque than metal.

Variations in radiopacities within a radiopaque area and the architecture produced by the variations are helpful in establishing the type of calcified tissue being visualized. For example, close inspection of a suspected retained root tip usually reveals evidence of pulp canal in the long axis of the radiopaque area.

The nature of the area immediately surrounding a radiopaque zone may be suggestive of a tooth follicle or periodontal space, thereby narrowing the possible diagnosis to a lesion of odontogenic origin. Osseous structures producing radiopacities are usually less well demarcated radiographically than odontogenic lesions.

Consideration of the foregoing factors will lead the examiner to a determination of the origin of the lesion. The possible origin of a radiopacity is much more limited and usually more easily determined than the origin of a radiolucency. The possible origin of a radiopacity is limited by the types of tissue in the body which are calcified. The origin of metallic foreign bodies is usually determined readily by the history.

Tumors.—Tumors visible as radiopacities include odontogenic and non-odontogenic.

Odontogenic Tumors.—Odontogenic neoplasms which produce an opaque image radiographically are the hard odontomas. The radiopacity is produced by a calcified mass made up of combinations of enamel, dentin, and cementum. (Fig. 207, A.)

The relative degree of radiopacity is variable throughout the mass in mixed odontomas due to the variation in radiopacity of the constituent calcified tissues. The enamel in the mass will be recorded as more radiopaque than either dentin or cementum.

The degree of involvement varies from masses of about 1 cm. to several centimeters in diameter. Odontomas do not seem to favor any particular location of the jaws. When they occur in close association with teeth, the result is usually failure of one or more teeth to erupt. Although the outline or margins of an odontoma are generally irregular, the margins are distinct. Frequently there is evidence of a follicle associated with the periphery of an odontoma, and there may also be evidence of a periodontal space.

Enamel pearls: Enamel pearls are misplaced spherical masses of enamel which appear at the cervical areas of teeth especially in the trifurcation and bi-

A   B

Fig. 207. *Osseous radiopacities.* **A,** Complex odontoma; note interference with eruption of central incisor. **B,** Hyperostosis, unilateral; etiology is unknown.

furcation areas of molar teeth. The pearls are of the same degree of radiopacity as the enamel on the crown of the tooth; however, they are rather distinct in outline due to their association with the root portion of teeth and their relatively greater opacity in comparison with dentin and cementum.

Cementoma: Multiple cementoma has been discussed previously under Periapical Radiolucency. In its final stage of development the cementoma is an irregular radiopaque mass involving the apex of one or more teeth.

Nonodontogenic Tumors.—The following nonodontogenic tumors are visible as radiopaque zones.

Bone whorls: Islands of compact bone, sometimes referred to as sclerotic bone or bone scars, are seen on routine periapical radiographs. Radiopacities of this general nature may occur without apparent cause or as the sequela of an inflammatory process such as a periapical abscess. Bone whorls are irregular in outline and are without clear-cut margins. They are of no significance as a radiographic entity, but areas of sclerotic bone are sometimes confused with odontomas or with root tips.

Enostoses and exostoses: Enostoses are inward growths of bone which appear radiographically similar to bone whorls and have the same significance as bone whorls. Exostoses are outward overgrowths of bone and include the tori of the maxilla and mandible. The most common exostosis seen radiographically is the torus mandibularis and appears as a well-circumscribed area of increased radiopacity superimposed on the roots of the mandibular bicuspids. A radiographic finding of exostosis bears little significance but should be confirmed during the clinical examination. Exostoses which occur on the buccal aspect of the alveolar processes do not show any remarkable radiographic change. Hyperostosis may produce a generalized radiopacity (Fig. 207, *B*).

Foreign Bodies.—Metallic objects and root tips are the most common foreign bodies seen in the periapical radiograph. Root tips are usually recognized rather easily due to their almost constant association with an edentulous area. Root tips which are well tolerated by the body may or may not be surrounded by a thin radiolucent line comparable to the periodontal space. When an inflammatory reaction occurs about a retained root tip, the surrounding area may show radiolucent changes; root tips seen with a surrounding radiolucent zone will be discussed under combined Osseous Radiolucency and Radiopacity.

In periapical radiographs of the complete mouth, metallic foreign bodies are a frequent finding in association with edentulous areas due to the frequent accidental deposition of amalgam in an extraction socket. In the extraction procedure the forceps fracture off varying sizes of amalgam particles from the restoration of the tooth being extracted. The silver amalgam fragments may appear as small granular radiopaque deposits or as large angular pieces. Silver amalgam is well tolerated by the body so the fragments are usually an isolated, incidental radiographic finding (Fig. 208). Amalgam in the tissue is frequently confirmed clinically by an area of bluish pigmentation of the oral mucosa at the extraction site.

Other metallic fragments may be observed as the result of accidental inclusion of metal in the soft tissues of the face and mouth. Shot residual from shot-

Fig. 208. *Osseous radiopacities.* Amalgam fragment in tissue at extraction site.

gun wounds, steel fragments, and a variety of other metallic objects may be seen radiographically and the diagnosis usually can be made on the basis of information about the event which caused the deposition of metal. Frequently metallic foreign bodies are superimposed radiographically on bone when in actuality the object is embedded in soft tissue. When foreign bodies are visualized radiographically, clinical examination should include inspection for scars and palpation of the involved soft tissue. Occasionally radiopaque areas which are the result of retained contrast media in sinus cavities or in the mouth are recorded on dental radiographs. A history of an examination requiring the use of radiopaque contrast media is sufficient to identify the foreign radiopacity.

Bone Dysplasias.—Dysplasias visible as radiopacities include, among others, leontiasis ossea and osteopetrosis.

Generalized Radiopacity of the Jaws.—Generalized obliteration of narrow spaces by osteosclerosis should suggest to the examiner that he is confronted with a generalized bone dysplasia such as leontiasis ossea or osteopetrosis. Confirmation of the existence of these processes requires the aid of a medical radiologist.

Combination of Osseous Radiolucency and Radiopacity

The following factors must be considered when periapical radiographic examination reveals an area or areas of combined radiolucency and radiopacity: (1) location and extent of the area in question, (2) relative degree of radiolucency, (3) relative degree of radiopacity, (4) variations in radiopacity within the radiopaque part of the area in question, (5) nature of the borders of the area in question, (6) apparent effect of the lesion on teeth and anatomic landmarks, and (7) possible origin of the lesion. These have been discussed under Osseous Radiolucencies and Osseous Radiopacities.

Neoplasms.—Benign and primary malignant neoplasms may produce a combination of radiolucency and radiopacity.

Benign Neoplasms.—Benign neoplasms include odontogenic and nonodontogenic.

Odontogenic neoplasms: Calcifying mixed odontogenic tumors show a varying degree of calcification in a radiolucent zone. The calcified portion is generally a mixture of enamel, dentin, and cementum which produces a variation in the radiopacity of the calcified portion of the lesion while the noncalcified portion results in an ill-defined margin. Mixed odontogenic tumors do not favor a particular location in the jaws and are marked by variation in degree of involvement and degree of calcification (Fig. 209).

Hard mixed odontomas may produce a combined radiolucency and radiopacity if the follicular epithelium associated with an odontoma undergoes cystic degeneration. When cystic change is associated with an odontoma, the combined radiographic features of both a cyst and an odontoma are evident.

The proliferative stage of multiple cementoma, as described previously, shows a combined radiolucent and radiopaque lesion (Fig. 210).

Nonodontogenic neoplasms: An ossifying fibroma has the same radiographic characteristics as a fibroma with the additional finding of ossification occurring in the radiolucent zone in varying amounts, depending upon the stage of maturity of the neoplasm.

Primary Malignant Neoplasms.—One neoplasm, osteogenic sarcoma, is outstanding in the category. Osteoblastic osteogenic sarcoma is characterized by rapid growth and bone production. Radiographically the area of involvement is usually extensive with no definite border. Radiopaque areas are visualized

Fig. 209. *Combined radiolucency and radiopacity.* Dilated odontoma.

Fig. 210. *Combined radiolucency and radiopacity.* Periapical osteofibrosis or multiple cementoma.

which show a "sunray" effect produced by divergent spicules of neoplastic bone. The "sunray" radiographic feature should suggest osteogenic sarcoma, although it may be seen in other neoplasms.

Bone Dysplasias.—Bone dysplasias which cause a combination of radiolucency and radiopacity are frequently generalized processes in the involved bone; however, single isolated lesions may occur.

Paget's disease, or osteitis deformans, is a generalized process which may affect the maxilla in its involvement of bones of the head. The radiographic appearance of bone which is produced in Paget's disease is frequently described as "cotton wool." Maxillary bone enlargement and hypercementosis or resorption of the teeth are seen when the maxilla is involved.

Fibrous dysplasia may be characterized radiographically by only a marked change in trabecular pattern. Single or multiple lesions may be seen, and the dysplasia may be confused with osteogenic sarcoma both radiographically and histologically by an inexperienced examiner.

Bone dysplasias which suggest a generalized process are not within the scope of dental treatment. Medical consultation should be sought for patients whose dental radiographic examination suggests that a generalized process is being manifested in the maxilla or mandible.

Osteomyelitis.—Chronic osteomyelitis is a productive infection. Areas of radiopacity representing bone production are seen in relation to radiolucent areas in long-standing osteomyelitis. Clinical manifestations suggest bone infection and confirm radiographic findings.

Foreign Bodies.—Root tips which are not tolerated by the body may be associated with radiolucent zones suggestive of a cyst or granulation tissue such as that seen at the apex of a devital tooth.

Other Dental Findings

Radiographs of the complete mouth are valuable in the evaluation of impacted teeth, the presence and position of supernumerary teeth, the tolerance

Fig. 211. *Other dental findings.* Impacted third molar; note that radiograph is inadequate for complete appraisal of root form.

A   B

Fig. 212. *Other dental findings.* **A,** Supernumerary mandibular bicuspid. **B,** Supernumerary tooth in anterior midline of maxilla.

of periapical bone to root canal fillings, and the presence of root irregularities; they are also of value in planning extractions and in planning for bridge and partial denture abutments.

Unerupted or impacted teeth are easily recognized radiographically. The radiograph is of value in planning the surgical approach to an impacted tooth (Fig. 211).

Supernumerary teeth are normal-appearing teeth in excess of the normal number of teeth in the mouth (Fig. 212). The most common location for supernumerary teeth is in the maxillary anterior region (Stafne). Occasionally a supernumerary tooth will be visualized radiographically parallel to the long axis of the x-ray film; this results in a confusing radiograph. Supplemental radiographs can be used to provide visualization of the long axis of the tooth. Supernumerary teeth are associated with a follicle which may undergo cystic change and produce a dentigerous cyst or rarely an ameloblastoma.

Careful evaluation or root canal fillings and periapical reaction to them are always included in the radiographic interpretation procedure. Newly placed as well as long-standing root canal fillings should be evaluated. Adaptation of the filling material to the walls of the root canal should be noted. Fillings which do not reach the apex of the tooth are of significance because of the frequent periapical radiolucency which is produced or which remains persistent at the apices when the root canal is incompletely filled. Overextension of the fillings into the periapical area is not uncommon. Such fillings are generally well tolerated by the periapical tissue of the tooth, but they may incite an inflammatory response.

POSTERIOR BITE-WING RADIOGRAPHS

The posterior bite-wing radiograph supplements radiographs of the complete mouth. It has limited use and should never be used as the only means of radiographic examination for a new patient nor for one who is returning for an examination and has not had radiographs of the complete mouth taken during the preceding one or two years.

Posterior bite-wing radiographs are used (1) to determine lamina dura continuity at the alveolar crest, (2) to estimate alveolar crest level in relation to the cementoenamel junction, (3) to evaluate tooth crown shape and formative defects of the tooth crown, (4) to determine pulp size and degree of pulpal calcification, (5) to evaluate existing restorations, (6) to locate calculus, and (7) to locate carious lesions.

Lamina Dura Continuity

Determining continuity of alveolar crest lamina dura may be less difficult in posterior bite-wing radiographs than in periapical radiographs which have been taken at steep vertical angulations in the posterior part of the mouth. The 8-degree vertical angulation used to obtain the bite-wing radiograph reduces the amount of superimposition of buccal alveolar crest image in a coronal direction which occurs in the periapical radiograph. Recognition of early periodontal disease is aided by careful inspection of the lamina dura for continuity. Interruptions of continuity can often be related to other findings in the interproximal area such as presence of calculus, overhanging margins, and open contacts (Fig. 213).

The width of the periodontal space associated with the cervical area of the tooth may be evaluated by means of posterior bite-wing radiographs; however, the evaluation is incomplete since the entire periodontal space must be evaluated by means of periapical radiographs.

Alveolar Crest Level

Within the limits of the coverage of posterior bite-wing radiographs, the level of the alveolar crest in relation to the cementoenamel junction can be determined accurately. Resorption of the crest to the point of bifurcation and trifurcation involvement of molar teeth is not always visualized in posterior bite-wing radiographs due to the limited amount of root which is included on the film (Fig. 213).

Fig. 213. *Posterior bite-wing examination.* **A,** Caries, overhanging restoration, normal bone level, and continuity of lamina dura over alveolar crest; interproximal caries indicated by arrows; overhanging restorations on lower second molars; and recurrent caries under restoration on distal aspect of lower right third molar. **B,** Auxiliary films to eliminate overlapping in molar area for visualization of interproximal caries. **C,** Loss of continuity of lamina dura at alveolar crest, caries, calculus, spacing of teeth, extrusion of maxillary third molar, and reduction of pulp size; calculus indicated by arrows; occlusal caries on upper and lower right first molars; and incipient interproximal caries on distal upper right second bicuspid. **D,** Pulp size, interproximal caries, spacing, and impaction; caries indicated by arrows.

Crown Shape and Formative Defects

In planning restorations of carious teeth, shape of the crowns of the teeth to be restored is often important in determining the best type of restoration and the best means of preparing a tooth to receive a restoration. The characteristics of the contact areas are easily determined in the bite-wing radiograph if the contact overlap areas have been eliminated by supplemental films at different horizontal angulations. The level of the contact point and the vertical length of the interproximal contact of adjacent teeth or the lack of a contact between two adjacent posterior teeth should be determined.

Local formative defects such as hypoplastic pits and alteration of crown form can be seen readily in posterior bite-wing radiographs. More generalized formative defects such as amelogenesis imperfecta, dentinogenesis imperfecta, and dentin dysplasia can also be recognized by the crown characteristics described under Radiographs of the Complete Mouth.

Pulp Size and Pulpal Calcification

Cavity preparation is performed with less possibility of pulp exposure if bite-wing radiographs are examined carefully to determine the size of the pulp of the tooth to be prepared. The degree of pulpal calcification represents the response of the pulp to occlusal function, restorations, and dental caries. The pulp size may be a determining factor in the type of restoration which can be placed in a tooth. Teeth of young individuals have large pulps and require more conservative types of preparation for restoration, while pulps which have undergone considerable calcification allow more room for extensive or radical restorations (Fig. 213).

Existing Restorations

Marginal fit, recurrence of dental caries, adequacy of contact points, and depth of involvement are important factors in examining restorations by means of posterior bite-wing radiographs. The reasons for replacing restorations are usually unsatisfactory function or recurrent caries which are determind by radiographic examination and confirmed wherever possible by clinical findings. Open and overhanging cervical margins of otherwise satisfactory restorations are important to recognize as contributory to periodontal disease. The effects of faulty restorations can usually be seen at the alveolar crest as resorption of the lamina dura (Fig. 213).

Location of Calculus

Interproximal subgingival calculus is quite well visualized on posterior bite-wing radiographs. It usually appears as a spurlike projection on the proximal surface of a tooth. Incompletely removed calculus following dental prophylaxis may present a rounded or flattened appearance on the bite-wing radiograph. Calculus occurring on the buccal or lingual surface of a tooth has the same linear appearance as it does in the periapical film (Fig. 213). Not all calculus can be seen radiographically; therefore, the bite-wing radiograph serves only to supplement thorough clinical exploration.

Location of Carious Lesions

Posterior bite-wing radiographs, together with radiographs of the complete mouth and clinical exploration, provide the complete procedure for location of carious lesions. Carious areas evident on bite-wing radiographs should be recorded numerically, and the combined findings by all three methods should be analyzed to produce a final list (see Chapter 5).

Interproximal carious lesions are well visualized in carefully taken posterior bite-wing radiographs when the lesions have progressed through the enamel and have involved the dentoenamel junction. Initial incipient carious lesions which have not entirely penetrated the enamel may be less easy to detect.

Carious lesions occurring in teeth without periodontal involvement are seen most commonly at the contact point or under the occlusal enamel at the apex of a developmental fissure. When periodontal disease is evident, the involvement of teeth by dental caries is frequently in the area of the cementoenamel junction.

Recurrent dental caries may be detected more readily in posterior bite-wing radiographs than in periapical radiographs due to the more favorable vertical angulation used for bite-wing radiographs.

Careful inspection for recurrent dental caries should be directed to the interproximal cervical margins of restorations and to the occlusal floor under the restoration. Recurrent caries are frequently indistinct and may present a poorly defined radiolucent line or zone at a restoration margin or wall.

The inspection of a bite-wing radiograph for carious lesions should be done in a routine manner so that all areas of the radiograph receive the same attention. All of the maxillary teeth should be inspected in sequence followed by the same procedure for the mandibular teeth (Fig. 213).

SUPPLEMENTAL RADIOGRAPHS

Radiographs of the complete mouth and posterior bite-wing radiographs are ordinarily sufficient to render a satisfactory diagnosis and treatment program for a patient. However, occasions arise when additional radiographs are extremely helpful. No special equipment or special training is required either in taking or interpreting supplemental radiographs.

TYPES OF SUPPLEMENTAL RADIOGRAPHS

1. Occlusal radiographs (Fig. 214)
   (a) Maxillary and mandibular topographical occlusal views
   (b) Maxillary and mandibular anterior occlusal views
   (c) Maxillary posterior occlusal views
2. Lateral views of the body of the mandible (Fig. 215)
3. Lateral views of the condyle
4. Temporomandibular joint radiographs (Fig. 216)

The selection of proper supplemental radiographs depends on the area which needs further radiographic investigation and the pathologic condition suspected by the examiner.

Supplemental radiographs are indicated (1) when a bone fracture is suspected, (2) when a salivary calculus is suspected, (3) when the extent of a radiographic lesion cannot be determined by means of periapical radiographs, (4) when the exact location of a radiographic lesion, foreign body, or tooth cannot be determined by periapical radiographs, (5) when the patient is unable to tolerate intraoral films, and (6) when there is suspicion of temporomandibular joint changes.

The location of fractures by the general practitioner of dentistry is limited to the mandible. Maxillary fractures require special radiographic technics which are best done in hospitals at the request of an oral surgeon.

Fractures tend to occur in specific areas of the mandible such as the symphy-

A   B   C

D   E

Fig. 214. *Supplemental radiographic examination.* **A,** Maxillary topographical occlusal view. **B,** Mandibular topographical occlusal view. **C,** Maxillary posterior occlusal view. **D,** Mandibular anterior occlusal view. **E,** Maxillary anterior occlusal view.

Fig. 215. *Supplemental radiographic examination.* Lateral view of body of mandible.

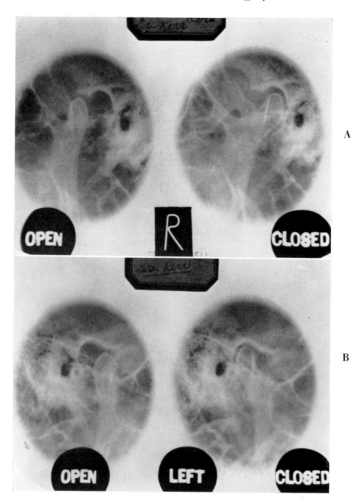

Fig. 216. *Supplemental radiographic examination.* Temporomandibular joint open and closed. **A**, Right. **B**, Left.

sis, the angle, or the head of the condyle. Lateral views of the body of the mandible, lateral views of the condyle, and occlusal radiographs may all be used to establish the presence or absence of a fracture.

Salivary calculi in Wharton's duct and Stensen's duct can usually be visualized radiographically. Calculi in Wharton's duct are best seen on mandibular topographic occlusal radiographs. Lateral films of the jaw are useful when a Stensen's duct calculus is suspected.

The limited area covered by periapical radiographs often does not provide a complete view of a pathologic process. Lateral films of the jaw or occlusal radiographs are usually large enough to provide a complete picture of most pathologic processes which occur in the jaws.

The exact location of pathologic areas, impacted teeth, or foreign bodies is simplified by utilization of the proper supplemental radiograph. Buccolingual relations of objects are easily determined by occlusal radiographs. Lateral views of the jaw are helpful in location of foreign bodies such as broken injection needles embedded in soft tissues; the insertion of landmark needles helps localize foreign objects on the radiograph.

Situations which prevent the use of intraoral x-ray film may be intense gag reflex, infection and swelling, or an extremely sore mouth. The selection of supplemental (or, in these patients, substitution) radiographs is limited to lateral films of the jaw and perhaps anterior occlusal views of the maxilla and mandible. The detail of the teeth is not as clear in the lateral view of the jaw as it is in the periapical radiograph, but the lateral film is sufficient to be used for diagnostic purposes in most cases where intraoral films are not obtainable.

Radiographs of the temporomandibular joint are of limited value since it is difficult to obtain a clear radiograph of the joint area and because seldom is anything of diagnostic importance recorded on the radiograph. Neoplastic involvement or bony ankylosis of the temporomandibular joint produces radiographic changes, and occasionally osteoarthritic changes with osteophyte formation are seen in the temporomandibular joint area. The vast majority of temporomandibular joint problems are the result of acute and chronic changes in the joint on a traumatic basis. The radiographic visualization of any important changes in traumatic temporomandibular joint arthritis which cannot be determined by careful clinical examination is doubtful.

Special Radiographic Procedures

It is not within the scope of the general practice of dentistry to carry out specialized types of radiographic examinations.

Cephalometry requires special equipment and is primarily of interest to the orthodontist. Sialography requires special equipment and materials. Contrast medium is a valuable radiographic aid in certain pathologic situations; however, special skills must be developed for its use. None of these procedures should be carried out without the special training required to interpret them accurately.

RADIOGRAPHS FOR CHILDREN

The radiographic examination of children differs from that of an adult in that the basic requirement is the posterior bite-wing radiograph supplemented by lateral films of the jaw and anterior radiographs (Fig. 217).

The interpretation of radiographs of children is the same as the interpretation of radiographs of adults with the additional concern for presence or absence of permanent tooth buds and position of permanent tooth buds in relation to normal position in the jaw and in relation to eruption sequence (see Chapter 5).

RADIATION HAZARDS

Radiation Hazards to the Patient.—It is well established that routine dental radiographs taken for diagnostic purposes do not endanger the patient. When a properly filtered x-ray machine, a diaphragm to limit the size of the x-ray beam, and fast x-ray film are used, the patient is exposed to an insignificant amount of x-rays. The Council on Dental Research of the American Dental Association has stated in effect that there is no justification for dental patients being concerned about being harmed by the use of x-ray examination and that curtailment of radiographic examinations would "impair proper diagnosis and treatment planning."

Radiation Hazard to the Dentist.—A dentist who takes many radiographs is subject to exposure of varying quantities of radiation, depending on the care he takes to protect himself from direct and scatter radiation. Whenever possible, a lead-lined shield should be installed in the office behind which the dentist will be completely protected from x-rays. A dentist should never hold x-ray film routinely for patients, nor should it ever be necessary for him to hold x-ray film for a patient since there are many devices available which enable the patient to retain the film under any circumstance.

A study by Richards shows some interesting data on the amounts of radiation to which a dentist is exposed in various positions in relation to the patient being radiographed. Adequate protection from exposure is easily obtained by

Fig. 217. *Radiographs for children.* **A,** Posterior bite-wing radiographs. **B,** Anterior occlusal films using No. 1 film. **C,** Anterior bite-wing radiographs. **D** and **E,** Lateral films of jaws.

proper shielding and proper use of the x-ray machine and should be the concern of every dentist who uses x-rays. Radiation badges should be worn by dentists who do not use a shield. Such badges are a good means of evaluating how much radiation is being received by members of a dental office staff, especially those who operate the x-ray machine.

ILLUSTRATIVE CASE

Summary of History and Clinical Examination

A 27-year-old Negro male presented with a chief complaint of vague pain on the left side of the face which had persisted for a period of three months. The patient had been examined by an internist and a neurologist without evidence of disease being found. The remainder of the medical history was noncontributory.

The dental history showed that the patient had received regular dental care; otherwise it was noncontributory.

Clinical examination revealed noticeable atrophy of the left temporal muscle. The oral mucosa was clear of lesions. The gingivae were uniformly pink and the gingival form was physiologic although there was evidence of recession of the free gingival margin and blunting of interdental papillae. The gingival sulcus depth was less than 3 mm. Teeth 15 and 16 were somewhat mobile and produced a dull percussion note. The existing restorations were functioning well and the carious lesions were minimal. The occlusal function was traumatic in the areas of the bridge abutments and in the right and left molar regions. The temporomandibular joints showed no significant findings. The clinical impression was as follows: (1) healthy mouth, minor caries, (2) dull percussion note on teeth 15 and 16 of questionable etiology, (3) occlusal trauma.

Radiographs of the Complete Mouth (Fig. 218)

1. Continuity and thickness of lamina dura
   A. The lamina dura at the alveolar crest lacks continuity between teeth 3-4-5, 6-7, 15-16, 19-20-21, 27-28-29, 31-32.
   B. The lamina dura is not visualized about the roots of teeth 15 and 16.
   C. The lamina dura shows increased thickness on the mesial aspect of tooth 11 and on the distal aspect of teeth 22 and 27.
2. Widening of periodontal spaces
   A. Periodontal space widening is evident on the mesial aspect of tooth 6, the mesial aspect of tooth 9, the mesial aspect of tooth 11, the mesial and distal aspects of tooth 28, the distal aspect of tooth 22, the distal aspect of tooth 27. The periodontal space is widened in the interradicular area of teeth 19, 31, and 32. The periodontal space is thickened at the apex of tooth 22.
   B. The periodontal space is not evident about the roots of teeth 15 and 16.
3. Level of the alveolar crest in relation to the cementoenamel junction
   Level of the alveolar crest on individual teeth expressed in millimeters apical to the normal level of 1 to 1½ mm. apical to the cementoenamel junction is as follows:
   Mesial aspect of tooth 5, 2 mm.
   Mesial aspect of tooth 6, 2 mm.
   Mesial and distal aspects of tooth 7, 2 ½ mm.
   Mesial and distal aspects of tooth 8, 1 ½ mm.
   Mesial and distal aspects of tooth 11, 1 ½ mm.
   Mesial aspect of tooth 19, 3 mm.
   Distal aspect of tooth 20, 3 mm.
   Mesial aspect of tooth 20, 1 mm.
   Mesial and distal aspects of tooth 21, 1 mm.
   Distal aspect of tooth 22, 1 ½ mm.
   Mesial aspect of tooth 22, 2 mm.

Fig. 218. See text.

Mesial aspect of tooth 27, 2 mm.
Distal aspect of tooth 27, 1 mm.
4. Periapical radiolucency
    A. Tooth 22 shows a small radiolucent area to the apex.
    B. Large area of relative radiolucency in the left maxillary tuberosity region with loss of trabecular detail and obliteration of the maxillary sinus outline.
5. Pathologic conditions of the teeth, none present; caries, none; calculus and overhangs, check tooth 8 clinically.
6. Pathologic conditions of the jaws
    A. Osseous radiolucencies—see area described in 4, B.
    B. Osseous radiopacities, none present.
7. Other dental findings—root canal fillings on teeth 11, 12, and 22 show good adaptation to the walls of the root canals; root canals are completely filled to apex.

Posterior Bite-wing Radiographs (Fig. 219)
1. Continuity of lamina dura at alveolar crest
    Lamina dura lacks continuity between teeth 1, 2; 3, 4, 5; 15, 16; 19, 20, 21; 31, 32.
2. Alveolar crest level expressed in same manner as in complete mouth
    Mesial aspect of tooth 1, 1 mm.
    Distal aspect of tooth 2, 1 mm.

Fig. 219. See text.

Between teeth 3, 4, 5, 1 mm.
Between teeth 11, 12, not determined.
Mesial aspect of tooth 19, 3 mm.
Distal aspect of tooth 20, 3 mm.
Mesial aspect of tooth 20, 1 ½ mm.
3. Tooth crown form and formative defects of crown
   A. Bell shape crown form.
   B. No formative defects.
4. Pulp size
   A. Pulp horns prominent in vital bicuspids.
   B. Prominent mesial pulp horn on teeth 14, 19, 31.
   C. Pulpal calcification to a minor degree.
5. Existing restorations
   A. Heavy cervical margin on restoration of tooth 12.
   B. No recurrent caries.
6. Calculus
   None visualized.
7. Carious lesions
   Teeth 28^2, 29^1 (both incipent), 19^5, 31^5.

Summary of Significant Findings
1. Questionable radiolucent area is associated with teeth 15 and 16 and involving maxillary tuberosity.
2. Evidence of localized areas of resorption of alveolar crest; possible bifurcation involvement of teeth 31, 32.
3. Evidence of occlusal trauma.
4. Significant caries involvement on teeth 19, 31.

Fig. 220. See text.

Additional Radiographs Required (Fig. 220)

Maxillary posterior occlusal view of left side; supplemental radiograph shows area of distinct radiolucency involving maxillary tuberosity and possibly hard palate; lamina dura is absent from roots of tooth 16.

Further Procedures Indicated by Radiographic Examination

Referral to an oral surgeon for biopsy of area producing radiolucency.

Results Reported From Oral Surgeon

Pseudoadenomatous basal cell carcinoma. Further medical investigation showed involvement of the left maxillary tuberosity, left pterygomaxillary fissure, left orbit, and base of skull by the neoplasm.

Comment

This case points out the significance of the procedures outlined in this chapter. The neoplasm might well have been overlooked if the loss of the lamina dura and the loss of anatomic characteristics of the tuberosity and maxillary sinus had not been noted. The sequence of examining radiographs and the notation of presence or absence of normal landmarks and details of bony architecture are extremely important in the recognition of many defects in radiographs of an apparently well-cared for patient.

REFERENCES

Barton, E. J.: Roentgenographic Evidence of Condylar Neck Fracture, Oral Surg. **8**:58-63, 1955.

Baumann, L., and Rossmann, S. R.: Clinical, Roentgenologic, Histopathologic Findings in Teeth With Periapical Radiolucent Areas, Oral Surg. **9**:1330-1336, 1956.

Björk, A.: Cephalometric X-ray Investigations in Dentistry, Internat. D. J. **4**:718-744, 1954.

Editorial: Safety of Dental Roentgenography Assured by Modern Technics and Equipment, J.A.D.A. **56**:113-114, 1958.

Eselman, J. C.: Is the Evidence on the Radiograph Reliable? J. D. Med. **11**:216-219, 1956.

Goldman, H. M., and others: Origin of Registration of the Architectural Pattern, the Lamina Dura, and the Alveolar Crest in the Dental Radiograph, Oral Surg. **10**:749-758, 1957.

Kronfeld, R.: Histopathology of the Teeth and Their Surrounding Structures, Philadelphia, 1949, Lea & Febiger.

McCall, J. O., and Wald, S. S.: Clinical Dental Roentgenology, ed. 4, Philadelphia, 1957, W. B. Saunders Co.

Peterson, E. E.: Roentgenologic Interpretation of Anatomic Lines of the Maxillary Sinus, J.A.D.A. 53:165-167, 1956.

Richards, A. G.: Roentgen-ray Doses in Dental Roentgenography, J.A.D.A. 56:351-368, 1958.

Richards, A. G.: X-ray Protection in the Dental Office, J.A.D.A. 56:514-519, 1958.

Robinson, H. B. G., and others: Radiographic Interpretation of Oral Cysts, Radiog. & Photog. 29:61-68, 1956.

Sherman, R. S.: Resume of the Roentgen Diagnosis of Tumors of the Jawbones, Oral Surg. 4:1427-1443, 1951.

Sonesson, A.: Odontogenic Cysts and Cystic Tumors of the Jaws, Acta. radiol. (suppl. 81), 1-159, 1950.

Stafne, E. C.: Dental Roentgenographic Interpretation Dealing With the Pulp Cavity and the Maxillary Sinus, J. Ohio D. A. 31:62-73, 1957.

Stafne, E. C.: Value of Roentgenograms in Diagnosis of Tumors of the Jaws, Oral Surg. 6:82-92, 1953.

Stafne, E. C.: Supernumerary Teeth, Den. Cosmos 74:653-659, 1932.

Thoma, K. H.: Oral Pathology, ed. 5, St. Louis, 1954, The C. V. Mosby Co.

Turner, J.: Injury to the Teeth of Succession by Abscess of the Temporary Teeth, Brit. D. J. 30:1233, 1909.

West, R. K.: Differential Diagnosis of Abnormal Dental Radiopacities, J.A.D.A. 53:271-285, 1956.

Witkop, C. J.: Hereditary Defects in Enamel and Dentin, Acta genet. (Basel) 7:236-239, 1957.

Supplementary examination aids

In addition to an adequate history, physical examination, and radiographic examination, supplementary diagnostic aids may be necessary to complete the examination of a patient. Such aids include bacteriologic studies, blood studies, serologic tests, urine studies, contact sensitivity tests, biopsy, pulp vitality tests, the articulation and surveying of study casts, and the use of disclosing solution. Clinical laboratory studies of occasional value to the dentist are bacteriologic tests, screening blood studies, and urinalysis.

Laboratory tests should not be considered routine examination procedures; they should be done only when indicated. In many instances too much emphasis is placed on the information expected from a battery of such tests. In reality there can be no substitute for a carefully taken and weighed history and the examination and observation of the patient by a competent clinician. Without these procedures, diagnostic laboratory aids cannot be intelligently utilized; in fact, a complete examination in most instances makes them unnecessary. Laboratory tests and radiographic observations are often important in confirming and establishing a diagnosis; however, they are not always employed with judgment. Of primary importance is the proper recognition of the need for laboratory studies; at no time should they become a substitute for an adequate history and examination of the patient. Dependence on laboratory aids and neglect and misinterpretation of the history and clinical findings often reveal a lack of understanding of the true value of laboratory studies. Such an approach is often conducive to errors in diagnosis and is an unnecessary expense to the patient. The examiner should not rely upon any one method of examination in his diagnostic procedure. Reliance should not be placed primarily on laboratory studies since, more often than not, a correct diagnosis can be more adequately determined by subjective and objective clinical symptoms alone than by laboratory studies alone.

The fact that many dentists do not use the services of a clinical laboratory for blood studies, urinalysis, and bacteriologic tests need not be interpreted as a failure of the dental profession to live up to the standards of the medical profession. For, while the literature is replete with laboratory tests for systemic disease, very few tests are practical for use in a dental office or dental clinic.

In addition, although the general practitioner may have laboratory facilities available to him where competent technicians can carry out the tests desired, very few dentists feel the need for auxiliary examinations or believe that they are qualified to interpret the results. In many instances the latter feeling is justified because of the infrequent need for laboratory study interpretation.

While the exclusion of an efficient and justified use of laboratory tests is not realistic, neither is the "shotgun" approach to laboratory diagnosis where the practitioner routinely uses multiple laboratory tests to supplement an obvious diagnosis of Vincent's infection, periodontitis, or herpetic gingivostomatitis. The expense of extensive laboratory studies showing vague changes in serum calcium, serum phosphorus, serum cholesterol, sugar tolerance curves, and dynamic action of proteins appears to be unjustified in the diagnosis of "precocious advanced alveolar atrophy." Such findings do not enhance the obvious clinical diagnosis since no etiologic or differential diagnostic problem is usually present nor do such studies generally aid in treatment planning or the evaluation of the progress of treatment of periodontal disease.

It is true that the practicing dentist should be informed of the clinical laboratory tests available for the conditions relevant to his field of endeavor. However, he should also be aware of his own limitations, the limitations of laboratory tests themselves, and the practicability and economic feasibility of performing the tests. The dentist's limitations should not be construed as an inability to interpret the laboratory findings, per se, but as an inherent drawback to the evaluation of such findings in view of the fact that the results of many tests are of little significance unless correlated with an examination of the whole body. Such an examination is in the province of the physician—not the general practitioner of dentistry. This in no way reduces the scope of dentistry or prevents the dentist from taking his place in a health service. It does mean that dental and medical cooperation must be encouraged by effective use of each profession's services. The limitations of the laboratory tests themselves must not be overlooked. There are tests, e.g., sedimentation rate, which are so nonspecific that they only indicate the existence of some disorder. The limitations of this test are so extensive and the sedimentation rate is influenced by so many variable factors that its use appears to be of very dubious diagnostic and prognostic value (Yardumian), especially in dentistry.

The practicability of laboratory studies being carried out by the general practitioner of dentistry is an important consideration, even when there are obvious indications for their use. The infrequent indication for laboratory tests on blood and urine does not appear to justify the equipment and procedures necessary to carry out these tests in a dental office. The collection of specimens in a dental office presents difficulties which are not easily overcome. Even though the alternative of sending the patient to a clinical laboratory or physician seems obvious, this procedure also has drawbacks. For example, a history of polyuria, polydipsia, polyphagia, and loss of weight and the examination findings of multiple periodontal abscesses are sufficient to make a presumptive diagnosis of the classical case of diabetes mellitus without laboratory assistance. However, since the diagnosis has to be confirmed, the dentist has two alternatives: (1)

refer the patient to a physician for further evaluation or (2) send the patient to a clinical laboratory for tests on the urine for "sugar" and on the blood for "sugar tolerance" or fasting blood sugar. In the first alternative the physician assumes all the responsibility for preparing the patient and evaluating the findings. In the second alternative the dentist assumes the responsibility for the interpretation and then the referral to a physician for confirmation and treatment of the diabetes. In many instances the physician will choose to do his own evaluating and testing. This is not only a "double" expense to the patient, it also discourages rapport between the dentist, the patient, and the physician. It must be pointed out that *occasional* interpretation of laboratory findings, especially of glucose tolerance curves, is not conducive to recognition of the many pitfalls which are inherent in such tests. The first alternative appears to be most rational.

The foregoing is not intended to discourage the use of laboratory tests; it is presented to point out the place of laboratory diagnostic aids in the practice of dentistry. There are many tests which are solely within the province of the dentist—not only for their interpretation, but also for their use in making a diagnosis and planning treament. Such laboratory tests include those of value in the diagnosis of mouth diseases of local origin and of those diseases whose treatment is the primary concern of the dentist. While this division of responsibility may appear to be rather vaguely defined at times, it will aid the general practitioner in determining what laboratory studies and their interpretations are in his field of endeavor.

The following situation is presented to point out the responsibility of the dentist in using laboratory diagnostic tests. A biopsy report indicates that a lesion is a giant cell tumor, and the pathologist has indicated that he has assumed that the patient has normal alkaline phosphatase and calcium levels of the blood. This reservation is made since the microscopic diagnosis of giant cell tumor does not rule out the possibility of osteitis fibrosa cystica generalisata. This report is an indication that the dentist should obtain the information needed to establish whether or not the lesion is of more than local significance. This is sufficient basis for determining the alkaline phosphatase and calcium levels of the blood. If the laboratory findings are abnormal, the dentist has a sound basis of referral to a physician for evaluation and treatment. While this situation appears to be quite similar to the one concerning diabetes mellitus, two important differences exist. The preparation of the patient and the interpretation of the laboratory findings in a presumptive case of diabetes mellitus have many more inherent problems than an interpretation of the laboratory findings related to alkaline phosphatase and calcium levels. The other difference is quantitative— in most instances the alkaline phosphatase and calcium levels will be within the range of normal, i.e., most giant cell tumors involving the jaws are of local origin and require only local treatment.

In other instances the indications for laboratory tests to be performed or interpreted by the dentist are even more apparent than the preceding situation. For example, a patient's history may strongly indicate a bleeding tendency; this is a positive indication for certain screening clinical laboratory tests to determine the presence or absence of a hemorrhagic disorder. The final evaluation and diagnosis should be left to the physician or hematologist.

It is not the purpose of this text to enumerate and describe all the tests which might be of diagnostic importance, especially those whose interpretation more rightly belongs to the physician or those which are impracticable to carry out or interpret in the office of the general practitioner of dentistry. The following list of clinical laboratory studies includes only those which are of practical value in oral diagnosis. The general dental practitioner should know when they are indicated and how to interpret the results. Although he may not carry out the tests in his office, he should know how to refer a patient to a clinical laboratory or a physician for the tests when they are indicated.

OUTLINE OF SUPPLEMENTAL EXAMINATION AIDS

Bacteriologic Studies

Antibiotic sensitivity tests
Wound, abscess, lesion, and surgical incision cultures
Caries activity tests
Root canal cultures
Fresh moist preparations and smears

Blood Studies

Hematologic diagnosis associated with anemia and polycythemia
    Red cell count
    Hemoglobin determination
    Hematocrit determination
Hematologic diagnosis associated with bleeding
    Bleeding time
    Coagulation or clotting time
    Clot retraction
    Tourniquet test
    Platelet count
    Prothrombin time
Hematologic diagnosis associated with infections
    White cell count
    Differential white cell count
Hematologic diagnosis associated with lymph node enlargement
Hematologic diagnosis associated with leukemias
Serologic tests
    Complement-fixation test
    Flocculation test
    Alkaline phosphatase, calcium, phosphorus, and serum protein determinations

Urine Studies

Contact Sensitivity Tests

Biopsy

Exfoliative Cytology and Aspiration

BACTERIOLOGIC STUDIES

Antibiotic Sensitivity Tests.—Occasionally it may become necessary to know which antibiotic is most effective against a particular strain of bacteria causing a patient's illness. Laboratory methods for determining the effectiveness of antibiotics are only suggestive since many variables that are present in vivo are not present in vitro. Since very few dental offices have the culture media and equipment necessary to culture a specimen, the specimen will have to be taken at the dental office and sent immediately to the clinical laboratory, or the patient will have to be referred to the laboratory or a physician for the collection of the specimen. If the specimen is sent to the laboratory, it must reach there in a condition suitable for cultivation. The following directions for collecting a specimen are recommended: (1) use regulation tubes or bottles (sterile), (2) use regulation plugs to stopper tubes, (3) use only one applicator per tube, (4) collect specimen on a sterile cotton swab, (5) place swab in sterile test tube, (6) seat plug firmly in place, and (7) send specimen to laboratory without delay.

A sterile technic is absolutely necessary. Those practitioners unaccustomed to the procedure should use the facilities of the clinical laboratory. An antibiotic sensitivity test may be made by disk or tube dilution methods. In the disk method a small disk of filter paper containing an antibiotic is placed on a Petri dish streaked with a culture of the specimen under consideration. The width of the zone of inhibited growth around the disk indicates the degree of sensitivity of the organism to the antibiotic. The limitations of the test should be well understood. Antibiotic treatment is usually instituted without waiting for the results of the test and then changed if the test indicates the organism is not within the spectrum of the antibiotic used.

Wound, Abscess, Lesion, and Surgical Incision Cultures.—When a wound, abscess, lesion, or incision site shows evidence of infection, it is sometimes advisable to identify the causative organism so that specific therapy can be instituted. It must be remembered that swelling following extractions and surgical procedures is not usually indicative of infection. Most wounds and surgical incisions are contaminated by bacteria; however, very few of them are infected. The significance of the culture will depend primarily on the clinical findings and the organisms present. Constitutional effects related to an infection must be evaluated; it may be necessary to establish the nature of the organism by laboratory examination of the blood. Since some types of bacteria do not survive changes in temperature or prolonged standing, it is impractical to send a specimen of venous blood to the laboratory to be cultured. A culture of venous blood should be inoculated directly into a culture medium.

In order to know what specific infecting agents to look for, it is necessary that the clinician be acquainted with a very wide variety of diseases and their symptoms. In addition to this, it is necessary that he be familiar with the laboratory methods of isolating and identifying the infective agent. In general, blood cultures are rarely indicated in dental practice; more often, but not frequently by any means, cultures of incision and drainage sites and discharges from lesions are necessary to isolate or demonstrate infective organisms. (Smears rather than cultures may be used in some instances to identify an offending organism.) The specimen to be cultured is collected on a swab and placed in a dry sterile test tube. An aseptic technic should be followed, and the specimen should be sent to the laboratory immediately. A report may take ten days;

however, preliminary reports may be available in twenty-four to thirty-six hours.

Caries Activity Tests.—Because of the association of lactobacilli to dental caries (Bunting), an estimation of the number of lactobacilli in the saliva is useful in determining the degree of caries actively present in caries-susceptible individuals.

The lactobacillus count, the Snyder test, and the Fosdick test are the most frequently used methods for determining caries activity. A method outlined by Hadley is generally used for a quantitative estimation of lactobacilli present per milliliter of saliva. This test utilizes various dilutions of saliva in glucose acid broth spread over the surface of tomato agar plates. The cultures are incubated at body temperature for four days and a quantitative estimate of the number of lactobacilli is made. Counts of between 1,000 and 10,000 lactobacilli per milliliter of saliva suggest a low caries activity. Counts of 50,000 lactobacilli per milliliter of saliva usually indicate a high caries activity. Rogosa and his co-workers have more recently devised a synthetic medium for the enumeration of oral lactobacilli which is used in many laboratories.

The Snyder test utilizes an acid medium containing bromcresol green which, when inoculated with saliva, indicates the degree of acid production. A change in color of the medium within twenty-four hours is generally considered to be indicative of a high caries rate. Color changes delayed from forty-eight hours to three days indicate less caries activity, while no color change within four days is considered to be indicative of no caries activity.

Lactobacilli counts require equipment not usually found in the dental office. However, saliva need not be freshly obtained and specimens may be mailed in suitable containers to a dental school or state public health laboratory where this test is carried out. Because of its simplicity, the Snyder test can be carried out in the dental office. Saliva specimens need not be freshly obtained for this test either.

Caries activity tests are used to determine the degree of activity. This information is useful in determining the effect of preventive measures instituted by the dentist. By periodically checking caries activity, the effectiveness of caries control measures can be evaluated. Such tests are of particular use in the control of caries by restriction of carbohydrate intake. Lactobacilli counts, and hence dental caries activity, can be reduced by periodically restricting the amount of carbohydrate in the diet (Jay).

Root Canal Cultures.—Cultures made from material obtained from root canals are valuable in determining the presence or absence of microorganisms. It is necessary that the dentist determine that a root canal is sterile before filling it. A culture is the best method for determining the presence of microorganisms in the root canal; radiographic findings of periapical involvement are not sufficient evidence to make a diagnosis of bacterial infection.

A culture consists of material taken aseptically from a root canal and inoculated directly into a suitable culture medium. Since a wide variety of organisms may be found in root canals, a culture medium must be used which is capable of growing the greatest variety. One of the best mediums for this and other requirements is glucose ascites medium. If penicillin is used in the treatment of the root canal, the bacteriostatic effect on the root canal sample can be over-come by the addition of penicillinase. Cysteine, semicarbazide, and sodium glycholate can be used in culture media to overcome the bacteriostatic activity of streptomycin and dihydrostreptomycin. There are no practical methods for the inhibition of such antibiotics as Chloromycetin, polymyxin, bacitracin, and neomycin. Camphorated parachlorophenol is not inhibitory after forty-eight hours (Sommer). Glucose ascites culture medium tubes can be purchased ready for use.

Root canal cultures may be done in the general practitioner's office. The incubation of cultures presents no serious difficulty since suitable incubators are quite inexpensive and occupy but little space. An aseptic technic for the col-lection and inoculation of the culture as described by Sommer, Ostrander, and Crowley is advocated. Paper points which have been inserted into the root canals are inoculated into the culture medium and incubated at 37.5° C. for forty-eight hours. Cultures should not be kept at room temperature for more than eight hours. Any cloudiness in the tube is an indication of the growth of micro-organisms.

True negative cultures should be obtained before filling canals. False nega-tive cultures may occur because of inadequate samples. The sample to be inoculated should be taken from the apex of the canal. More than one negative culture should be obtained since the initial culture may not show evidence of microorganisms existing under dormant conditions. Three to four treatments of the canal may be necessary to obtain two successive negative cultures.

Fresh Moist Preparations and Smears.—These tests are useful occasionally in confirming the presumptive diagnosis of oral moniliasis (thrush), tuberculosis, and actinomycosis. Their use in necrotizing gingivitis is of dubious value since fusospirochetal organisms are present in the mouths of most individuals. Their use in solitary lesions of Vincent's angina and cancrum oris (noma) is of oc-casional value.

The examination of the discharge from a lesion suspected of being actino-mycotic can be accomplished by the use of a moist preparation. So-called "sulfur granules" which are characteristic of actinomycosis should be searched for in the pus or discharge. They can be seen best by washing the discharge with a saline solution in a Petri dish. The "sulfur granule" should be placed on a slide in a drop of saline solution and crushed with a cover glass. When examined under a microscope with the low-power objective, an entire fungus can be seen contained in a hard, sandlike "granule." Macroscopically the granule may appear white, yellow, or black. Microscopically the crushed "granule" will show a mass of radiating filaments with "clubbed" ends. When stained with Gram stain, the central filaments will appear gram-positive, while the "clubs" will appear gram-negative.

If the clinical findings are positive for actinomycosis but the smear and/or biopsy is negative, an anaerobic culture technic using blood agar should be employed.

The material taken from suspected monilial (thrush) lesions can also be examined microscopically using a moist preparation. The heavy white growth

Fig. 221. *Thrush* involving soft palate and tongue.

(Fig. 221) can be removed from the mucous membranes with a scraper. The scrapings are placed on a glass slide with a 10 per cent solution of KOH and heated gently and are examined under a low-power objective for round spores and short mycelia. This test may come into more clinical use with the widespread use of antibiotics.

It is not common for the general practitioner to have a microscope in his office. However, obtaining specimens presents no difficulty and they can be sent to a clinical laboratory for evaluation. From a practical standpoint, the actual staining of smears in a dental office appears to be outside the province of the general practitioner. Smears obtained from suspected tuberculous lesions should be fixed by gently warming the slide or by air drying and should be sent to the laboratory for an evaluation of the material for acid-fast organisms. Even though the smear is found to be negative, if the clinical findings are positive, guinea pig inoculations and biopsy procedures should be performed before ruling out tuberculosis. Smears are probably the least valuable in the diagnosis of a tuberculous lesion. Smears are also of little value in determining the presence of fusospirochetal organisms and necrotizing gingivitis. The clinical evidence is of much greater value than a stained bacteriologic smear. However, the smear may be of some value in a negative sense since necrotizing stomatitis does not occur in the absence of fusospirochetal organisms.

BLOOD STUDIES

Occasionally the general practitioner may find it necessary to evaluate certain clinical signs and symptoms of disease by examination of the blood. Of particular importance to the dentist are the principles of hematologic diagnosis associated with anemia and polycythemia, bleeding, infections, lymph node enlargement, and leukemias. It must be pointed out that the presence of the signs and symptoms of diseases responsible for changes in the blood, blood-forming tissues, and the lymph nodes are the main indications for blood studies. Therefore a presumptive diagnosis derived from the history and physical examination should indicate the need for a screening hematologic examination.

Pallor, anemia, bleeding, lymphadenopathy, and the cardinal manifestations of inflammation are only symptoms of disease, and their evaluation may require a thorough and complete examination of the body. The primary concern of the dentist should be the detection of the presence of such symptoms by the history and examination (to the degree his examination may extend). Inasmuch as most general practitioners will refer patients with these symptoms to a physician, the collection, examination, and evaluation of the blood should be left to the physician. This procedure may not be indicated in a few instances in which the presumptive diagnosis is not sufficiently clear to warrant a referral without a screening examination of the blood. In other instances a patient may be referred to a dentist by a physician for an evaluation of gingival bleeding. The dentist's findings may suggest the necessity for an examination of the blood. In this situation a hematologic screening examination for a hemorrhagic disorder should be instituted by the dentist. Frequently a patient gives a history of prolonged bleeding, and this information should be evaluated before dental treatment is instituted. Not infrequently a history is given of extensive hemorrhage following extraction of a tooth. In most instances, such bleeding is due to trauma of blood vessels; however, each case must be evaluated individually. Further questioning and a special search for signs of a hemorrhagic tendency should be carried out. A hematologic screening examination may be necessary to determine the presence or absence of a bleeding tendency. If the screening examination and the clinical findings correlate, the patient should be referred to his physician for a complete evaluation and diagnosis.

Hematologic Diagnosis Associated With Anemia and Polycythemia

The presence of an anemia is usually suspected by the dentist because of the subjective symptoms obtained in the interview of the patient and because of the presence of objective symptoms such as pallor, smooth tongue, Plummer-Vinson syndrome, and abnormal tongue sensations. Headache, vertigo, faintness, increased sensitivity to cold, tinnitus, weakness, and irritability are common subjective symptoms associated with anemia. Of particular importance to the dentist are anemias associated with excessive destruction of the blood, chronic diseases, plumbism, irradiation, and leukemias.

A simple anemia and polycythemia can be detected from the red cell count, the hemoglobin content, or the hematocrit determination. Since the objective and subjective findings referable to anemia may not be clear cut, these laboratory examinations of the blood may be necessary. However, these tests are only screening in nature; if the red cell count, hemoglobin content, or hematocrit findings are abnormal and substantiate the clinical findings, the patient should be referred to an internist so that the degree of polycythemia or anemia, the activity of the bone marrow, the morphology of the blood cells, changes in the white cells and platelets, and the cause of the anemia can be determined.

In a normal adult male the average red cell count is 5.5×10^6 per cubic millimeter; in the female the average count is 4.8×10^6 per cubic millimeter. The normal adult range of hemoglobin as determined by hemoglobinometry is 16 ± 2 grams per 100 ml. of blood in the male and 14 ± 2 grams per 100 ml. in the female. The normal hematocrit range for women is from 37 to 47 per cent; for men, from 40 to 54 per cent (Wintrobe). More extensive measurements of red blood cells take into consideration such characteristics as size, shape, and hemoglobin content; however, such measurements should be left to the hematologist. For screening purposes, the red cell count and hemoglobinometry or the hematocrit determination may be used. Since many errors are possible in the determination of an anemia or polycythemia by red cell count and hemoglobinometry, the hematocrit determination should be used as a screening test. It is suggested that the reader review standard clinical laboratory diagnostic texts for a complete presentation of the characteristics of red cells and their hemoglobin content. Such a review will serve to point out the limitations of a screening examination and the complexity of evaluating extensive blood studies.

In a normal individual the clinical laboratory findings might be indicated as follows: hematocrit, 45 per cent; red blood cell count, 5 million per cubic millimeter; hemoglobin, 15 grams per 100 ml. (red cells are normocytic as indicated by a normal mean corpuscular volume of 90 cubic microns). In a severe pernicious anemia there is macrocytosis indicated by an increased mean corpuscular volume; hematocrit, 14 per cent; and a red cell count of 1 million per cubic millimeter. In a severe hypochromic anemia, the red cell is microcytic as indicated by a reduced or low mean corpuscular volume, hematocrit 14 per cent, and a red cell count of 2 million per cubic millimeter. These latter findings warrant referral of a patient to a physician for complete evaluation, diagnosis, and treatment.

Hematologic Diagnosis Associated With Bleeding

The indications for hemorrhagic study include consideration of a history of a bleeding tendency and the presence of petechiae, ecchymoses, and spontaneous bleeding from the mucous membranes. A history of prolonged bleeding can be quite well evaluated on the basis of previous episodes of unusual bleeding following extractions, cuts, and operations; ease of bruising; prolonged use of antibiotics and anticoagulants; and the presence of systemic disease such as nephritis, tuberculosis, or leukemia. A positive history of "easy bleeding" should indicate the need for a thorough examination of the lymph nodes for enlargement and of the mucous membranes for evidence of hemorrhage.

A screening examination of the blood of a patient with suspected hemorrhagic disease should include bleeding time, coagulation or clotting time, clot retraction time, tourniquet test, white cell count, differential white cell count, platelet count, and hematocrit determination. While the performance and interpretation of these tests for screening purposes are within the dentist's responsibility, in most instances he will elect to refer the patient to a clinical laboratory or a physician for the tests and their interpretation. A screening examination may be useful to the general dental practitioner if it is needed to enhance a presumptive diagnosis of a hemorrhagic disorder so that a sound referral to a physician can be made. The routine use of blood screening studies is not indicated; such tests should be performed only when the findings of the clinical examination do not furnish sufficient evidence to warrant a referral without further evidence of disease. More complete examinations should be left to the physician since their evaluation may require examination procedures outside the scope of the dentist's responsibility. For example, patients receiving Dicumarol and related anticlotting agents for the control of thromboembolic disease (coronary thrombosis) should not have teeth extracted until the prothrombin concentration is brought to an effective level. Since the anticlotting therapy is supervised by the physician, the determination of the prothrombin concentration is the physician's responsibility. Teeth should be extracted only when the dentist and the physician believe that the effective level of prothrombin concentration is such as to allow safe extraction of the teeth.

To further emphasize the limitations of a presumptive diagnosis of hemorrhagic disease based on clinical findings and a blood screening examination performed by the dentist, the answers to two basic questions should be considered in making the final diagnosis: (1) Is a primary disease present which is complicated by hemorrhagic manifestations? and (2) Are the manifestations of the hemorrhagic disease primarily an abnormality of vascular response and clot formation? It is outside the scope of general dentistry to answer these questions completely. Thus, besides a history, an oral examination, and a blood screening examination, a minimal examination of a patient with a hemorrhagic disorder must include a complete physical examination, including examination of the stool and urine. Extensive clinical examinations and special tests relative to vascular disease and abnormalities of clot formation may be necessary to make a diagnosis.

With these considerations in mind it would be well at this time to determine what part the dentist should play in the evaluation of hemorrhagic diseases. First, the limitations of the oral examination must be considered; the dentist is not trained to make a complete physical examination of a patient. Second, the evaluation of urine and stool studies should be left to the physician making the complete physical examination; the infrequent need for such an evaluation does not justify the time required to "keep up" on all the ramifications of the results of such tests. Thus, the primary role of the dentist is to predict a tendency of a patient to bleed during or following a dental operation and to cooperate with the hematologist or physician in evaluating the operative risk of patients who have a history and the signs of a primary or secondary hemorrhagic disorder. For example, a patient with the signs and symptoms of a hemorrhagic disorder may present to the dentist for treatment of spontaneous hemorrhage in the mouth, extraction of teeth, or treatment of gingival disease. If the presumptive diagnosis is borderline and if the clinical findings of the dentist hardly warrant a referral to a physician for evaluation but do warrant further evaluation, the dentist can carry out screening tests related to vascular response and clot formation. If the results of these tests are positive, the dentist has a sound basis for referral to a physician for a complete work-up of the patient. Dentists interested in collecting blood specimens and carrying out the laboratory procedures should consult detailed accounts of the procedures. It should be borne in mind that the history and examination are more important in the prevention of hemorrhagic problems than laboratory tests. The limitations and interpretation of basic screening laboratory tests for abnormal vascular response and clot formation should be understood by the dentist if such tests are to be used by him.

Bleeding time is the time required for hemostasis to occur in a standard wound of the capillary bed. With the Duke method the normal range of time is 1 to 6 minutes. Many difficulties are encountered in producing a standard wound. Poor tissue tone resulting from senile changes, altered vascular response, and abnormal clot formation can prolong the bleeding time. Bleeding time is prolonged in thrombocytopenic purpuras but variable in nonthrombocytopenic purpuras. It is normal in hemorrhagic states such as scurvy and allergic non-thrombocytopenic purpura since the only abnormality is a decrease in capillary resistance.

Coagulation time or clotting time is a screening test to determine plasma coagulation defects and anticoagulation activity. The normal time depends on the test method used. The normal range of the clotting time as determined by the Lee-White method is 4 to 12 minutes. Coagulation time measured by the capillary tube method is unreliable and should not be used. A prolonged clotting time does not indicate a specific abnormality and should be used only in relation to plasma coagulation defects. An increased clotting time does not in itself indicate specifically an absence of fibrinogen, a deficiency of prothrombin accelerator, or the presence of hemophilia, since many factors must be evaluated in the interpretation of a prolonged coagulation time.

Clot retraction time is a test of the ability of the clot to retract adequately in a given interval of time. Coagulation time takes into account the time required for the clot to form, whereas clot retraction time takes into account its ability to retract and capability of closing a wound. Clot retraction occurs normally in one hour. Good clot retraction is usually associated with normal platelet counts. Clot retraction may be affected by platelets, decreased fibrinogen, anemia, polycythemia, and hyperglobulinemia.

The tourniquet test is a measure of capillary fragility. This test is considered to be a test of the vascular factors in hemostasis. It is performed by applying positive pressure methods with a tourniquet or blood pressure cuff which produces an increased venous pressure for 5 minutes halfway between systolic and diastolic pressure. The cuff is placed above the elbow. If no petechiae appear after 5 minutes, the pressure is raised to 100 mm. and continued for another 5 minutes. The test should be discontinued if numerous petechial spots begin to appear. In normal subjects only a few scattered petechiae may appear. This test does not indicate a specific diagnosis. It may be positive in scurvy, severe primary or secondary thrombocytopenia, and other systemic vascular abnormalities.

In addition to these tests, a white cell count and a white cell differential count should be a part of the screening examination. A leukopenia in severe cases of hemorrhage is highly suggestive of an abnormality of the marrow.

These screening examinations will serve to point out a hemorrhagic diathesis. Additional special tests are necessary to determine the precise defects causing the hemorrhagic conditions, viz., a deficiency of platelets, a deficiency of one or more of the factors of plasma necessary for coagulation, and circulatory anticoagulants. The latter has practical significance to the dentist who is contemplating the extraction of teeth or other procedure likely to produce hemorrhage. The measurement of prothrombin activity is of diagnostic and prognostic significance not only in diseases of the liver and hemorrhagic diathesis, but also in the control of the prothrombin level when Dicumarol is being used in the treatment of thromboembolic disease. While the hematologist or physician may be responsible for testing the prothrombin activity and instituting treatment, the dentist should be informed on the limitations and interpretation of the tests in order to have a better understanding of the problems involved. The prothrombin test is valuable in detecting the absence of prothrombin as a cause of hemorrhagic diathesis and in the study of response to vitamin K therapy. The prothrombin level should be determined whenever disease of the liver or biliary system is present and surgical procedures are contemplated.

Two methods of determining prothrombin activity in terms of its concentration in per cent of normal are used: the one-stage procedure of Quick and the more complete but less practical two-stage procedure. The interpretation of prothrombin time requires a knowledge of the factors other than prothrombin deficiency which may cause prolongation and a knowledge of the sources of error in the test. By the Quick method the prothrombin time is prolonged in afibrinogenemia and in deficiencies of "prothrombin accelerators." The prothrombin concentration is usually normal in other hemorrhagic diseases. In order to prevent thrombotic accidents, the prothrombin time is usually maintained at approximately 30 to 40 seconds or the prothrombin concentration between 4 and 8 per cent of normal (Ham). Since individuals may vary widely in their response to Dicumarol therapy, periodic estimations of prothrombin activity are necessary.

No attempt has been made to mention all the hemorrhagic diseases. The patient's history and the clinical findings are usually sufficient to alert the examiner to the possibility of the presence of such disease. Thus, the stress should be upon the detection of the signs and symptoms rather than on blood studies necessary to make a diagnosis since the latter is rightly in the field of the hematologist. It might be mentioned that unexpected hemorrhage occurring during surgical procedures is more often due to leukemia, aplastic anemia, or systemic disease that has been overlooked than to a primary hemorrhagic disease such as hemophilia (Miller).

An uncommon hemorrhagic diathesis of interest to the dentist is scurvy. The clinical manifestations of hemorrhage occurring from the mucous membranes of the mouth, especially the gingivae in the presence of local traumatic factors, are not particularly specific. Therefore, if scurvy is suspected, the diagnosis can frequently be made on the basis of the history of an inadequate diet. Bleeding time and all other special tests are normal except capillary fragility. Thus the history and the cessation of bleeding following ingestion of orange juice and vitamin C are of primary consideration in the diagnosis of scurvy. Quantitative determinations of the cevitamic acid content of the blood and urine appear to be unnecessary except in rare instances.

Hematologic Diagnosis Associated With Infections

Blood studies are occasionally indicated in the presence of fever. An elevation of temperature in patients seen by the dentist can usually be related to tissue injury. In most instances the cause of the fever will be clinically evident—necrotizing gingivitis, herpetic gingivostomatitis, abscesses, and dry socket. Only rarely will the dentist see patients with fever from a drug sensitivity reaction, neoplasia, generalized infections, or immunity reactions. A white cell count and white cell differential count should be made when a fever is present in the absence of distinctive clinical signs of disease, and when the systemic reaction exceeds that expected for the degree of tissue injury present.

In the adult, the normal range of circulating leukocytes is between 5,000 and 10,000 cells per cubic millimeter. The leukocyte count is affected by many factors other than tissue injury. Leukocytosis associated with exercise, paroxysmal tachycardia, pain, and other factors such as physical and mental rest can usually be differentiated from that associated with tissue injury by the increase in young cells which accompany the latter.

The leukocytosis most commonly seen in oral disease is that of neutrophilic leukocytosis. Pyogenic infections due to coccal organisms are likely to produce neutrophilia. The extensive destruction of tissue and liberation of protein as well as the presence of organisms may produce leukocytosis in acute necrotizing gingivitis (Vincent's infection). Leukopenia is much less likely to be observed in relation to diseases seen in the practice of dentistry. Changes in the eosinophilic leukocyte count may be manifest in allergic disorders, angioedema, skin diseases (with oral manifestations), or parasitic infections. An increase in the number of lymphocytes occasionally occurs in diseases with associated oral manifestations. An increase in the number of monocytes occurs in bacterial infections such as tuberculosis and in such disorders as Hodgkin's disease.

Hematologic Diagnosis Associated With Lymph Node Enlargement

Blood studies may occasionally be indicated in lymph node enlargement of the neck and submaxillary region. Most instances of enlargement seen by the dentist can be related to regional tissue injury.

Blood studies are indicated if lymphadenopathy is thought to be related to primary lymph node disease or lymphoma, leukemia, or syphilis. An examination of the peripheral blood will generally distinguish the lymph node enlargement of the lymphomas from the leukemias because of the characteristics of the blood cells of the latter. A serologic test for syphilis is indicated when lymphadenopathy (bubo) is present and accompanied by the characteristic lesions of syphilis—chancre and mucous patches. In the chronic forms of lymph node enlargement, especially in the differentiation of lymphomas, a biopsy of the node may be necessary. If lymphadenopathy is not related to infection in the mouth such as syphilis, herpetic stomatitis, and necrotizing gingivitis, and the peripheral blood is not characteristic of leukemias, lymph node enlargement should be considered as the result of metastatic neoplasm or lymphoma until proved otherwise.

Hematologic Diagnosis Associated With Leukemias

The most common symptoms of leukemia seen by the dentist are referable to gingival changes (enlargement and hemorrhage) and enlargement of lymph nodes. Acute and chronic forms of leukemia differ considerably in their clinical manifestations; however, very little clinical difference in the various forms of acute leukemias or the chronic leukemias may be seen.

The onset of acute leukemia is usually abrupt, and not infrequently the first obvious sign of the disease is gingival bleeding or prolonged bleeding following the extraction of a tooth. The initial symptoms may arise from leukocyte infiltration of the gingivae and lymph nodes. Lymph node enlargement is usually not so obvious as that seen in chronic leukemia. Gingival enlargement due to infiltration of immature leukocytes occurs in response to local irritation. Ulceration and superimposed Vincent's infection may be present. Differentiation of the various types of acute leukemia cannot be made on the basis of clinical symptoms alone and is frequently difficult even with a blood examination. The blood examination will generally reveal a severe anemia, decreased platelet count, prolonged bleeding time, poor clot retraction, and a positive tourniquet test. The leukocyte count may reach 100,000 cells per cubic millimeter but may be less than 10,000 cells per cubic millimeter.

The onset of chronic myelocytic leukemia is insidious; the most common symptoms are related to anemia, loss of weight, weakness, slight fever, and, later, a tendency to bleed. Lymph node and gingival enlargement from leukocyte infiltration is seldom apparent. The blood picture early in the disease is primarily one of leukocytosis of the myeloid series with a "shift to the left." As the disease progresses, myelocytes predominate. The leukocyte count may range from 100,000 to 500,000 cells per cubic millimeter. Anemia may be absent in the earlier stages but becomes profound as the disease progresses. The platelet count is usually normal except in the terminal stages when hemorrhagic manifestations and the signs of thrombocytopenic purpura are found.

The clinical findings in chronic lymphocytic leukemia are enlargement of the lymph nodes and manifestations of anemia. The blood picture is that of an overwhelming increase in lymphocytes. Sometimes the level may reach 250,000 cells per cubic millimeter. As with myelocytic leukemia, the platelet count decreases as the disease progresses and hemorrhagic disorders may develop (see Chapter 4).

Hematologic Diagnosis Associated With Chemotherapy

Many patients with neoplastic disease are being treated with a variety of chemotherapeutic agents. This form of therapy is being most intensively used in the treatment of leukemia, but other types of neoplastic disease are being treated by this method. Agents such as nitrogen mustard, urethan, cyclophosphamide, and many others are being used for this purpose.

All of these drugs have a depressant effect upon bone marrow, so the patients develop an agranulocytosis which has early manifestations in the oral cavity. The mucosa becomes smooth and shiny with some intensification of color. The changes progress rapidly to superficial ulcerations of the type typical of neutropenia. (Fig. 222). Superficial ulcers are present in the vestibular mucosa, and there are also gingival ulcerations associated with the palatal aspect of the upper central incisors (Fig. 222, A). A copy of the patient's chart shows the white blood cell count in the left column; the administration of the nitrogen mustard is re-

A

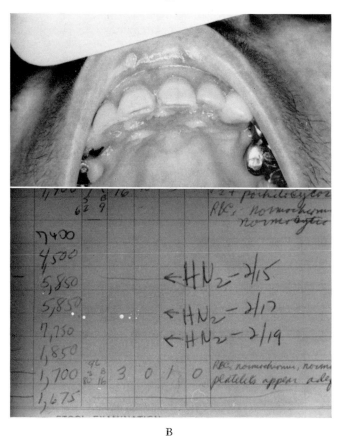

B

Fig. 222. *Neutropenia.* **A,** Mouth of a patient on chemotherapy. **B,** Chart indicating drug administration.

corded on the right side with the dates indicated (Fig. 222, *B*). The correlation of drug administration and the fall in the white blood cell count is apparent.

Serologic Tests

The clinical diagnosis of syphilis, except in the most typical cases, is unreliable. Even when a syphilitic chancre is suspected by its clinical characteristics and from the history, clinical laboratory procedures are the most reliable and valuable methods for a positive diagnosis. These procedures include smears from the lesion, cultures, biopsy, and serologic tests.

In the presence of a lesion with the characteristics of a primary chancre (Fig. 15, *A*), the examiner should take precautions against infection by wearing rubber gloves. The test to be used depends upon the stage or localization of the disease. The presence of syphilis can be detected by finding the *Treponema pallidum* in the discharge from the lesion (dark-field examination), recognizing rather characteristic tissue changes, identifying the causative organisms by biopsy, and recognizing immunologic responses by serologic methods.

Early syphilitic lesions of the skin and the demonstration of the spirochetal organism by dark-field examination or dry smear may be the only proof of a primary syphilitic infection. Mucous patches (Fig. 99, *B*) may show organisms regardless of the stage of the disease. In the secondary stage of the infection, complement fixation or precipitation tests are the most valuable. Primary chancres of short duration, up to one week, will rarely give a positive serologic test. In tertiary syphilis, serologic tests are almost always positive. False negatives are possible in any stage. Biologic false positive serologic tests may be present in yaws, leprosy, certain febrile diseases, malaria, and collagen diseases.

Complement Fixation and Flocculation Tests.—A correct serologic diagnosis of syphilis is usually based on two approved tests. Specimens to be evaluated are sent to public health laboratories. If the dentist is accustomed to collecting blood specimens, he may send them directly to the nearest public health laboratory. In other instances a referral to a clinical laboratory or physician for the test may be made. Whether or not the tests used are based on complement fixation (Wassermann) and/or flocculation (Kahn) is less important than their execution and interpretation. While serologic tests were originally reported as negative or positive (1+, 2+, 3+, or 4+), this scheme of reporting led to erroneous interpretation. Recent qualitative reporting of reactions are signified by negative, doubtful, or positive. Quantitative reporting is based on the greatest dilution at which the tested serum produced a positive reaction. For example, a serum which gives a positive reaction in the undiluted state is reported as 1:1; if the highest dilution of the serum with saline is 1:32, the reaction is reported as 1:32. Contraction of the term dilution to dil is sometimes used and the 1 dropped; e.g., a 1:32 dilution would become 32 dils.

Alkaline Phosphatase, Calcium, Phosphorus, and Serum Protein Determinations.—The dentist is sometimes called upon to interpret the values for serum calcium, phosphorus, and phosphatase in relation to diseases of the jawbones. It is assumed that the reader is familiar with basic concepts of the metabolism of calcium and phosphorus in bone.

Alkaline phosphatase is elevated whenever bone matrix is being formed in excess and when diseases of the liver and biliary system prevent the excretion of bile. Thus the presence of liver disease must be considered and evaluated in the presence of changes in the serum concentration of alkaline phosphatase, calcium, and inorganic phosphorus. The dentist is primarily interested in the changes of the concentration of these factors in relation to diseases of the bone, more especially the jawbone.

The serum alkaline phosphatase activity of normal adults is 1.5 to 4 Bodansky units. A Bodansky unit is equivalent roughly to 2.5 King-Armstrong units and 0.8 Gomori unit. The level in children from 2 years of age to late childhood ranges from 5 to 14 Bodansky units. The activity of serum alkaline phosphatase should be considered in conjunction with the serum levels of phosphorus and calcium.

Inorganic phosphorus is found mainly in bone in combination with calcium.

The level of serum inorganic phosphorus is influenced by the functional state of the kidney, by the parathyroid and growth hormones, and by vitamin D. Renal disease may produce phosphate retention; Parathormone increases the excretion of phosphorus and mobilizes calcium and phosphorus from the bone; vitamin D aids in the absorption of calcium from the gastrointestinal tract and the excretion of phosphorus by the kidneys. The normal adult level of serum inorganic phosphorus is 3 to 4.5 mg. per 100 ml. Children tend to have a slightly higher concentration.

Calcium is found principally in bone. It exists mainly in two states in the blood serum—ionized calcium and protein-bound calcium. The concentration of serum calcium in normal individuals varies from 9 to 11.5 mg. per 100 ml. Approximately 5 mg. per 100 ml. are ionized and most of the remainder is

Fig. 223. *Paget's disease.* Diffuse nature of the radiographic findings suggests systemic disease.

present as protein-bound calcium (a small amount, 0.25 to 0.5 mg. per milliliter, is also present in the form of an un-ionized but diffusible citrate). A change in the concentration of serum calcium may be due to a rise in protein-bound or ionized calcium.

The serum concentration of calcium, total serum protein, inorganic phosphorus, and alkaline phosphatase activity should be determined in individuals who show radiographic evidence of bone disease and clinical evidence of systemic disease. The radiographic findings alone may suggest the diagnosis and the need for blood studies. Not infrequently the dentist is the first to see bone lesions. The radiographic findings correlated with the history may be the basis of a presumptive diagnosis of a bone disorder. Occasionally bone lesions will be biopsied when the history and radiographic findings do not obviously suggest a systemic disorder of bone metabolism. Such a situation occurs in giant cell tumors of the jaws. The histopathologic features of the lesion as determined by biopsy may be the first indication that the lesion is other than of local origin. Therefore a diagnosis of giant cell tumor of the jaw requires that the blood

Fig. 224. *Advanced periodontal disease.* Blood and urine studies are not indicated on basis of radiographic findings of periodontitis.

studies mentioned be carried out to determine whether or not the lesion is local or systemic in origin, i.e., giant cell tumors associated with hyperparathyroidism.

Metabolic disorders of bone such as Paget's disease and diseases characterized by increased serum proteins such as multiple myeloma and sarcoidosis generally show clinical evidence of systemic disease and/or diffuse radiographic pictures suggestive of a systemic disorder (Fig. 223). These findings should suggest the need for clinical laboratory examination of the blood. Blood and urine studies are not indicated in periodontitis (Fig. 224).

• • •

The dentist's responsibility regarding the patient has been discussed previously. The dentist should be familiar with the interpretation and implication of the results of the blood studies. The reader is referred to texts on clinical medicine, oral medicine, and clinical laboratory diagnosis for the complete details of decreases and increases in alkaline phosphatase, inorganic phosphorus, and serum calcium in diseases of the bone. The final diagnosis of systemic bone disease should be left to a competent physician, since a complete physical examination, radiographic examination, blood study, and urinalysis may be necessary.

URINE STUDIES

Urinalysis should not be considered a routine part of the examination of a patient. The dentist only rarely will have occasion to require urinalysis and then only as a screening procedure.

Probably the most frequent use of urinalysis by the dentist relates to a suspicion of diabetes mellitus. However, the dentist who believes that a negative or positive test for "sugar" in the urine is an appreciable evidence that his patient does or does not have diabetes mellitus might better obtain the knowledge for proper interpretation before he uses the test. Not infrequently the clinical examination and history may warrant the presumptive diagnosis of diabetes mellitus. Occasionally a dentist may feel that he should obtain a clinical laboratory report on the patient's urine for "sugar" to substantiate the diagnosis. Unfortunately the presence or absence of melituria alone cannot be depended upon as an indicator of diabetes mellitus. While persistent melituria will most often be found to be glycosuria and a manifestation of diabetes mellitus, it also occurs in the presence of a lowered renal threshold associated with otherwise normal subjects, in pregnancy, and in patients with chronic renal disease. Transient glycosuria occurs frequently in persons without diabetes under conditions of stress or after ingestion of a high-carbohydrate meal. Even glycosuria associated with ketonuria is not always pathognomonic of diabetes mellitus.

If it is observed that a urine contains substances capable of reducing copper or ferricyanide solutions, glycosuria is suggested. It must be determined that the reducing substances are sugar, and diabetes mellitus must be considered. The diagnosis can be made only after a high fasting blood sugar of 150 mg. per cent or more or an impaired glucose tolerance has been demonstrated. It must be pointed out again that many patients with diabetes mellitus exhibit only minor symptoms and do not excrete sugar in the urine. Thus a urine screening test for sugar may overlook a significant number of persons with this disease. However, if a screening procedure for blood sugar is used, more adequate coverage can be expected. An effective screening test consists of determining the blood glucose level on a single sample of blood taken three hours after ingestion of a breakfast containing 100 grams of carbohydrate. If the value is within normal limits (70 to 110 mg. per 100 ml. of blood), diabetes mellitus is excluded (Thorn and Forsham). This is merely a "screening" test. If positive, the patient must be referred to a physician for additional tests and evaluation. The question of referring the patient to the physician in the first place instead of after tests are performed has been discussed previously.

CONTACT SENSITIVITY TESTS

Patch tests for agents producing contact stomatitis are of little practical value. The simplest method for determining the presence of an agent causing a contact mucositis of the mouth is to refrain from using the suspected agent. If the stomatitis disappears after withdrawal and reappears when the agent is used again, it is reasonably established as the offending agent. Only rarely is it necessary to actually patch test the oral mucosa to determine what components of an agent may be responsible for stomatitis. It is fairly well known that some part of a denture, or certain ingredients of tooth paste, mouthwash, or almost any substance, for that matter, may be responsible for an untoward reaction. A history of their use, the clinical appearance of the reaction of the tissues to the agents, and remission after withdrawal of the agent make the identification possible.

Patch testing of the skin is not reliable as a substitute for testing the oral mucosa since the oral mucosa and the skin very often differ widely in their response to sensitizing agents. It must be kept in mind that such a simple procedure as skin testing may result in untoward systemic effects in susceptible subjects. Scratch tests of the skin have no general practical or important value in the general practice of dentistry. They are unreliable in many instances, and severe systemic reactions can occur. Unless the dentist is prepared to meet these emergencies in his office, he should refer the patient to a competent allergist.

Patch testing is of no value in determining the causative agent in stomatitis medicamentosa. Cessation of the stomatitis when the suspected agent is withdrawn is fairly good evidence of the nature of the agent. Readministration of a drug to observe the possibility of a recrudescence may produce severe systemic reactions. This method of testing should be used with caution.

BIOPSY

Of the various supplementary diagnostic aids, biopsy is one of the most valuable. Because histologic changes provide the basis for a high degree of accuracy in determining the nature of a lesion, biopsy is frequently used to confirm a presumptive diagnosis made on clinical and radiographic findings.

Some clinicians have the impression that biopsy is used only as a means of recognizing neoplastic disease and therefore use it only to a limited degree.

However, it may be used to verify the presence of specific inflammatory or granu-lomatous processes, blood dyscrasias, certain metabolic disorders, developmental disturbances, reactive lesions, etc. It is also of value in determining the type of treatment to be instituted in certain diseases and in evaluating the progress of treatment. Further, it is a valuable self-teaching diagnostic aid. The repeated microscopic verification or correction of clinical impressions improves diagnostic acumen.

Biopsy should always be used to verify the presence and nature of neo-plastic disease. Since the type and extent of treatment of a neoplasm are dictated by the microscopic findings, biopsy is therefore imperative before treatment is instituted.

Taking a biopsy is relatively simple, inexpensive, and painless. The removal of tissue to be examined microscopically can be accomplished in a dental office with a limited armamentarium by anyone who has basic surgical training and an understanding of the anatomy of the area from which the specimen is to be removed.

The armamentarium needed for biopsy consists of the following:

1. Antiseptic to apply at the injection and biopsy sites
2. Local anesthetics and syringe
3. Scalpel
4. Small pointed scissors
5. Tissue forceps
6. Surgical hemostats
7. Sponges
8. Sutures
9. Needle holder
10. Wide-mouthed bottle containing 10 per cent formalin 15 times the volume of the specimen
11. Periosteal elevator ⎤
12. Bone bur   ⎥
13. Bone chisel   ⎬ for intraosseous lesions
14. Mallet   ⎦
15. Curettes
16. Syringe for aspiration (10 to 20 ml. capacity and large-bore needle)
17. Biopsy punch—rarely used in dental practice

Specific Indications for Biopsy.—Specific indications for biopsy are as follows:

1. Any ulcer which has not shown evidence of healing in a period of three weeks.
2. Any tumescence suspected of being a neoplasm.
3. Any persistent hyperkeratotic lesion.
4. Any tissue surgically excised.
5. Any tissue spontaneously expelled from a body orifice.
6. Material from a persistent draining sinus, the source of which cannot be readily iden-tified, together with some of the lining of the sinus.
7. Any intraosseous lesion which cannot be positively identified radiographically.

Precautions and Contraindications for Biopsy.—Permission to take a biopsy should always be obtained from the patient. This is usually not difficult if the value of the biopsy procedure is explained. The following precautions and con-traindications should be observed:

1. Pigmented lesions which suggest the presence of melanin should never be removed by the incisional method. They should be excised, with a wide margin of the normal tissue surrounding the lesion.
2. Lesions which are purplish in color and appear to be filled with blood are probably vascular in origin, and incision would result in extensive hemorrhage. Consequently, such lesions should not be biopsied as an office procedure. When possible, the entire lesion should be removed in the initial procedure.
3. The specimen should be removed with a minimum of manipulation of the area.
4. Local anesthetics should never be injected into the lesion.
5. The lapse of time between taking the specimen and reporting the diagnosis should be as short as is possible and practical. If the lesion is suspected of being a neoplasm, provision for treatment immediately after receipt of a positive report is imperative.

Some observers have suggested that the removal of tissue from a neoplasm may cause dissemination of the cells, resulting in early metastasis; others have shown that this is not true. However, unnecessary rough manipulation and palpation of a lesion is much more dangerous than performing a biopsy. Certainly the minimal dangers incident to removal of a biopsy specimen far outweigh the dangers of attempting any type of treatment without definite diagnosis. Under no circumstances should the treatment of a neoplasm be attempted without a positive diagnosis by microscopic means whether the lesion is far advanced or in early stages of its development.

Selection of the Biopsy Specimen.—The tissue specimen should be removed from a site and in such a manner as to provide the pathologist with a representative piece of tissue in a state suitable for microscopic examination. The following rules should be observed in obtaining a biopsy specimen:

1. From the standpoint of the pathologist, the whole lesion provides the most desirable specimen. This should pertain in all cases where the lesion is small and where removal of an adequate specimen would take practically the entire lesion.
2. In large lesions the specimen should be removed from the most easily accessible area and from an area that represents the characteristic portion of the lesion.
3. Thin deep sections taken from the substance of the lesion across the border into the normal tissue are more desirable than large shallow specimens taken from the surface. Surface specimens often provide only necrotic tissue or crust and do not represent the deeper, more typical character of a lesion.
4. If several lesions are present, the specimen should be taken from the most representative.
5. If the lesion is intraosseous, the cortical plate of bone should be removed and, along with the material curetted from the interior of the lesion, submitted for examination.

Removal of Tissue.—The tissue specimen may be obtained by any one of the following methods:

Complete Excision
When a lesion is small, it can be excised in its entirety with some of the surrounding tissue; thus the entire lesion serves as the biopsy specimen.

Incision
When a lesion is extensive and complete removal would entail a complicated surgical procedure, an adequate specimen for observation of the pathologic character of the entire lesion can be obtained by the removal of a small portion of the lesion and some of the surrounding tissue by incision.

Aspiration

This method is used for large masses which are relatively inaccessible and for lesions whose clinical character suggests that they are soft or semifluid in consistency. Aspiration is done by inserting a large-gauge needle into the softer parts of the mass. Strong negative pressure is created which draws fluid and cells into the needle. More than one sample may be necessary to demonstrate positively the character of a disease process.

Paracentesis

This is withdrawal of fluid from a body cavity through a large needle by negative pressure.

Punch

A tissue punch is inserted into the center of a lesion and a small plug of tissue removed. This method is sometimes used for lesions which are surgically inaccessible.

Curettage

This is the removal of small bits of tissue with a sharp instrument. Curettement is used to remove tissue from a bony cavity, a sinus tract, or a body space such as the maxillary antrum.

Tissue Smears

Smears from tissue surfaces are sometimes used when a lesion is ulcerated and surgically inaccessible. They can be taken on Gelfoam or similar material which can be fixed and sectioned without disturbing the material obtained.

The method chosen for obtaining the tissue specimen is dependent on the size, location, and character of the lesion. A small lesion elevated above the surface in a region in which the tissue is flexible, such as in the buccal mucosa, can be removed by complete excision as shown in Fig. 225. This leaves a small oval-shaped defect which can be closed easily with a couple of sutures.

In a small, elevated lesion in an area in which the tissue is not flexible, such as the gingiva or palate, two elliptical-shaped incisions (which surround the lesion) should be made at such an angle that they meet beneath the base of the lesion and the specimen removed with tissue forceps. The resulting wound can be closed smoothly with a few sutures. The removal of gingival tissue for biopsy of gingival enlargement is best accomplished by elliptical incisions. The specimen should include the interdental papilla, free gingival margin, and base of crevice (Fig. 226). The wound may be dressed with Ward's surgical dressing.

It is desirable that the specimen removed from a large lesion be thin, deep, and ellipsoidal in shape. The incisions should converge deep in the lesion and extend to its full depth if possible. The specimen should be removed with tissue forceps, and it should be grasped lightly in only one location to prevent crushing. The resulting wound should be closed with sutures. (Fig. 227.)

In a large friable fungating lesion in which the site of tissue removal would be difficult to close with a suture, the specimen can be removed with an electric scalpel. However, the specimen must be larger than that obtained with a steel scalpel to compensate for coagulation which takes place at the margin of the specimen.

In an intraosseous lesion, an incision should be made through the periosteum, the periosteum stripped away to expose the cortex, and the cortex of bone over the lesion removed by the use of bone burs, chisels, or a combination bur and chisel, with care taken to prevent disturbing the underlying tissue. A portion of

Fig. 225. *Excisional biopsy* of lesion involving soft tissue.

Fig. 226. *Gingival biopsy*. Elliptical incision for removal of interdental papilla, free gingival margin, and base of crevice.

the lesion then is removed through the cortical opening with sharp curettes. The soft tissue should be sutured over the defect.

In aspiration biopsies a large needle is inserted into the center or softer part of a lesion and strong suction created to bring material into the needle or syringe. The small amount of material obtained can be expressed from the needle onto a piece of Gelfoam for ease in handling. If the quantity of fluid is large, it can be expressed into a test tube containing a fixative. If cultures are also desirable, some of the material should be placed in a sterile plugged test tube or in a Petri dish.

Handling of the Tissue Specimen.—In the laboratory the material is usually sectioned by the paraffin embedding method which can be completed in twenty-

Fig. 227. Incisional biopsy. Specimen includes normal and pathologic tissue.

Fig. 228. *Aspiration of cyst.* Slightly compressible bulging of buccal plate over first molar, indicating a possible cyst. Aspiration with exfoliative cytology may be helpful in establishing true character of intraosseous lesion.

four hours. Calcified material will require decalcification and will take a longer period to prepare. If immediate diagnosis is necessary, the material can be prepared by the frozen section technic in ten minutes. This method produces extensive distortion and is much less accurate than the paraffin method and is rarely required for oral specimens. The following instructions should be followed:

1. The tissue should be removed with a sharp instrument and with a minimum of manipulation. If tissue forceps are used, they should not grasp that portion of the lesion selected to show the character of the process. The specimen should not be grasped more than once since crushing with forceps distorts the cells and makes the tissue unsatisfactory for microscopic examination.

2. The specimen should be placed immediately into a fixative. It should not be left in the air to dry.
3. The container for the fixative should have a wide mouth to permit the specimen to be dropped into the fixative. A specimen should never be placed in a dry container and the fixative poured over it, since it may adhere to the side of the container and prevent the fixative from penetrating the adhered surface.
4. Ten per cent formalin (4 per cent formaldehyde) is a good universal fixative. Bouin's solution, mercuric chloride, or other special fixatives may be used.
5. The specimen container should have a leak-proof cap and should be clearly labeled with the patient's name.
6. If more than one specimen is removed from a patient, they should be placed in separate, clearly identified containers.
7. A history bearing the patient's name, age, and sex, name of operator, and pertinent information about the lesion should be attached to the outside of the specimen container.
8. The specimen should be sent or mailed to the pathology laboratory immediately.

•   •   •

Any abnormal tissue removed from the oral cavity should be biopsied to verify clinical impressions. In many instances what appears to be a lesion of little significance is found to be one of a more grave nature when the histologic features are studied. When the more exact nature of the lesion is known, proper therapy which benefits the patient and protects the operator can be instituted. For patients who have a cancer phobia, the histologic examination provides a means of eliminating the phobia. Legally the treatment of a lesion without the aid of biopsy can be construed as malpractice.

EXFOLIATIVE CYTOLOGY

Numerous writings extol the use of exfoliative cytology as a simple and reasonably accurate method for the detection of oral disease. The exfoliative cytology technic has been used effectively as a means of detecting disease in remote areas of the body not accessible to biopsy as well as a screening technic for cancer of the cervix. It also has been suggested as a method for the diagnosis of oral disease. The use of exfoliative cytology as a diagnostic technic has advantages and disadvantages. The advantages include the following:

1. A limited amount of equipment is needed.
2. The procedure is simple and can be accomplished without anesthetic or surgical instruments.
3. The time involved is much shorter than that in any other method.
4. It does not provide the same degree of anxiety or arouse intense fear of cancer in the patient.
5. It is a simple and inexpensive laboratory procedure.

The disadvantages of exfoliative cytology are the following:

1. It detects only surface lesions.
2. If the surface of the lesion is heavily keratinized, the typical character of the lesion will not be demonstrated by the limited material.
3. Treatment cannot be predicated on a positive smear—a biopsy is still necessary to verify the positive lesion.
4. There are many disease processes other than cancer which produce "white lesions" that are not precancerous, nor can they be diagnosed from exfoliated cells.

5. In other areas of the body exfoliated cells are retained in body secretions, but in the oral region they are continually washed away.
6. The technic, although simple, frequently is not adequately accomplished so that material is not representative.
7. A negative report on such material provides a false security of having adequately surveyed the area or lesion.
8. A positive smear indicates the need for a biopsy; the negative smear means very little.
9. Exfoliative cytology is inadequate as a screening procedure.

Materials.—The materials needed in the office include the following:

1. Ethyl alcohol, 95 per cent
2. Glass slides (preferably full-surface frosted slides)
3. Paper clips
4. Plain lead pencil
5. Metal or wooden spatula or cotton-tipped applicator
6. Mailing container

Although 95 per cent ethyl alcohol is the ideal fixative, 70 per cent alcohol may be substituted if the need arises. Wooden spatulas or cotton-tipped applicators should be moistened before use, preferably in physiologic saline solution. Any type of cardboard or plastic mailing container is satisfactory if it is adequate to protect the slides en route to the cytology laboratory. Several types of containers are available commercially.

Method.—If exfoliative cytology is to be used as a diagnostic procedure, the following method of obtaining and handling the material is recommended.

1. The patient's full name should be written on one end of each of two slides, and a paper clip should be placed on that end of the slide.
2. If cellular debris and exudate are excessive, the lesion should be wiped moderately clean with a piece of gauze.
3. The lesion should be scraped with the instrument of choice (a metal spatula and a cotton-tipped applicator moistened in a saline solution) and the material should be spread immediately on the slide.
4. If the spatula is used, the material should be placed on one slide and another drawn across it. If the cotton-tipped applicator is used, the material should be smeared on both slides with the applicator.
5. As soon as the material is placed on a slide, it should be immersed immediately in fixative, since the slightest air drying will cause distortion of the cells and will make interpretation difficult or impossible. The slides should be fixed for at least thirty minutes and then air dried.
6. Next, the slides are prepared for shipment together with the clinical information available. This information should include, at least, the name and address of the sender and of the patient, the age, sex, and race of the patient, the duration and location of the lesion, and its description.

Aspiration.—Aspiration is a means of obtaining material from a body cavity, a cystic space, or a lesion containing fluid. The fluid obtained through a large-bore needle by negative pressure will provide varying numbers of individual cells or aggregates of a few cells. The material so obtained may be handled in a variety of ways to permit the study of cellular detail for diagnostic purposes.

The obtained material may be smeared on a slide and treated in the same manner as the smears prepared for exfoliative cytology. The material, if abundant, may be fixed and then centrifuged. The compressed sediment may then be

processed as solid tissue and sectioned for study. When the material is of limited quantity, it may be placed on a piece of cellulose sponge or some other
similar porous material which will be unaffected by tissue-processing procedures. The material can be processed and cut by the same method as tissue with
the cells entrapped in the mesh of the sponge. This procedure in reality is a type
of exfoliative study and provides the same aid to diagnosis.

PULP VITALITY TESTS

The excitability of the dental pulp is related to the physiologic state of this
tissue—the principle upon which the determination of abnormalities of the pulp
has been based. Clinical procedures utilizing mechanical, chemical, thermal,
and electrical stimuli have been used. Each method has certain basic limitations.
Mechanical stimulation with an explorer or bur is difficult to evaluate and is
considered to be unreliable. Chemical stimulation has even greater drawbacks
and has never been widely used. Both thermal and electrical excitation have
been used with considerably more success in determining the biologic state of
the dental pulp. These two methods can be regulated fairly well and are of
considerable value when their limitations are well understood.

Several types of electric current have been used: faradic, galvanic, alternating, and condensor discharge current. Serious attempts have been made by
diagnosticians to assess the physiologic condition of the pulp accurately by the
establishment of a positive and direct correlation between the quantitative exciting factors (voltage, current, frequency, wave form, etc.) and the irritability
of the pulp tissue. However, the clinical use of a pure quantitative factor and
the determination of the excitability of the dental pulp have not progressed
to the point of consistent results. It is not surprising that many instruments have
been designed in an attempt to relate voltage and/or current accurately with
the irritability of the pulp tissue.

The physiologic basis for the use of electrical stimulation is based upon the
fact that pain is a specific sensory experience mediated through nerve structures
which are separate from those which mediate other sensations such as touch,
pressure, heat, and cold. No sensation other than pain can be elicited from the
dental pulp. Electrical pulp testing is an algesimetric method based upon the fact
that pain can be elicited from the pulp by electrical stimuli. Procedures for determining pain threshold of the teeth are difficult to evaluate because the methods used do not closely associate the stimulus with the tissue changes causing
the pain.

The minimal stimulus necessary to cause excitation of the free nerve endings
and to register pain is called a *threshold stimulus*. The response or reaction
of a patient to an excessive stimulus is a subjective sensation; it is a complex
physiopsychologic process involving the cognitive functions of an individual and
represents an emotional and physiologic expression resulting from the perception
of pain. The dual aspect of pain—threshold stimulus and reaction to pain—is
of experimental value only; it is of no clinical value because of the intricate
relationship between the two factors. Hence, under clinical conditions it is
better to consider only the factor which can be easily measured—*pain perception*

threshold. This factor is defined as the lowest perceptible intensity of pain caused by a pain threshold stimulus; this is the amount of stimulus necessary to induce threshold pain (Bonica).

Under normal circumstances the threshold for the perception of pain is approximately the same in the same subject at varying times of the day. It must be remembered that while this threshold does not vary appreciably, the threshold for reaction to pain varies widely. The patient's mentation and attitude may cause the reaction threshold to vary considerably. Age, sex, emotional security, fatigue, drugs, and race may also alter it.

The following conditions are necessary for a reaction to a stimulus to occur: (1) there must be an adequate stimulus that transcends the excitement threshold of the free nerve endings; (2) the stimulus must be conducted by the nerve tracts to the brain; and (3) the tissue must be capable of being excited. Obviously the blocking of the nerve transmission caused by anesthetics, nerve resections, nerve injuries, or nerve lesions will prevent the stimulus from producing a painful sensation. Changes in the excitability state of the nerve tissue may result from injury to the pulp. Probably other factors may be related indirectly to the excitability of the teeth. The teeth of young persons, especially maxillary central incisors with apices which are open, may fail to show response to what might ordinarily be considered painful stimuli. The reaction of the patient to pain varies greatly and may be only slightly correlated with the intensity of the stimulus. It is apparent that the electrical stimulus of choice should be the one which is the most indicative of stimulus intensity.

The problems of electrical pulp testing are numerous. They include high resistance and variations of resistance in the teeth, periodontal membrane reaction, difficulty in determining the difference in pain perception and reaction to pain, limitations of the testing apparatus and its clinical application, and inability to establish a direct relationship between the threshold value and the pathologic process viewed microscopically.

Attempts have been made to separate the response of the periodontal membrane from the response of the pulp by utilizing the difference in the frequency necessary to stimulate the two contiguous tissues and the difference in the excitation thresholds of the teeth and periodontal membrane. Under normal conditions the threshold of excitation of the periodontal membrane is about 200 to 400 microamperes (Bjorn) and the excitation threshold of pulp is about 15 to 20 microamperes. Ziskin and Wald considered that frequencies between 1,000 and 5,000 cycles per second separated the pulpal and periodontal responses in some instances. The use of ultrahigh frequency alternating current for the stimulus is of no value. An increase in the frequency of excitation current produces a rise in the pain threshold to the point that no excitation occurs (Bjorn).

In order for an electric pulp tester to be completely effective in correlating pathologic pulp changes and changes in the excitability of the pulp, it is necessary that the tester indicate induced pain without tissue damage by a stimulus whose intensity can be accurately measured and which can be used in a predictable manner accomplished by means of a relatively simple neuroreceptive conductive and perceptive mechanism.

As previously mentioned, several problems make this goal difficult, if not impossible, to obtain at the present time. Serious attempts, directed toward both instrument design and instrument use, have been made to eliminate most of the problems.

One of the principal problems in instrument design is related to the construction of an instrument which will be simple, easy to use clinically, and safe. Many types of apparatus have been developed to apply and measure an electrical stimulus to the tooth for the purpose of determining the excitability state of the dental pulp tissue. The two most practical accepted methods are measurement of the current or measurement of the voltage necessary to produce the lowest perceptible intensity of pain. Accordingly, the pain threshold is considered to be raised when more stimulus energy is required to induce threshold pain; conversely, when less energy is required, the pain threshold is said to be lowered. Thus the rationale for using an electrical pulp tester as a diagnostic aid in determining the state of the pulp depends on two important factors: (1) in order for the determination of the threshold stimulus to be of value, the stimulus (current or voltage), must be exactly defined and (2) there must exist predetermined physiologic and/or pathologic states to correlate with alterations in the threshold stimulus; this implies that the stimulus be standardized and that normal thresholds of other teeth be known or be determined.

The excitation of the teeth by electrical stimulation is dependent upon the current passing through tissue which is capable of responding to a stimulus. Hence excitation depends on current density; this varies with the total current, the placement and size of the electrodes, and the conductivity of the tissues. It becomes obvious that the absolute threshold of excitation of the pulp is obscure at best. The duration of the stimulus is also related to the excitation. In general, the shorter the duration of the exciting stimulus, the greater the intensity required to produce a response. The time of the application of the stimulus must be a certain minimum for a given current; otherwise there is a possibility of producing tissue damage. Electrical stimuli of reasonable intensity do not produce tissue changes, and repeated applications of the stimulus are possible without loss of uniformity of response—all other factors remaining equal (Goetzel). However, prolonged stimulation at high current intensity results in irreversible damage to the tooth (Hardy). The current in a pulp tester should be utilized according to its form, strength, and duration. For uniform results the form should be easy to define and constant and the current duration should not be so short that the strength is unnecessarily high nor so long that excessive amounts of energy are applied to the tissues.

The physiologic effect of an electrical stimulus depends upon current strength. This factor is related to the voltage and the electrical resistance in the current circuit. There is considerable variation in the resistance of teeth and in the resistance between the pulp tester electrode and the tooth. Measurement of voltage would then tend to measure the resistance of these two factors rather than simply the threshold stimulus. Pulp testers utilizing voltage measurements are of clinical value when the operator is familiar with the necessity for keeping conditions under which the tests are made as nearly uniform as possible. While there appears to be little agreement among investigators as to which aspect of an electrical stimulus should be measured to indicate stimulus intensity, Bjorn and Ziskin and Wald consider current strength to be the important decisive factor.

In order to eliminate the variations in the resistance of the dental tissues and the resistance between the electrode and tooth and also to protect the tooth against accidental excessive current, pulp testers generally are constructed so as to have a high internal resistance. In these instruments it is the voltage applied that determines the current strength and not changes in the external circuit. This is possible because resistance changes in the external circuit are minor when compared to the high resistance of the internal circuit of the pulp tester.

In general, whenever an electrode of a pulp tester is applied to the lip, finger, gingiva, or cheek, a stimulus is usually felt at a very low threshold. The threshold for excitation of the finger or lip is more than fifty times that of many teeth; however, the electrical resistance of the skin is very low compared with that in the teeth and the stimulus is usually felt at a very low intensity. Inasmuch as the dental pulp has only specific stimuli receptors for pain and the cheek and lip and periodontal structures have other receptors present for cold, heat, and pressure sensations, it is to be expected that certain current strengths may produce two sensations. Therefore, it is possible that a current may produce only a tickling sensation in soft tissues of the lip and cheeks whereas the same application may produce pain in the dental pulp. As was previously pointed out, current voltage, wave form, frequency, and other factors play a considerable part in what the reaction and threshold of stimulus will be for any given instrument. The proper use of an electrical pulp tester dictates that the patient respond only to those stimuli which produce pain—not to those which produce tickling sensations or other types of responses.

Pulp Testers in Use.—The Burton Vitalometer is an electrical pulp tester which employs an interrupted high frequency wave produced by a mechanical generator. This tester provides for an internal circuit resistance of over 3,000,000 ohms, which limits the actual current in the external circuit to about 4 micro-amperes. An applied interrupted voltage which is used to stimulate the pulp may be increased or decreased by sliding an indicator along an arbitrary scale; this sliding indicator operates the secondary coil of an inductorium. A mechanical magnetic breaker system in the primary coil of the inductorium alters the output of the tester from 60 cycles to 50,000 cycles per second. The Burton Vitalometer is connected in the manner indicated in Fig. 229. The patient holds the capacitor and the operator manipulates the inductorium (sliding scale) while holding the electrode on the tooth. The vibrator mechanism is actuated when the contact button is pressed. The contact button is moved from the lowest point on the scale to that point which first elicits a response from the patient. The arbitrary scale is numbered from 1 to 16. The value of each figure must be calibrated for each tooth being tested by comparing it with that of adjacent teeth or with similar teeth on the opposite side of the arch. Low readings on the scale are usually indicative of a hyperexcitable pulp; high readings usually indicate

Fig. 229. *Types of Burton Vitalometers.* The Vitalometer on the right is a new model (No. 205MB) that eliminates the patient-held electrode, **B,** by incorporating the capacity tube, **B,** into the tooth electrode. **A,** Tooth electrode. **Aa,** Tooth electrode with included capacity tube. **B,** Patient's hand electrode. **C, Bb,** Inductorium. **D, Ce,** Power generators. (Courtesy Burton Manufacturing Co., Santa Monica, Calif.)

Fig. 230. S. S. *White pulp tester No. 2A.* (Courtesy The S. S. White Dental Manufacturing Co., Philadelphia, Pa.)

a hypoexcitable or "dead" pulp. The significance of each reading cannot be fully evaluated without the correlation of clinical findings.

The S. S. White pulp tester No. 2A is a low-frequency pulp tester which operates between 1,000 and 5,000 cycles per second (Fig. 230). It contains a voltage transformer, the primary coil of which is connected to a source of alternating current. The secondary coil of the transformer furnishes current for the pilot light on the instrument panel and for an adjustable high resistance potentiometer which controls the current applied to the external circuit. The amount of current in the circuit is indicated by a microammeter. The patient and the microammeter are protected against accidental short circuits and excessive current through a protective resistance of 100,000 ohms. A separate metal hand electrode is used by the patient. The tooth electrode is so constructed as to utilize a wood plug about 2 mm. in diameter that protrudes about 1 mm. beyond the electrode. The wood is soaked in a saline solution for better adaptation to the tooth surface and to ensure a good electrical circuit. This pulp tester is used by having the patient hold the hand electrode while the examiner places the wood plug electrode on the teeth; the operator then varies the voltage control knob to apply current in the patient's circuit. The current is increased gradually and smoothly until

Fig. 231. *Ritter pulp tester.* (Courtesy Ritter Co., Inc., Rochester, N. Y.)

pulp stimulation results. The microammeter will reveal the amount of current in microamperes flowing through the pulp-testing circuit. In anterior teeth the normal range of reading will be from 1 to 10 microamperes. Readings in excess of these usually indicate hypoexcitability or a devital tooth.

The Ritter pulp tester (Fig. 231) delivers a current of about 20,000 cycles per second of short duration to a tooth electrode. The intensity of the current can be regulated by a circular dial attached to the handle of the instrument. An arbitrary scale of 0 to 10 is afforded to indicate the degree of current tolerated by the patient. A neon light is present in the circuit to indicate whether or not current is being delivered to the tooth. The operator holds the handle of the pulp tester in one hand and completes the circuit by contacting the patient with the other hand. The manufacturer recommends that a drop of tooth paste rather than water be applied to the tooth electrode tip to ensure adequate electrical contact. The electrode is maintained in constant contact with the tooth, and the regulating dial located on the top of the instrument handle is moved slowly from 0 upward until the patient indicates a tingle or a sense of warmth. Readings in the region of 10 without eliciting a response indicate a hypoexcitable or devital pulp.

The Parkell Dentotest Vitalometer is a fully transistorized, battery-operated instrument. The source of power is a 4-volt mercury battery with an operating life of about 90 hours. A rheostat varies the current applied to the tooth from 20

Fig. 232. *Parkell Dentotest Vitalometer.* (Courtesy Parkell Products, Inc., Long Island City, N. Y.)

microamperes to 220 microamperes. The Dentotest operates on a frequency of 9,000 cycles per minute (Fig. 232).

Test Considerations.—The following considerations should be taken into account when testing with an electric pulp tester.

1. The patient should be informed of the nature of the test.
2. The teeth to be tested should be dried.
3. Adequate electrical contact between the tooth and the electrode must be made.
4. An excessively applied stimulus is likely to result in a false positive test because of leakage.
5. The electrode should be placed on sound tooth structure.
6. The electrode should not touch or be in close approximation to the gingiva.
7. Molar teeth may require tests at more than one point.
8. Electrical conduction through proximal inlays and continuous bridgework should be avoided.
9. Teeth with full gold, porcelain, or acrylic coverage cannot be tested with an electrical stimulus.
10. Pulp tests should substantiate the findings from the history and clinical examination.

The patient should be fully informed of the nature of the test. Since many patients are apprehensive of electrical apparatus, they are likely to respond to the test prematurely. Excessive pain is to be avoided. The tooth should be thoroughly dried to prevent leakage of the current to the soft tissues. When leakage occurs, the patient incurs an unnecessary painful experience and false positive readings can occur. The electrical contact between the electrode and the tooth may be enhanced by wetting the electrode with a saline solution. Unless an adequate electrical contact is made, an excessive current may have to be applied and a false hypoexcitable or devital pulp may be suggested by the test.

The electrode should be placed on sound tooth structure—never on restorations (Fig. 233). Placing the electrode on undermined enamel should be avoided. Occasionally large restorations may extend beneath the outer surface of the

A   B

Fig. 233. *Pulp testing.* Application of Vitalometer tip on tooth with restoration.

Fig. 234. *Pulp testing.* Vitalometer tip is placed well away from gingiva to prevent gingival response.

Fig. 235. *Pulp testing.* Rubber dam for isolation of tooth to be tested.

tooth being examined—the electrode should not be placed over these areas but over areas where sound tooth structure exists between the pulp and the surface of the tooth.

The electrode should be placed so as to avoid leakage to the gingiva (Fig. 234). Placement close to the gingiva may result in a leakage via the small amount of moisture left on the surface of the tooth, especially if the electrical resistance path to the pulp is greater than that to the gingiva. Leakage is quite likely to occur when the electrical stimulus is intense.

Multirooted teeth may have to be tested at more than one point since the pulp may be vital in one portion of the tooth and devital in another. It should be remembered that larger teeth, viz., molar teeth, generally require more stimulus to elicit a painful response than smaller teeth. Comparisons of vitality readings should be made between the same kind of teeth.

Occasionally the electrical resistance between adjacent teeth will be less than that of the tooth being tested because of approximating restorations. This occurs frequently when large restorations are present. This situation can be avoided by use of a rubber dam to isolate the tooth being tested (Fig. 235). While this shortcoming cannot be overcome with fixed bridgework, it can be minimized by proper placement of the electrode, viz., on exposed surfaces where abutment teeth are three-fourths crowns.

All tests should be correlated with the clinical findings. If a tooth appears to be involved apically as indicated by the radiographic examination but the electrical test is positive, the examiner should review his technic to assure himself that leakage or other shortcomings have not occurred. The shortcomings of electrical vitality tests should be well known to the examiner. In most instances, false positive or false negative tests are the fault of the person making the test, not the testing device.

Thermal Tests.—Thermal tests are frequently of value in testing changes in the pulp. Since the patient may experience pain in the pulp upon drinking hot coffee or cold water, thermal tests may be more effective in duplicating the natural cause of the pain than electrical tests. They are especially useful for teeth with full gold, porcelain, or acrylic coverage.

The correlation between pain caused by thermal stimulation and the state of the pulp is not specific or constant. Teeth which are sensitive to heat may not be sensitive to cold; those sensitive to cold may not be sensitive to heat; teeth may be sensitive to both heat and cold. To correlate these changes with histopathologic changes of the pulp is often misleading. Irrespective of the type of stimulus used, the clinical findings must be correlated with the pulp test findings.

Heat thermal tests may be accomplished by heating a small ball of guttapercha on the end of a plastic instrument and touching it to the tooth being tested (Fig. 236). The tooth should be wet to prevent the gutta-percha from sticking. The material should be applied lightly to the surface until the degree of tolerance by the patient can be determined. Since conduction of heat is slow but accumulative, it is possible for excessive heat to be applied unless the examiner is careful, especially in the presence of large restorations.

Fig. 236. *Pulp testing.* Thermal test using hot base plate gutta-percha.

A   B

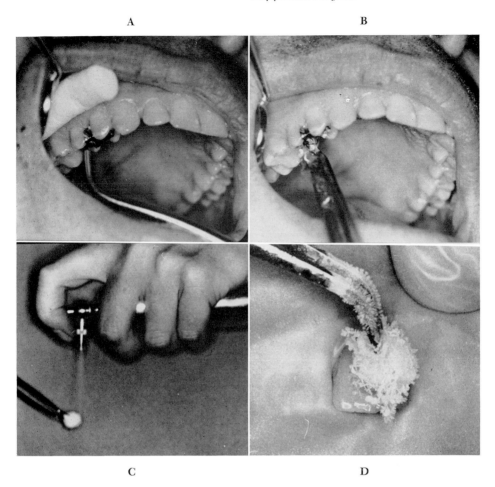

C   D

Fig. 237. *Pulp testing.* **A,** Thermal pulp test with cold air. **B,** Thermal pulp test with ice. **C** and **D,** Thermal pulp test with ethyl chloride applied to cotton pledget; ethyl chloride should not be sprayed directly on the tooth.

Cold thermal tests may be performed with cold air, ice, or cotton soaked in ethyl chloride (Fig. 237). Ethyl chloride should never be sprayed directly on the teeth. Since the transfer of heat away from the pulp is delayed, the application of the cold should be accomplished slowly to avoid excessive cold and a severe painful stimulus. Probably the most specific relationship that exists between the state of the pulp and the reaction to thermal change is that associated with an acute suppurative pulpitis or acute alveolar abscess. In these conditions the patient will experience severe pain when heat is applied and gain relief when cold is applied. In most instances he has discovered this for himself and is treating the pulp symptomatically by keeping ice on the offending tooth and avoiding heat.

Interpretation of Pulp Tests.—The principles of interpreting pulp tests are the same for both electrical and thermal stimulation. Because of the individual variations that exist in the response of a diseased pulp to any kind of painful stimulus, no specific histologic picture can be anticipated clinically or microscopically even if the tooth is extracted for study. Thus, it must be emphasized that it is impossible to make a differential diagnosis of the histopathologic features of pulp disease on the basis of pulp tests and clinical radiographic examinations alone. The clinical diagnosis is made on the basis of history, physical examination, radiographic examination, and the findings from the electrical and/or thermal tests. If all of these are used correctly, an accurate diagnosis of devital or vital pulp usually can be made. The diagnosis of hyperplastic pulpitis (pulp polyp) is obvious clinically. Aside from the common clinical findings relative to acute suppurative pulpitis and acute alveolar abscess already mentioned, no other unequivocal clinical diagnosis of pulp disease can be made without exposure of the pulp.

The acuteness of pulp disease for practical purposes must be based on the severity of the pain and the suddenness of onset. This does not imply any particular degree of pulp damage, for the symptoms of partial pulpitis may be the same as those of total pulpitis. From a practical standpoint, acute clinical symptoms of pulp disease in adult teeth with closed foramens generally indicate the death of the pulp. As far as pulp testing results are concerned, it is well known that pulp destruction from severe inflammatory or circulatory disturbances will produce a rise in the threshold of excitation. It is also well known that the threshold of excitation may be lowered in the early stages of inflammation. However, it should be remembered that the threshold value may be affected by factors having nothing to do with the excitability of the tooth per se (Bjorn).

The diagnosis of chronic pulp disease can only be made clinically on the basis of a history of chronicity or recurrence and the absence of acute symptoms. A history of an acute episode of pulpitis followed by less severe episodes may also occur. In some instances a state of mild, chronic, recurrent, or latent pulpitis may be detected on the basis of history alone. On occasion a tooth will suddenly give signs of pulp disease after it is restored or used as an abutment tooth. Not infrequently the exacerbation of such latent disease will be due to the occlusal trauma. In many of these situations acute exacerbations result in failure of extensive reconstructions. This can be avoided many times by a complete history, physical examination, radiographic examination, and vitality test of the teeth prior to reconstruction. Unfortunately not all cases of latent pulpitis can be determined in advance.

Summary.—These salient features of pulp testing should be kept in mind:

1. A maximum stimulus without reaction is always indicative of a partial or totally necrotic pulp, and root canal therapy is indicated (assuming the pulp test is correlated with the clinical findings and the tests are accurately done).
2. A "normal" reaction to pulp testing either by electrical or thermal stimulation may not necessarily indicate a healthy pulp, since retrogressive changes may not affect the threshold of excitation.
3. A raised threshold of excitation does not necessarily indicate a diseased pulp.

Some of the confusion arising from the diagnosis of pulp changes and excitation threshold can be eliminated by taking an adequate history and making a careful physical and radiographic examination. Thus, no one method of examination should be done to the exclusion of all others.

STUDY CASTS

Study models can be an important aid in diagnosis and treatment planning when the patient is away from the dental office. Articulation of study casts will materially aid the examiner in evaluating occlusal function and allow trial adjustments to be made and the effect noted before actually carrying out the procedure in the mouth. Articulation of models and the preparation of a grinding chart may be quite valuable in the occlusal adjustment of a difficult case. The mounting of casts in an articulator is also helpful in studying the preparation of the mouth for prosthetic appliances. The examination of unmounted casts by visual inspection and by a surveying instrument may reveal factors that will interfere with the seating of fixed appliances or with the insertion and removal of removable appliances. This information will help the examiner decide what appliance is most appropriate and what changes should be made during the preparation of the mouth to more effectively utilize a particular appliance. Study casts can be surveyed by the use of a paralleling surveyor to determine the most advantageous path of insertion and removal of an appliance; the amount and location of retention can be determined by the use of a surveyor. Further, study casts serve as excellent visual aids in informing a patient of his dental problems.

Articulation of Casts

The articulation of study casts on an adjustable articulator is an important procedure in the functional analysis of occlusal relations. While errors of reproducing the complicated movements of the human jaws are inherent in any method of mounting, the simple procedure presented here will be of considerable value in diagnosis and treatment planning in spite of its limitations. A clinical functional analysis of occlusal relationships should be carried out prior to mounting study casts. This analysis has already been described (see Chapter 5).

The mounting procedure should be as follows:

1. Determination of the conventional hinge axis
2. Preparation of the bite fork with wax
3. Positioning of the bite fork in the mouth
4. Positioning and locking of the face-bow
5. Transfer of the face-bow to the articulator and mounting of the maxillary cast
6. Preparation of wax recording of centric relation
7. Transfer of the recording to the articulator and mounting of the mandibular cast
8. Preparation of protrusive wax recording
9. Transfer of the recording to articulator and adjustment of condylar guidance

Conventional Hinge Axis.—Determination of the true hinge axis cannot be determined without the use of a kinematic face-bow. If used properly, the Hanau face-bow is sufficiently accurate to record a hinge axis which is reasonably close to that of the true terminal hinge axis. Such a hinge axis is called a conventional hinge axis. The error between a true hinge axis and a conventional hinge axis may be kept to a minimum if the opening between the teeth is limited to ½ to 1 mm. If marked premature occlusal interferences prevent this, a preliminary adjustment of these areas should be made. Since the determination is also dependent upon the ability of the patient to relax his muscles during hinge axis closure, muscle spasms, pain in the teeth, and temporomandibular joint pain will have to be relieved before the registration can be accomplished. Symptomatic treatment with muscle relaxants may be of value.

The conventional hinge axis is determined by measurement (Fig. 238, A). A millimeter rule is placed on the face so that it forms a line from the middle of the tragus of the ear to the corner of the eye, and the axis is marked 13 mm. in front of the anterior border of the tragus. After marking the point, it should be evaluated for accuracy by palpation of the condyle while the patient makes small up-and-down movements of the mandible.

A   B

C

Fig. 238. *Articulation of casts.* **A,** Location of hinge axis. **B,** Placement of face-bow. **C,** Mounting maxillary cast on articulator.

Use of Bite Fork.—The Hanau bite fork is made for use with occlusion rims which may hinder its use with natural dentition; therefore it should be related to the study casts to determine whether or not it will cause an interference. Modification of the center prong and shape of the fork may be necessary to avoid impingement on the teeth.

The bite fork is wrapped with two or three layers of medium hard base plate wax that has been softened. The thickness and form of the wax should be related to the study cast to determine if sufficient wax is present to prevent the teeth from going through to the metal fork. Marked overbite and convex occlusal planes require more wax than straight occlusal planes to prevent impingement on the metal fork. The wax should be uniformly soft throughout; this can be accomplished by placing the waxed fork in warm water. The fork is positioned in the mouth so that its handle is sufficiently displaced laterally to avoid contact with the incisal pin of the articulator when the cast is mounted and the patient is instructed to bite until sufficient occlusal imprints have been made to provide stability. The waxed fork is then chilled thoroughly and removed, and all excess wax and soft tissue impressions are removed with a sharp knife. The waxed fork is placed on the casts to determine stability. Rocking of the models on it indicates an improper relationship and the bite should be taken again. The wax should be trimmed along the incisal and buccal surfaces of the teeth. The waxed fork is chilled and placed back in the patient's mouth in its original position, and the patient is instructed to hold it while the face-bow is centered (Fig. 238, *B*). The ends of the condyle pins of the face-bow should be centered on the ink markings which have been previously made on the face to mark the conventional hinge axis. They should just touch the surface of the skin and no pressure should be exerted on the tissues. Their position should be checked after the face-bow has been fixed in position since movement may occur during the tightening procedure. The face-bow is then transferred to the articulator and the maxillary cast is mounted (Fig. 238, *C*). Since the ordinary face-bow does not have an infraorbital pin for orientation to the Frankfort horizontal plane, the occlusal plane is set arbitrarily. The bite fork is leveled with the notch on the incisal pin.

Registration of Centric Relation.—Centric relation may be registered with plaster or wax. Wax is more commonly used because of its ease of manipulation and because of the margin of error between the cast and wax bite that can be tolerated. Plaster is quite accurate but it cannot clear undercuts. It flows into the embrasures and requires considerable trimming before the impression can be seated on the casts. One distinct advantage of plaster warrants mention. When it is used there is less tendency for the patient to displace the jaw than when wax is used because plaster offers no resistance to closure of the jaws. While displacement of the jaw can be minimized when wax is used if the wax is uniformly soft, the difficulty with the plaster flowing into undercuts and requiring considerable trimming cannot be minimized easily. Whether or not wax or plaster is used is primarily up to the clinician. The use of wax will be discussed here merely because of its more common usage.

In addition to the disadvantage of wax mentioned are its tendency to harden before the registration can be completed and the difficulty in chilling it completely before removal. The latter can be partly overcome by the use of a wax containing aluminum. This type of wax tends to heat more evenly, retain heat longer, and chill more quickly. The experienced operator may find that ordinary plate wax with a medium hard base serves his requirements as well.

In order to register centric relation, the patient's muscles must be relaxed as completely as possible. Trial movements of the mandible in hinge axis closure should precede the actual registration so that the patient may be trained to assist in the procedure. When this has been accomplished, the wax registration can be made.

The wax to be used is prepared by making a narrow roll (½ inch) of two or three thicknesses of base plate wax. The form of the wax can be determined by softening the roll and adjusting it to the curvature and length of the maxillary cast. The roll is immersed in warm water until it is uniformly warm throughout; it is then positioned in the patient's mouth.

A   B

C   D

Fig. 239. *Articulation of models.* **A,** Wax in position to record centric relation. **B,** Trimming excess wax. **C,** Completion of wax bite. **D,** Positioning mandibular cast on articulator with wax bite.

Fig. 240. *Determination of correct wax bite.* **A,** Series of casts in acquired centric occlusion. **B,** Series of casts showing incorrect wax bite; note discrepancy in comparison lines; these points of reference must be compared with the mouth. **C,** Series of casts showing correct wax bite. Posterior displacement on both sides of the mouth should be the same for two consecutive bites. Center line deviation, if any, should be the same for two consecutive wax bites.

The mandible is guided and controlled by light pressure on the patient's chin in the direction of the joint in order that there be no displacement from hinge axis movement during the final one to one-half inch of closure (Fig. 239). Centric relation registration should be recorded with 1 to 0.5 mm. of wax or space between the teeth just prior to initial occlusal contact. As soon as the operator is satisfied that this position has been reached in the wax bite, he should trim the excess wax from the teeth so that the labial and buccal incisal edges of the maxillary teeth are visible (Fig. 239). The wax should then be chilled and removed from the mouth, and any wax that has touched soft tissue should be removed. At least three recordings should be taken for a comparison of results. The amount of wax used and the interocclusal space present just prior to initial occlusal contact should be relatively the same.

A method for visualization and comparison of wax bites is demonstrated in Fig. 240. The casts are marked with vertical lines on their anterior and posterior parts. The casts should be in maximum occlusal contact—acquired centric. The operator should compare the position of the midline in the mouth in centric relation and in acquired centric occlusion. If deviation of the midline occurs on opening 1 to 0.5 mm., the amount should be indicated on the mandibular cast. If two wax registrations are identical, the most posterior displacement of the lines on the mandibular teeth will be the same for the two wax bites. The amount of displacement is not important since the thickness of the wax may alter the actual linear displacement. The important consideration is that the displacement posterior to the mandibular lines be proportioned on the same sides for two wax registrations. In general, if the closure is within 1 to 0.5 mm., the variation in the width of the wax bite will be of no significance. Therefore, if true centric relation is registered in two different registrations, the most posterior displacement of the mandibular lines on like sides of the cast will be the same. Any change from this will indicate a displacement of the mandible from true centric relation during closure.

No wax pattern should be used which shows perforation of the wax since this indicates that the initial occlusal contact has been recorded and some displacement of the mandible probably has occurred. There is no simple and completely accurate way in which to determine whether or not a wax bite has recorded true centric relation. A comparison of wax bites is of some assistance, but even then an experienced operator may have difficulty in obtaining a proper registration. Even the experienced operator may on occasion have to remount his cases several times before being satisfied that he has the proper centric relation recorded. For the beginner the mounting of a case for study may present a problem, but some of the sources of error may be eliminated by careful attention to details. The stone models must be as nearly perfect as possible, and all extraneous plaster and imperfections should be removed. The patient should be thoroughly relaxed and trained in the method of centric relation closure, and the wax should be uniformly soft throughout.

Protrusive Registration.—The wax roll is prepared in the same manner as for centric relation registration. The thickness of the wax roll may have to be increased in the molar region to compensate for a large interocclusal space due to a pronounced overbite of the maxillary incisors.

The patient should be trained to bite straight forward about 4 to 5 mm. Lateral displacement or Bennett movement should be avoided. After the patient is trained to bite in the desired position, the uniformly soft wax roll is inserted in the mouth. The closure should be stopped 1 to 0.5 mm. short of initial tooth contact. The wax is chilled and trimmed the same as in centric relation registration.

Mounting of the Mandibular Casts.—The accepted centric wax registration is used to position the mandibular cast to the maxillary cast. It may be held in position by wax or string (Fig. 239, *D*). Before the mandibular cast is fixed to the mounting ring, the incisal pin of the articulator is adjusted sufficiently (2 to 3 mm.) to compensate for the thickness of the wax registration. The centric lock is closed and locked to prevent displacement of the articulator arm. The mandibular cast is then fixed to the mounting ring (Fig. 241). After the plaster has set, the next step is to transfer the protrusive bite recording to the articulator.

Fig. 241. *Articulation of casts.* **A,** Centric relation. **B,** Protrusive relation. **C,** Centric relation without wax bite in place; note the posterior displacement of reference line on the mandibular cast; condyle axis is locked, and teeth are occluding on premature contacts only. **D,** Acquired centric occlusion. Difference in position of casts in **C** and **D** represents slide in centric.

Adjustment of Condylar Guidance.—The centric lock is opened, the condylar guidance screws are loosened, and the incisal pin is raised or removed. The protrusive registration is then positioned and fitted firmly to the maxillary and mandibular casts. The condylar guidance adjustments are moved forward and backward while the maxillary and mandibular casts are held firmly in position in the wax. The movement of the condylar guidance will cause the maxillary cast to rock in the wax. The condylar guidance should be locked in a position half-way between its forward and backward position where no rocking of the cast takes place. Each side is checked individually and then rechecked after the first position on each side is determined. The variation in the condylar guidance angulation should not vary more than 2 to 4 degrees from one side to the other if the temporomandibular joints are normal. Negative readings are generally the result of an inadequate registration. The lateral guidance is computed using the formula on the undersurface of the base of the Hanau articulator.

If the centric lock is tightened, the incisal pin raised, and the casts brought into contact, it will be found that the casts are in centric relation, and the initial occlusal contact should be the same as that seen in the mouth (Fig. 241). With the centric locks free the casts should articulate in the acquired centric occlusion (Fig. 241, *D*). If the articulation is closed in centric relation, incomplete occlusal contact is made until sliding of the maxillary cast on the articulator occurs; this represents a slide in centric.

When the mounting has been completed, the operator should determine whether or not he has a reasonably accurate centric relation registration. The most frequent sign of an improper registration is the presence of space between the molar teeth without the presence of any initial contact even in the position of habitual centric occlusion. Lateral movements should be made with a comparison of the excursions of the teeth with facets worn on the teeth. When the teeth do not occlude in any position or with these worn facets, it is apparent that the mounting is incorrect. The comparison of these excursions on the facets can be best seen in working relationship.

• • •

A functional occlusal analysis can be made by an experienced clinician without the aid of an articulator; however, many of the details can be analyzed more conveniently when the patient is not in the dental chair. Occasionally the occlusal interferences may be so complex as to require a more detailed study than can be accomplished when the patient is in the dental chair. The articulation of casts may make it possible to determine if satisfactory treatment can be achieved by grinding alone or if other forms of treatment will be necessary. In some instances the clinician may wish to make the occlusal adjustment on the models before the treatment is carried out on the patient so that the extent and limitation of the grinding may be determined. When occlusal rehabilitation is being considered, articulation of casts is very advantageous in planning the proposed reconstruction. It may be helpful in the preparation of abutments, in the trial use of pontics and facings, and in the determination of the type of restoration which can be used. Occasionally when orthodontic treatment is indicated, articulation of the casts is helpful in determining what the alignment of the teeth will be after orthodontic treatment and what the functional possibilities are. Thus, the articulation of stone casts can be used (1) as a diagnostic instrument, (2) as a planning instrument, and (3) as an instrument for carrying out technical work in connection with prosthetic occlusal reconstruction or full dentures.

USE OF SURVEYOR

No attempt will be made to present all the details of the use of a surveyor. A few of the principles of its use as they relate to diagnosis will be given. It is suggested that the reader consult suitable references at the end of this chapter for the application of the surveyor to specific cases.

The surveyor is primarily used to determine what preparation of the mouth will be necessary to reduce to a reasonable limit the amount of interference to the insertion of an appliance (Fig. 242). Thus, the cast may be used in a preliminary survey to determine the degree of nonparallelism of surfaces to be used. Surveying of the cast may indicate the necessity for reduction of tooth contours by disking, the placement of parallel restorations, the extraction of excessively malposed teeth, and the surgical correction of connective tissue and bone that present severe undercuts (Applegate).

A   B

Fig. 242. *Cast survey.* Surveying casts to determine parallelism prior to preparation of the mouth for prostheses; this procedure aids in formulating the treatment plan.

In addition, the surveyor is important in determining the path of insertion and removal of appliances. The position and type of clasp which may be used should be designed with the aid of a surveyor to determine the proper amount of retention to avoid excessive lateral movement of the retaining teeth during insertion and removal of an appliance. The surveyor is also used to determine the position and placement of adequate guiding planes. Guiding planes on opposing parallel tooth surfaces are necessary to assure that the appliance will be given a positive direction for removal and insertion.

The principles of the use of a surveyor for diagnostic purposes are centered around the advisability of using a particular appliance with the conditions present which affect retention, path of insertion and removal, and the alignment of the teeth and surfaces relative to parallel guiding planes. This information is necessary before treatment planning can be undertaken. Since the preparation of the mouth for a prosthetic appliance should be planned in advance, a survey of the casts will greatly facilitate this part of treatment. The survey as it relates to the preparation of the mouth should be an integral part of treatment planning.

DISCLOSING SOLUTION

Disclosing solution is a valuable aid in detecting the location of plaques on the teeth, in demonstrating the presence of plaques to patients, in determining the efficiency of home-care procedures, and in detecting irregular and rough surfaces that habitually take up stains. Various types are available. Most contain iodine in some form. The reader is referred to *Accepted Dental Remedies* for complete details of their constituents. The following disclosing solution contains no iodine, and no known sensitivity reactions to it have occurred.

Bismark brown	3 Gm.
Alcohol	10 ml.
Glycerin	120 ml.
Anise	1 drop

A   B

Fig. 243. *Disclosing solution.* **A,** Before application. **B,** After application; showing areas of plaques.

The disclosing solution is placed on the teeth with a cotton applicator. The patient is instructed to rinse his mouth with water to remove the excess solution. The solution will stain readily all the tooth surfaces on which soft mucinous plaques are present (Fig. 243). Margins and porous cracks, imperfect margins, and rough porous acrylic and silicate restorations are often temporarily stained.

REFERENCES

Accepted Dental Remedies, ed. 23, Chicago, 1958. American Dental Association.

Applegate, O. C.: Essentials of Removable Partial Denture Prosthesis, Philadelphia, 1954, W. B. Saunders Co.

Applegate, O. C.: Use of a Paralleling Surveyor, J.A.D.A. 27:1397-1407, 1940.

Bjorn, Hilding: Electrical Excitation of Teeth and Its Application to Dentistry, Sv. Tandl.-Tidsk. (suppl.) vol. 39, 1946.

Bonica, John J.: The Management of Pain, Philadelphia, 1953, Lea & Febiger.

Broshear, A. D.: Innervation of the Teeth, J.A.D.A. 23:662, 1936.

Bunting, R. W., and Parmerlee, Faith: The Role of Bacillus Acidophilus in Dental Caries, J.A.D.A. 12:381, 1925.

Fosdick, L. S., Hansen, H. L., and Epple, C.: Enamel Decalcification by Mouth Organisms and Dental Caries. A Suggested Test for Caries Susceptibility, J.A.D.A. 24:1275, 1937.

Goetzl, F. R., Burrill, D. Y., and Ivy, A. C.: A Critical Analysis of Algesimetric Methods With Suggestions for a Useful Procedure, Quart. Bull., Northwestern University M. School 17:280-291, 1943.

Hadley, F. P.: A Quantitative Method for Estimating Bacillus Acidophilus in Saliva, J. D. Res. 13:415, 1933.

Ham, T. H. (editor): A Syllabus of Laboratory Examinations in Clinical Diagnosis, Cambridge, 1950, Harvard University Press.

Hardy, James D., Wolff, H. G., and Goodell, Helen: Pain Sensations and Reactions, Baltimore, 1952, Williams & Wilkins Co.

Jay, P.: The Reduction of Oral Lactobacillus Acidophilus Counts by the Periodic Restriction of Carbohydrate, Am. J. Orthodontics (Oral Surg. Sec.) 33:162, 1947.

Kaletsky, T., and Furedi, Anna: Further Studies on the Reliability of Various Types of Electric Pulp Testers, D. Cosmos 78:732-742, 1936.

Koss, L. G.: Diagnostic Cytology and Its Histopathologic Bases, Philadelphia, 1961, J. B. Lippincott Co.

Miller, S. E. (editor): A Textbook of Clinical Pathology, ed. 4, Baltimore, 1952, Williams & Wilkins Co.

Oral Exfoliative Cytology, Veterans Administration Cooperative Study, 1962, Washington, D. C., 1963, U. S. Government Printing Office.

Pfaffman, C.: Afferent Impulses From the Teeth Due to Pressure and Noxious Stimulation, J. Physiol. 97:207, 1939.

Reiss, H. L., and Furedi, A.: Significance of the Pulp Test as Revealed in a Microscopic Study of the Pulps of 130 Teeth, D. Cosmos 75:272-281, 1933.

Rogosa, M., Mitchell, J. A., and Wiseman, R. F.: A Selected Medium for the Isolation and Examination of Oral Lactobacilli, J. D. Res. 30:682-689, 1951.

Sandler, H. C., and Stohl, S. S.: Exfoliative Cytology as a Diagnostic Aid in Detection of Oral Neoplasms, J. Oral Surg. 16:414, 1958.

Selbach, G. J., and von Haam, E.: The Clinical Value of Oral Cytology, Acta cytol. 7:337-345, 1963.

Snyder, M. L.: A Simple Colorimetric Method for the Estimation of Relative Numbers of Lactobacilli in the Saliva, J. D. Res. 19:349, 1940.

Sommer, R. F., Ostrander, F. D., and Crowley, M. C.: Clinical Endodontics, Philadelphia, 1956, W. B. Saunders Co.

Todd, J. C., Sanford, A. H., and Stilwell, G. G.: Clinical Diagnosis by Laboratory Methods, ed. 11, Philadelphia, 1948, W. B. Saunders Co.

Thorn, G. W., and Forsham, P. H.: Diabetes Mellitus. In Harrison, T. R. (editor): Principles of Internal Medicine, Philadelphia, 1950, The Blakiston Co., chap. 59.

Wolff, H. G., and Wolf, S.: Pain, Springfield, Ill., 1948, Charles C Thomas, Publisher.

Yardumian, K.: Physiochemical Factors Influencing the Red Cell Sedimentation Rate, Am. J. Clin. Path. 7:105-119, 1937.

Ziskin, D. E., and Wald, A.: Observations on Electrical Pulp Testing, J. D. Res. 17:79, 1938.

CHAPTER 8

Diagnosis and treatment planning

DIAGNOSIS

The term *diagnosis* (from the Greek word meaning to distinguish or to discern) means the identification of a disease by investigation of the signs and symptoms. The exact meaning is obscured by the many ways in which the term is used: clinical diagnosis, laboratory diagnosis, physical diagnosis, radiographic diagnosis, deductive diagnosis, exclusion diagnosis, etc. Use of the word diagnosis with a qualifying adjective connotes an awareness of the meaning of observations made by particular methods. It does not necessarily signify identification of a disease by these methods. The term diagnosis, without a qualifying adjective, is used in this discussion to mean identification of a disease by a systematic synthesis of all its manifestations. This identification not only signifies the identification of the disease but the process by which the identification is derived.

Differential diagnosis is a determination of the one of several diseases from which a patient is suffering by systematically comparing and contrasting their symptoms. In the final analysis all diagnosis is probably differential diagnosis. It is easy to enumerate the symptoms of an acute pulpitis, but to present a system of diagnosis whereby the conditions which simulate pulpitis may be excluded easily is difficult. Specialists in oral diagnosis sometimes find it difficult to commit their methods of reasoning to writing. Teachers of oral diagnosis usually rely on two methods of teaching differential diagnosis: the chair side or demonstration clinic and the clinical pathologic conference. These methods are not without drawbacks. Usually the student will hear little of the reasoning or methods involved in arriving at a diagnosis. Such demonstrations should not become mere deductive diagnostic clinics, but rather times for teaching methods of reasoning. Neither a perusal of lists of symptoms of disease nor referrals to treatises which enumerate the various diseases which give rise to a specific sign or symptom can develop an adequate concept of the process of synthesis which must be used in solving diagnostic problems.

OUTLINE OF DIAGNOSTIC METHOD

1. Collecting the facts
   a. Clinical history
   b. Clinical examination
   c. Supplementary examinations when indicated by analysis of collected facts from (a) and (b)
2. Analysis of the facts
   a. Critical examination of the collected data
   b. Consideration of the alteration of anatomic and physiologic systems that may give rise to the signs and symptoms
   c. Determination of the relative importance of the findings
   d. Review of the positive and negative findings to determine if it is necessary to collect more information
3. Synthesis of examination facts and of descriptive features of disease
   a. Selection of the central features of the collected facts (those features most directly related to the disturbed physiologic processes responsible for the signs and symptoms of the disease)
   b. Correlation between collected facts and those diseases which may account for important significant findings
   c. Establishment of cause and effect relationship, where rational and practical
   d. Evaluation of the possibility of the presence of more than one disease
   e. Listing of diseases in which the same significant features are present
4. Making the diagnosis
   a. Selection of the disease which best explains the collected facts and the apparent and/or proved disturbed physiologic processes
   b. Significance of the diagnosis

The greatest stumbling block to students of diagnosis lies in the collection and evaluation of the facts. Collection of the facts is difficult because of the student's inadequacy in systematic observation and his failure to realize that the same disease may present itself in many forms. More often than not he is accused of poor judgment when the chief problem is a lack of training in interviewing and examination procedures. All too often he has forgotten his basic science and has little conception of its value in the practical solution of diagnostic problems.

The examiner should seek to select objective features which will serve to orient the analysis. The beginning student in oral diagnosis usually has difficulty in determining the significance and relative importance of some finding and is led up a blind alley. Normal variations, insignificant shadows in radiographs, minor complaints, and changes secondary to primary disease are frequently given undue consideration. It is only through trial and error that the student learns to arrange the facts in proper perspective.

While many times the signs and symptoms may appear to be the same as those described for many diseases, this does not necessarily mean that more than one disease is present. Neither does it mean that the selection of the disease with the greatest number of signs and symptoms common to the disease in question will be the true diagnosis. Where several diseases are suspected, the final diagnosis may ultimately be that of a disease which has the fewest number of signs and symptoms present which are common to the disease being evaluated. The signs and symptoms of many diseases usually indicate an alteration of an anatomic and/or physiologic system. For example, an alteration of the blood may reflect changes in the respiratory, neuromuscular, digestive, and cardiovascular systems. Further, an alteration of the digestive system may show ultimately the same signs and symptoms as those seen in the disturbance of the blood. More specifically, the symptoms of temporomandibular joint disease may be pain, restricted movements of the mandible, referred pain, and paresthesia. The same symptoms may be present in disease of the pulp of a mandibular molar tooth. While the symptoms given are the same for both disturbances, the diagnosis is entirely different. These examples serve to point out that the relative importance of each symptom to the disease has to be fully evaluated and, in such instances, more facts are needed to make the correct diagnosis. It must be remembered that, when dealing with a system or a group of systems which are as intimately related as those that comprise the body, a disturbance in one area or one system may reflect on other areas or systems.

Facts obtained by interviewing and examining the patient are the primary requirements for making a diagnosis. Without adequate facts no progress toward a diagnosis can be made. During the examination the examiner must be constantly aware that additional supplementary procedures may be required. He will learn by experience when such procedures are necessary. An analysis of the facts collected as a result of the clinical examination serves to determine the reliability of the history so that proper significance can be placed on the signs and symptoms noted in the history.

Collecting the Facts

The history and clinical examination will provide the essential facts necessary to make a diagnosis. The procedures for interviewing and for making a clinical examination have been presented in the foregoing chapters. Also, the value of laboratory diagnostic aids has been pointed out. If the results of laboratory tests do not correlate with the facts obtained from the history and examination, they should be considered as subsidiary in importance. When collecting the facts, it must be borne in mind that they may well represent the natural history of a disease whose manifestations are being recorded. The examiner should be alert to the usual pattern of development of diseases as well as to their manifestations. If a pattern of disease appears to be unfolding during the history and examination, all the facts pertaining to the natural history of the disease should be positively or negatively correlated.

Frequently the dentist is called upon to render a diagnosis after the disease has been in progress for variable lengths of time and after treatment of one form or another has been rendered. He should attempt to analyze the facts in light of the passage of time and the treatment rendered. He must also remember that he may be called on to make a diagnosis before all the facts have become apparent in the course of the disease. In most instances it is necessary to make an early diagnosis to prevent further inroads of the disease. In a few instances a period of observation may be necessary before the final diagnosis can be made and correct therapy instituted. An example will serve to illustrate this point: Upon the initial examination of a lesion of the oral mucosa which has no particular orienting features, a presumptive diagnosis of traumatic ulcer is rendered with reservations on the possibility of its being of neoplastic origin, and the patient is requested to return in a week or two for re-examination and evaluation since a lesion of traumatic origin will have had time to heal in that time whereas one of neoplastic origin will not heal. If the lesion heals, the diagnosis of traumatic ulcer is confirmed by exclusion. However, if the lesion fails to heal and begins to show some signs of a neoplastic growth, biopsy should be considered. In this example the facts necessary to render a final diagnosis could not be collected before more information was available.

Analysis of the Facts

The examiner should begin his analysis by determining the reliability and significance of the information obtained from the history and examination. For example, a negative serologic test in a patient with a lesion suggestive of syphilis may be of no significance if carried out before dissemination of the organisms. The negative test does not constitute valid grounds for ruling out syphilis. By the same reasoning occlusal interference in itself is not sufficient evidence to warrant the assumption that occlusal trauma is present and a toothache cannot always be attributed to the presence of a carious lesion. In analyzing the information regarding a toothache, the examiner should be aware that pulpitis may be primary or secondary in origin and may, for example, result from sinusitis. To record the fact that the patient has a toothache is not a significant finding unless additional information about the cause is brought out. Thus a critical evaluation of the collected facts in relation to the over-all picture of the complaint is necessary in order to arrive at the correct diagnosis.

An attempt should be made to analyze the findings in terms of disturbed physiologic processes. This will aid in correlating seemingly unrelated symptoms. For example, an inability to carry out certain mandibular movements should be analyzed in terms of the known normal functions of the components of the masticatory system. Inability to perform certain movements may be due to disturbances in occlusion, joints, or the neuromuscular system. Positive or negative correlative data should be collected and analyzed with regard to the function of all the components of the system. If the abnormality is considered to be neuromuscular, the facts should include information relative to the status of the nerves and muscles usually concerned with the movement which cannot be performed. In analyzing gingival bleeding the examiner must relate it to the state of the blood and vascular system if possible. While such bleeding is most often the result of local factors and inflammation, it is occasionally associated with a hemorrhagic diathesis. Gingival bleeding and positive findings from screening blood tests do not constitute an adequate collection of the facts if the information that the patient is on Dicumarol therapy is overlooked in the history. Thus, an analysis of the completeness of the collected facts should also be considered. Similarly the method whereby the information is collected should be analyzed; e.g., a blood sugar analysis is of little value if the patient is not in the prepared fasting state before the test is done.

Importance of Findings.—One of the difficult features of analyzing the information obtained from the history and examination lies in determining the relative importance of each fact. As mentioned previously, the beginning student has difficulty in separating the wheat from the chaff, and only through practice in assessing the importance of signs and symptoms can their proper perspective be determined. For practice the student can list his signs and symptoms in the order in which they are found in the history and examination. To illustrate, assume that a 9-year-old girl has been referred to a dentist by a physician and the following list of symptoms is forwarded to the dentist: sore mouth, high fever, anorexia, dysphagia, lymphadenopathy, sialorrhea, ulceration of gingiva, fetor ex ore, coated tongue, dental caries, and poor oral hygiene.

The problem of assessing the importance of each of these may be reduced by placing those symptoms which occur rather frequently in most individuals low on the list of importance. Another consideration in establishing the importance of a sign or symptom is the correlation between the degree of the subjective complaint and the extent of the objective sign of disease. Thus, mild localized tissue destruction does not generally produce marked constitutional reactions unless the disease is infectious in nature. On the other hand, marked tissue destruction is accompanied by a rather marked constitutional reaction in many individuals. Those related facts which give a good degree of correlation between themselves should be placed high on the list. Still another means of determining the relative importance of the collected facts is the grouping together of signs and symptoms that are usually associated with each other in a disease. These findings may be placed under one heading: e.g., sialorrhea, poor oral hygiene, coated tongue, and fetor ex ore might accompany any disease of the mouth; high fever and anorexia usually occur together; sore mouth and ulceration might be expected to be associated; and lymphadenopathy might be expected to be found secondary to infection in the mouth. Finally, lesions should always be placed high in importance. Revision of the foregoing list in order of importance might appear as follows:

Ulceration (an expression of sore mouth)
Lymphadenopathy (frequently associated with extensive oral lesions)
High fever (anorexia to be expected with fever and sore mouth)
Dysphagia (possibly related to lymphadenopathy)
Sialorrhea
Fetor ex ore (commonly related to poor oral hygiene)
Dental caries

It is apparent that these are the symptoms of more than one disease and that additional information is necessary before a diagnosis can be made. The ulcerative lesions and lymphadenopathy are important symptoms and require detailed evaluation.

The evaluation of soft tissue lesions should follow a systematic procedure. Lesions of the mouth may be primary or secondary in nature and may be the manifestation of local or systemic disease. The following outline suggests the facts which should be collected in the history and examination to relate lesions of the soft tissues to a descriptive knowledge of disease.

METHOD FOR EVALUATION OF LESIONS

I. Case history
    A. Inquiry into the general health of the patient and a review of the body systems whose altered function may be related to the lesions present
    B. Inquiry into the subjective symptoms associated with the lesions
        1. Cause
        2. Manner of onset
        3. Duration
        4. Constitutional symptoms
        5. Treatment, if any

II. Clinical examination of the lesions
    A. Location
    B. Arrangement—coalescing, discrete, irregular, grouped, linear, circinate, etc.
    C. Elevated or depressed
    D. Consistency—firm, soft, hard, etc.
    E. Character of base—broad, infiltrated, narrow, pedunculated, stalked, indurated, depth of involvement
    F. Involution—ulceration, resorption, atrophy
    G. Color of lesion and surrounding mucosa and/or skin
    H. Sequelae—pigmentation, scarring, etc.
    I. Cause

If these facts are known, it is then possible to extend the scope of the information regarding the disease in the hypothetical case mentioned:

Ulceration

Unknown cause; began as small vesicles but rapidly formed into ulcers; all the mucosa of the mouth affected, but gingival involvement most pronounced; few scattered ulcers elsewhere; sudden onset; duration—two days; initial lesions described as small blisters by patient; few lesions present on the lips—termed "cold sores" by patient; latter dry with a crustlike surface exuding serum and yellowish-white in color; ulcers in the mouth are shallow, present a ragged edge, a membranelike yellow base, and an erythematous halo; a few of the lesions show healing without scar formation.

Lymphadenopathy

Difficulty in swallowing and "sore throat" prior to lesions in mouth; lymph nodes in neck painfully swollen prior to lesions.

Fever

Fever preceded oral lesions; increased salivation, cachexia, and anorexia commenced with fever and became pronounced with the oral lesions; temperature 103° to 105° F.

Dysphagia

Difficulty in swallowing present early in course of the disease; throat not actually sore; dysphagia actually related to lymphadenopathy.

Sialorrhea and fetor ex ore are nonspecific findings and may accompany many forms of oral disease. Sialorrhea is of importance in metallic intoxications but never of a degree to be considered as an orienting or central finding. Dental caries resulting in sharp and badly broken teeth may be of significance in traumatic ulcers. The diffuse nature of the ulcers and the presence of fever and lymphadenopathy rule out this consideration.

After the facts have been evaluated and listed in the order of importance, it is desirable to select the central or outstanding features necessary to orient the examination.

Synthesis of Examination Facts and of Descriptive Features of Disease

It is sometimes difficult to select the central and most important feature of a disease. It is best to select the symptom that logically explains the disturbed physiologic process. In the example used and in other instances, the selection of a single item will be impossible. In this case a summary of one or more features that are logically related should be listed. For the preceding case the following summary is suggested: Vesicular eruptions with secondary lesions (ulcerations) present; constitutional factors and lymphadenopathy occur prior to the eruptions.

These are the central features of the disease and must be correlated with diseases which produce similar symptoms. The vesicular phase of the disease may well be overlooked, and for this reason it is generally best to select two features that have potential value. It is not wise to overlook the possibility that without the presence of vesicles being established, the oral manifestations presented and the lymphadenopathy might represent lesions secondary to a primary systemic disease.

At this time it is well to list the diseases which might account for the signs and symptoms collected. It would be impossible to list all the diseases that might produce ulcerations in the mouth. However, it is possible to list diseases that have this feature plus the other symptoms presented. In order to be brief, yet not overlook logical possibilities, only the most common diseases likely to produce the clinical impression given in the case presented will be considered.

Those diseases *most commonly* producing fever, lymphadenopathy, and ulcerations of the mouth are herpetic gingivostomatitis, necrotizing gingivitis (Vincent's infection), and erythema multiforme.

The same symptoms may also be secondary to leukemia and chickenpox, but far less frequently. The possibility that more than one disease is present must be evaluated, viz., Vincent's infection superimposed on leukemia.

There are several approaches to the problem of selecting the disease which best explains the facts collected: (1) select several diseases, each of which best explains some of the facts; (2) review all evidence with the most likely diagnosis that is in mind; (3) from a knowledge of the natural history of the diseases considered, determine what additional facts might be present which have been overlooked; (4) consider the possibility of more than one disease process being present; (5) give careful consideration to the negative findings in light of the usual positive findings attending certain diseases; (6) re-evaluate the information that is considered to be the most significant; and (7) select an outstanding feature of the facts collected that may serve to orient the synthesis.

In making the differential diagnosis from the choices mentioned, the examiner will have little difficulty in separating herpetic gingivostomatitis from necrotizing gingivitis if the presence of *vesicles* has been recognized. From a practical standpoint, this orienting or central feature is frequently overlooked, and the disease is diagnosed as acute necrotizing gingivitis (Vincent's infection).

However, even if the vesicles are not discovered, the natural history of the disease as well as the character of the ulceration will make the differential diagnosis possible. (See Chapters 2 and 5 for descriptions of the lesions of herpetic stomatitis and necrotizing gingivitis.) It should be noted that the natural history of herpetic gingivostomatitis is rather characteristic in that the constitutional symptoms, lymphadenopathy, and "sore throat" begin prior to the formation of the lesions. In acute necrotizing gingivitis the constitutional symptoms and lymphadenopathy, when present, occur after the onset of the ulceration. Another feature of Vincent's infection is the age at which this disease is likely to occur. Vincent's infection rarely, if ever, occurs in a 9-year-old child; primary herpetic gingivostomatitis occurs frequently in young children.

A descriptive knowledge of erythema multiforme is necessary to evaluate this disease. No definite characteristic lesions are present. The multiplicity of lesions encountered assists in making the diagnosis. Erythema multiforme is an acute process with a sudden onset. The lesions may be macules, papules, nodules, vesicles, or bullae, may be vesicular in appearance, or may appear as hives and urticaria. They usually start as small macular or papular lesions but expand rapidly, with the center becoming blue and violaceous on an erythematous base—"bull's-eye type of lesion" (iris type). There is some tendency to undermine. In herpetic lesions the erythematous halo develops after rupture of vesicles, whereas the halo precedes the vesicle formation in erythematous lesions. The lesions subside in a three- to four-week period. There are exacerbations and remissions without cause. Severe acute manifestations last for two to four weeks.

Making the Diagnosis

The diagnosis in the hypothetical case presented is evident from the facts collected and their identification with the symptoms of herpetic gingivostomatitis. Since this is a self-limiting disease, the diagnosis can be confirmed when the disease subsides. A bacteriologic smear should reveal the absence of overwhelming numbers of Vincent's organisms which might be expected in acute necrotizing gingivitis. However, a bacteriologic smear presents little evidence of the etiology of the lesion. It must also be remembered that Vincent's organisms are present in most mouths, and a smear is of little positive diagnostic value. For those who wish to further substantiate the diagnosis by clinical laboratory methods, scrapings from the lesions can be used for intracerebral inoculation of mice or to show diagnosable corneal scarification of an inoculated rabbit. These tests are cumbersome, and the disease is usually abated by the time the results from the laboratory studies are known.

A tentative diagnosis is sometimes made on the basis of the facts available at the time of examination. Treatment can then be instituted before the final diagnosis is established. The tentative diagnosis need not be expressed in specific terminology. A description of the disease may be all that is possible. Students are frustrated many times because of an inability to call something by name. This implies that all disease processes have a specific name and that the ultimate in diagnosing ability is to be able to affix a name tag to a disease. This is unfortunate since the emphasis is in the improper place. A name of a disease is merely shorthand for the signs and symptoms of a diseased state. Emphasis should be placed on recognition of the facts collected and not on the name of the disease.

Diagnosis of Neoplasms

The dentist in general practice assumes the responsibility for recognizing neoplasms which may arise in or about the mouth. The dentist must make the decision as to the malignant or benign nature of soft tissue lesions. The ability to recognize clinically the nature of a lesion of the mouth is usually directly proportional to the diagnostician's training and experience in the field of oral pathology. The diagnostician who has limited training and experience must rely on the most positive procedures available to diagnose soft tissue lesions. The uncertainty of the clinical nature of a soft tissue lesion of the mouth cannot be eliminated by observation of the lesion for a period of time. During prolonged observation, growth and extension can occur to the extent that the lesion is untreatable and can prove fatal. Immediate determination of the histologic features of a soft tissue lesion may be ascertained by biopsy. This procedure will prevent delay in diagnosis and thus improve prognosis.

Soft tissue lesions have characteristics which are helpful in determining their nature. In general, they may be thought of as being developmental in origin, inflammatory, systemic in origin, or neoplastic. When a soft tissue lesion can be characterized unequivocally clinically as one of the three non-neoplastic lesions, biopsy is unnecessary. Since biopsy is impractical for every soft tissue lesion of the mouth, some clinical judgment must be exercised; it should be based on the recognition of tissue characteristics. Still, a safe rule is—when in doubt, biopsy.

Developmental lesions are limited in number and maintain rather constant characteristics. Fordyce's disease and median rhomboid glossitis are two developmental lesions which may vary in size or area of involvement; however, the location in which they occur and their general appearance are quite constant. Dermoid cysts and teratomas occur only rarely and usually produce a change in contour of normal tissue, which simulates neoplastic disease, and therefore require biopsy.

Inflammatory lesions are most likely to be confused with neoplastic lesions. Blastomatoid lesions are reactive in nature; they are well named since they produce a clinical picture similar to neoplasia. Many times the diagnosis is not known until the lesion is seen microscopically. Blastomatoid lesions such as mandibular and palatal tori are common enough to be readily recognized even by dentists with limited experience. Traumatic fibromas and giant cell tumors, on the other hand, often simulate neoplasia by their persistence and growth characteristics. Traumatically induced ulcers of the tongue often present perplexing problems in diagnosis, particularly when an ulcer is deep, secondarily infected, and of long standing. Ulceration elsewhere in the mouth also requires close attention to tissue characteristics. The evidence of an inflammatory halo and tenderness is not always sufficient to permit the clinical diagnosis of inflammatory reaction.

White lesions in the mouth which are reactive in origin often simulate the premalignant process of leukoplakia. The chronicity and appearance of white lesions are seldom indicative of their true nature. Extensive clinical experience with white lesions of the mouth is helpful but not a positive means by which to decide the benign or malignant character of the lesion.

Systemic reactions in the mouth are secondary to a generalized process, and therefore their recognition is extremely important. The varied causes and appearances of these reactions make it impossible for anyone to immediately recognize them all. Since systemic reactions only occasionally simulate neoplasia, they are not a major consideration. The occasional appearance of leukemic lesions, amyloidosis, hyperparathyroid tumors, and multiple myeloma may be dealt with by referral to the proper specialists for diagnosis.

Neoplasms are commonly characterized by their persistence, continued growth, and increase in size. Benign neoplasia in the mouth is not extremely common, but its recognition is nonetheless important in differentiating a benign growth from a malignant growth. Benign lesions on soft tissue are frequently slow growing and noninvasive in character. Benign neoplasms of bone may be well demarcated, or, in the case of ameloblastomas, locally invasive in character.

The characteristics of malignant neoplasms vary according to the type of tissue undergoing neoplastic change. Carcinomas originating on the surface of the soft tissues should be evident to the careful examiner; however, early lesions are not infrequently overlooked by the casual examiner. Lip lesions are important when they have been present for a period of several weeks without signs of regression. Deformity of the lip, induration, ulceration, or extension to deeper structures should be considered signs of carcinoma until proved otherwise. The same characteristics may be stated for carcinomas on the mucous membrane; a white surface or granular base may be an additional finding. Salivary gland carcinomas arise beneath the mucous membrane and produce focal swelling which should not be interpreted clinically as primarily an inflammatory reaction although inflammation may accompany such swellings.

Sarcomas arise in connective tissues and present frequently as unexplained swelling of the jaws or focal swelling under the mucous membrane surface. Lymphomas are known to involve the mouth and may appear as innocent localized swellings which cannot be explained on the basis of trauma or infection. Focal swellings of the mucosa which tend to appear bluish and which have overlying telangiectases should be considered seriously as malignant connective tissue neoplasms or lymphomas on the basis of clinical findings. Giant cell tumors that recur may on rare occasion prove to be malignant neoplasms and may rapidly involve a wide area of jaw even though the histologic features are typical of benign giant cell tumors. This should not change one's confidence in histologic examination but should stimulate prompt treatment of all giant cell tumors.

Examination of lymph nodes of the neck and face which reveal evidence of lymphadenopathy should be investigated thoroughly for the causative factor. Positive intraoral findings must be related to lymphadenopathy to determine if lymph nodes are enlarged as the result of inflammation in the mouth or throat, neoplastic disease in the mouth and pharyngeal area, or a generalized neoplastic process involving lymph nodes primarily.

The detection and prompt diagnosis of neoplasms are two of the most important services a dentist offers to a patient even though malignant neoplasms may not be seen frequently in the average dental practice. The dentist should be able to recognize neoplasms in the mouth when they are in the early stages and while treatment can still be effective. Success in recognition of neoplasms is more a matter of developing a thorough examination procedure and inquisitive mind in regard to minor and major soft tissue abnormalities than it is a matter of learning to recognize specific types of neoplastic disease.

Prognosis

The prognosis of a disease should be expressed in terms of time and tissue response. It is not enough to state that the disease can be eliminated in a certain length of time; the degree of tissue damage, loss of function, and susceptibility to recurrence must be considered. All too frequently patients believe that the cure of Vincent's infection will restore their gingival tissues to normal. However, the tissue lost from extensive interdental necrosis will not and cannot be made to return to its original form. Furthermore, the altered form poses an added burden for the patient in maintaining adequate oral hygiene to prevent recurrence of the disease. The dentist is obligated to point out these facts in the prognosis of acute necrotizing gingivitis.

TREATMENT PLANNING

Successful dental treatment is always based on careful planning. Regardless of how simple or complex therapy may be, it cannot be carried to a successful conclusion without a planned procedure. Dental treatment has become more complex with the development of specialties and with the improvement of technics. It is no longer possible for treatment to be planned at each appointment without denying the patient the possibility of receiving the benefits of long-range treatment planning and maintenance of oral health.

Rationale and Outline for a Treatment Plan

Rational treatment is dependent on an accurate diagnosis. An accurate diagnosis in dentistry includes a consideration of all oral structures. Oral diagnoses are seldom concerned with one disease and one treatment; they frequently result in a series of various types of treatment for different areas of the mouth. For example, a dentist cannot proceed with gingival treatment in a patient who has a suspicious lesion on his lip nor place extensive fixed bridges on teeth that show evidence of periodontal disease. There are many examples which can be cited in which one type of treatment requires priority over another or in which one phase of treatment depends on completion of another phase.

A rational treatment plan is made with these considerations in mind: the urgency of treatment, the sequence of treatment, and the result expected from treatment. Diagnosis of a condition of an urgent nature compels the dentist to carry out treatment which, if not done first, may result in unnecessary discomfort to the patient or even endanger his life. The sequence in which therapy progresses may mean the difference between success and failure of dental treatment. A well-organized sequence of treatment prevents many false starts, repetition of treatment, and, in some cases, waste of energy, time, and money. Dental treatment is never directed toward the cure of one disease; it should be directed toward the prevention and correction of all forms of oral disease. Unless the treatment plan is made with the end point visualized, therapy cannot progress to a satisfactory end point.

In developing a rational plan of treatment, even the most experienced dentists follow a pattern of organization of treatment. A pattern or outline, broad in scope, is essential in developing the sequence of treatment with the total needs of the patient in mind. An outline which is broad in scope serves as a reminder of the phases of treatment which must be considered. The following outline is suggested for general treatment planning.

OUTLINE FOR TREATMENT PLANNING

I. Systemic treatment
   A. Referral to a physician for systemic evaluation and treatment as indicated by history and clinical findings
   B. Appraisal of the influence of systemic treatment on the dental treatment plan
   C. Premedication with antibiotics or sedatives as indicated by the history
   D. Corrective therapy for oral infection
II. Preparatory treatment
   A. Oral surgery
   B. Endodontic therapy
   C. Caries control
   D. Periodontal therapy
   E. Orthodontic treatment
   F. Occlusal adjustment
III. Corrective treatment
   A. Operative dentistry
   B. Prosthetic dentistry
IV. Periodic recall examinations and maintenance treatment

Systemic Treatment

The dental profession is well aware of the influence of systemic disease on dental treatment. Such disease may be suspected in the course of examining a patient, and a past history of systemic disease may influence the way in which a patient is cared for. A patient undergoing medical treatment who also needs dental treatment may present special problems in treatment planning. The inter-relationship of dental and medical treatment should be fully appreciated by both physicians and dentists and a cooperative plan of treatment worked out for the benefit of the patient.

Significance of Systemic Disease in the Treatment Program.—The importance of the recognition of the presence of systemic disease and the significance of systemic disease to the dental patient cannot be overemphasized. It is imperative that the individual outlining a program of treatment for a patient take into consideration all facets of the information obtained in taking the history and examining the patient. The correct diagnosis and a rational therapy can be provided only when information regarding all aspects—biologic, physiologic, psycho-logic, and sociologic—of the patient has been obtained, correlated, and evaluated. Each facet provides something of importance in the proper plan of therapy.

All of the relationships of systemic factors to therapy cannot be discussed in this text, but some of the relationships between systemic disease and therapy will be considered.

Consider, for example, the patient who presents with a systemic disease which is terminal, but whose chief complaint concerns his oral symptoms. Some therapy is therefore indicated. This may be the patient with terminal cancer who has lost a restoration because of recurrent caries with resultant pulp exposure. Extraction without replacement is indicated, of course, because of the short life expectancy of the patient. On the other hand, the patient may be in the terminal stages of leukemia with gingival ulceration and bleeding and a periodontal abscess. In this instance, extensive dental therapy is not indicated because of the short life expectancy, the possibility of producing severe, uncon-trollable hemorrhage, and the possibility of initiating septicemia. Nevertheless, the individual's chief complaint is oral and he must be provided with palliative therapy within the limits permitted by his systemic disease. It is necessary that the dentist recognize the limitations imposed by the systemic disease and develop an effective and palliative treatment plan for this patient. The dentist must be capable of evaluating the systemic status in relation to the treatment needs of the patient and know the limitations imposed by the biologic state so that he can carry out a beneficial palliative therapy.

Another example of a patient with a systemic disease is the patient who presents with a history of rheumatic heart disease, sensitivity to penicillin, and a moderately advanced periodontitis with early bifurcation involvement of molar teeth and 5 mm. to 6 mm. pockets on the anterior teeth. Because of the nature of the patient's systemic disease and his dental disease and the requirements for periodontal therapy, the patient is not a candidate for periodontal therapy. The presence of periodontal disease which cannot be eliminated will leave residual areas of infection to produce intermittent bacteremia associated with oral physio-therapy or with vigorous chewing. This situation provides a precarious life for the patient, with subacute bacterial endocarditis existing as a constant hazard. Any other program of therapy would not give adequate consideration to the evaluation of the patient's history and the examination findings.

Another example of the effect of systemic disease on treatment is demon-strated by the "brittle" diabetic patient who presents with moderately advanced periodontitis and a history of recent frequent periodontal abscesses. It is well recognized that the effect of the dental infection may make stabilization of blood sugar difficult and may be responsible for the patient's "brittle" character. The elimination of the infection is therefore an important part of the treatment of the systemic disease. On the other hand, it may be difficult to alter the activity of the periodontitis while the patient has only limited control of blood sugar. The cooperation of physician and dentist to achieve optimum control of systemic disease and dental disease is significant, and the success of this initial therapy will determine the future course of treatment. If the patient's blood sugar level can be maintained at a normal level, he can be treated as a normal patient. Treatment of the periodontal disease must result in complete elimination so that recurrence will not rob the individual of his controlled blood sugar level. Although the patient with controlled diabetes responds normally to treatment and is a candidate for periodontal therapy, he must receive definitive, positive therapy which does not temporize with complete elimination of periodontal infection. The treatment for such a patient may be limited by his physiologic status.

In the patient with newly discovered diabetes there is no way to evaluate the nature of the patient's response to the periodontal disease or to predict the degree of success of medical treatment. In such instances it is necessary to eliminate the acute oral disease and then evaluate medical therapy. After full control of the systemic disease is achieved, the patient may then be adequately evaluated for dental therapy.

Another example of the effect of systemic disease on treatment plan may be observed in the patient who has scleroderma. The patient presents with moderately advanced periodontal disease and a history and evidence of advanced and progressive scleroderma with fixation of the face resulting in a small, inelastic oral orifice. The extent of periodontal disease indicates that treatment will be unsuccessful but not impossible. It is evident that if the disease progresses to any extent, the patient will be unable to insert or remove a denture. In this case the systemic disease dictates the temporizing dental therapy which is necessary to provide a temporary usable dentition for this patient. His systemic disease dictates the temporary type of therapy.

Finally, dental disease may dictate the nature of dental treatment. For example, a patient who presents with moderately advanced periodontal disease which would necessitate periodontal surgery with the resultant exposure of root surface and who also has evidence of moderate caries susceptibility, especially of exposed root surfaces, is not a candidate for periodontal therapy. Exposure of root surfaces is a condition which frequently results from chronic necrotizing ulcerative gingivitis. Restoration of extensive carious lesions on the roots of teeth under such circumstances may be impractical.

The situations proposed are only a few of the possible situations in which the total information about the patient is necessary to outline an effective, rational, healthful therapy. There is no substitute for total information with accurate correlation of all factors to determine the physiologic requirements for the achievement of a biologically acceptable therapy which will provide a status of total body health.

Referral to a Physician.—Whenever a patient's history or findings of the clinical examination are suggestive of systemic disease, the dentist should refer the patient to a physician.

This may be done by means of a letter of referral containing a precise statement of those symptoms or signs suggestive of systemic disease and a specific request for information from the physician relative to the dental aspects of the disease.

Systemic Treatment Already in Progress.—It may be necessary to consult the physician of a patient who is receiving medical treatment at the time dental treatment is being planned so that any forms of medical therapy that may be potentially hazardous to the patient can be discussed.

A patient receiving medical treatment for an illness which is expected to terminate fatally in a relatively short time will require special treatment planning by the dentist. In such a patient he may elect to plan treatment on an emergency basis. On the other hand, much can be done to avoid oral disease in such patients by carrying out preventive measures.

Preventive Therapy.—Premedication by antibiotics prior to oral procedures which cause bleeding is important in treatment planning when there is a history of rheumatic fever, rheumatic heart disease, or congenital heart disease. Insofar as possible, treatment which causes bleeding (e.g., scaling) should be carried out in one appointment rather than several to avoid the necessity for repeated premedication. In such instances the treatment plan may call for longer appointments than usual.

Apprehensive patients should be given a suitable sedative prior to treatment. This type of premedication should be freely discussed with the patient when his treatment plan is presented to him.

Corrective Therapy.—Systemic therapy with antibiotics and other drugs for oral infections is generally of an emergency nature. However, before such treatment is instituted, the patient should be questioned regarding a history of sensitivity to certain drugs.

Preparatory Treatment

Preparatory treatment is the type of treatment employed in preparing the mouth for corrective treatment. While many of the procedures presented in the following paragraphs may be considered corrective in nature, they nevertheless prepare the mouth for the final corrective restorative and reconstructive procedures. This portion of the treatment plan is discussed to emphasize the necessity for completion of certain phases of treatment before proceeding to the next phase.

Oral Surgery.—The surgical eradication of soft tissue lesions often receives priority in dental treatment planning. Small lesions which are amenable to excisional biopsy should be considered early in the plan. Larger lesions, particularly neoplasms, may take priority over any other form of oral treatment.

Extraction of teeth on an emergency basis because of infection or pain should be given early attention in treatment planning. Teeth which have advanced carious lesions or are impacted should also be given early consideration. Those which are hopelessly involved with periodontal disease may be extracted early, but in some instances extraction may be delayed so that function may continue until the treatment is further along. Sequence of extraction may be planned in certain types of periodontal disease in order to maintain as much edentulous ridge as possible. Extraction of maxillary teeth preparatory to the insertion of a complete maxillary denture may be delayed pending completion of a partial mandibular denture which the complete maxillary denture is to oppose.

Correction of anatomic tissue defects must be completed prior to complete and partial denture construction.

Endodontic Therapy.—Endodontic therapy is carried out early in the treatment plan due to the emergency nature of the condition in many instances. However, the condition of the remaining teeth should be considered so that treatment is not carried out on teeth which are ultimately to be extracted. When there is any question concerning retention of a tooth, pain relief and control of infection should be instituted until the condition of the mouth is completely evaluated and the fate of the tooth determined.

It is desirable to remove carious dentin from deeply involved teeth early in the course of treatment so that the necessity for endodontic treatment may be determined well in advance of corrective treatment.

The placement of temporary restorations is desirable when the carious involvement of a tooth has progressed to a point where the pulp might be involved if the process is not interrupted before other treatment is continued.

Caries Control.—An evaluation of the rate at which dental caries is likely to progress is an important part of every treatment plan short of complete dentures. Lactobacilli counts should be done when it is evident that some means for control of caries is necessary to preserve the teeth and the proposed restorations. Institution of a caries control diet should be considered seriously for patients who show a desire to cooperate and reduce the progress of caries.

Periodontal Therapy.—Periodontal therapy on a conservative basis and on a preventive basis is within the scope of the general practitioner of dentistry. More advanced periodontal treatment may require referral to a specialist. In any case, periodontal treatment should be done prior to corrective treatment. Only when periodontal therapy has been completed can there be any assurance that the supporting structures of the teeth will withstand the additional stress placed on them by prosthetic appliances. Not until periodontal treatment is completed is it possible to determine which teeth are to be retained and which will require replacement.

Orthodontic Treatment.—The orthodontist is best qualified to plan orthodontic treatment; nevertheless, the dentist in general practice must consider orthodontic treatment not only for young individuals, but also for certain adults. There are many instances in which a better result could be obtained in restoration of a dental arch if tooth position were more favorable. Orthodontic consultation should be obtained and should be indicated where it is best suited in the over-all treatment plan.

Occlusal Adjustment.—Occlusal equilibration is a technic which should be mastered by every dentist who includes bridges and partial dentures in his treatment plan. The removal of occlusal interferences, the establishment of a satisfactory occlusal plane, and the improvement of occlusal function should precede any reconstruction of the dentition. The failure of bridge abutments and partial denture abutments is frequently the result of improper occlusal relations that might have been corrected by occlusal adjustment.

The improvement of occlusal function by occlusal adjustment in the treatment of temporomandibular joint disorders which result from trauma should also be considered at this point in the treatment plan. Acute temporomandibular joint problems receive first priority in treatment planning, but the relationship of a complete treatment plan to the acute problem should not be overlooked. While the control of acute symptoms may be obtained by occlusal adjustment, the completion of a treatment plan is necessary to prevent recurrence.

Corrective Treatment

When the treatment plan has provided for adequate preparation of the mouth for corrective measures, the corrective measures may be carried out with assurance that the supporting structures and functional relations of the teeth are at an optimum for the particular case. When corrective measures are carried out in a mouth which is poorly prepared, they merely become temporary stopgaps prior to complete dentures.

Operative Dentistry.—Restorative treatment of individual teeth requires careful planning so that restorations can be placed first on teeth that show the most carious involvement and each appointment can be used efficiently so that operations can be performed on adjacent teeth in the same quadrant of the mouth whenever possible.

The choice of restorative material must be included in the treatment plan and is dependent on the functional requirements of the proposed restoration and on the esthetic result desired.

Restorative treatment should not be planned without reconstructive treatment in mind. Partial denture abutments present special requirements for their restorations. Fixed bridge abutments may be temporarily restored with cement or even temporary crowns while the treatment progresses in other areas. Temporary restorations may be required to prevent further carious involvement or to maintain proper occlusal relations.

Prosthetic Dentistry.—The choice between fixed and removable bridges and between clasp type and precision attachment partial dentures is largely dependent upon the treatment plan up to this point. Without entering into the controversial subject of advantages and disadvantages of clasp and precision attachment partial dentures, it may be said that the indications for either type are important considerations during the reconstructive phase of treatment planning. In either fixed bridge or partial denture treatment the selection of abutment teeth and the requirement for splinting in order to make use of multiple abutments are largely dependent on the diagnosis of root form and periodontal involvement of proposed abutment teeth. Abutment teeth with root canal fillings may require special care during preparation due to the type of filling material if a post type abutment restoration is required.

Periodic Recall Examinations and Maintenance Treatment

At the time a treatment plan is presented to a patient and also upon completion of the plan, the dentist should impress upon the patient the necessity for periodic examinations and maintenance care at frequent, regular intervals. Many dental treatment failures result from lack of regular maintenance care.

Much complicated and expensive dental treatment could be avoided if patients took advantage of regular dental care.

The final consideration in the plan is preventive treatment based on semi-annual examinations. Very few patients can be allowed to go one year between examinations without meeting some difficulty eventually. When they are taught by the dentist that maintenance treatment is preventive treatment, they will usually accept the responsibility for obtaining periodic examinations and care eagerly.

Principles for Outlining a Treatment Plan

Importance of the Chief Complaint.—A good "rule of thumb" in treatment planning is this: Treat the patient's chief complaint before trying to present plans to him for full-mouth rehabilitation. When a new patient presents with a chief complaint of pain or discomfort, his only thought is for relief. An uncomfortable patient is not psychologically oriented to receive a presentation of his dental difficulties and their proposed treatment unless the presentation is concerned directly with his chief complaint. The present complaint should provide some information relative to the importance he attaches to his complaint and his expectations from treatment. If the findings indicate the need for further treatment following immediate care of the chief complaint, such treatment should be suggested to the patient.

Consideration of Past and Present Systemic Diseases.—The influence on the dental treatment plan of systemic disease which is expected to end fatally is quite evident. In certain fatal illnesses, relief of discomfort is all that can be accomplished, while in other instances much can be done to improve oral function. Cooperation with the physician treating the fatal illness is mandatory.

While no attempt will be made here to point out all the important systemic diseases which require special consideration in planning dental treatment, a few which are directly related to dental treatment will be mentioned. The importance of the prevention of oral infection in patients with diabetes mellitus should be kept in mind because of the significant number of such patients encountered in most dental practices. The recognition of bleeding problems and their discussion with the patient's physician in order to prevent serious complications from surgery is obviously important. A reminder of the importance of a history of rheumatic fever and congenital heart disease is not out of order. Patients being treated with anticoagulants, patients with hypertension, and patients with cardiac disease should be given special consideration in treatment planning. There are many instances in which consultation with a patient's physician will allow the dentist to complete a treatment plan with the assurance that the cooperative effort of the physician and the dentist will provide the patient with safe and important dental treatment.

Influence of the Personal, Social, and Economic History on the Treatment Plan.—The personal history contains information about the patient's personal oral hygiene habits. Poor oral hygiene habits may be the result of a lack of instruction in oral hygiene or may be the result of a careless attitude toward oral health. Treatment planning for patients with poor oral hygiene habits should be contingent upon the improvement of mouth care by the patient.

The social and economic history of a patient should provide information on his occupation, family, and income. This information may have an important bearing on the type of dental treatment prescribed since patients with limited incomes and large family obligations are unable to assume the expenses which may be incurred in the course of certain types of dental treatment.

Treatment planning in patients whose occupations require precise articulation of sounds, such as public speakers and singers, should be given special consideration relative to retention of teeth and the type of reconstructive measures to be carried out in order to retain natural teeth for stability of prostheses and in order to interfere least with articulation.

Effects of Past Dental Treatment on the Treatment Plan.—An accurate account of past dental treatment may be important enough, at times, to decide between a treatment plan calling for additional treatment and one calling for complete extractions. Uncontrolled dental caries, rapidly progressing periodontal disease, or failure of a patient to show an interest in maintaining oral health, in spite of extensive treatment, would not permit consideration of further extensive treatment. Many times a prediction of the success of future dental treatment can be based on the success of past dental treatment.

It is not safe to jump to the conclusion that failure of past treatment is the fault of the patient. In some cases it may be the result of faulty treatment or the dentist's failure to inform the patient of the rewards of maintenance treatment.

The nature of past dental treatment may provide a favorable outlook for future treatment. This is particularly true in patients who show minimal periodontal destruction in spite of the presence of overhanging restorations, "built-in" occlusal trauma, and calculus which was never completely removed.

Needless to say, the patient who has received good dental care on a regular basis is a patient who will desire continued regular dental care.

Significance of the Disease Process and Its Etiology to the Treatment Plan.— In general, diseases of the oral soft tissues which the dentist treats are developmental, inflammatory, or neoplastic in nature; the diseases of the teeth which he treats are the result of caries, trauma, and developmental disturbances.

In planning treatment for soft tissue diseases of the mouth, the dentist is primarily interested in the nature of the process. Once the nature of the process is determined, the etiologic factor is more easily identified. Developmental disturbances such as cleft lip and cleft palate are beyond the scope of general dentistry; however, the dentist may assist the oral surgeon and orthodontist in the maintenance of teeth and construction of a prosthesis. Cleft lip and cleft palate are examples of oral problems which require careful cooperative treatment planning between the dentist, oral surgeon, orthodontist, and speech therapist. Minor developmental disturbances of soft tissue usually do not require specific treatment; rather the dentist may only reassure the patient of the benign nature of the condition.

Inflammatory processes of the oral soft tissues and gingiva make up the bulk of the soft tissue lesions treated in general dental practice. An inflammatory process should be considered from the standpoint of whether it is the result of local irritation, infection, or systemic reaction. Occlusal trauma, sharp teeth, ill-fitting dental appliances and restorations, habitual cheek biting, and calculus are common etiologic factors to be considered in planning correction of local irritation. Planning treatment for infections of the mouth depends on the causative organism. In primary herpetic gingivostomatitis, treatment must be planned to keep the patient comfortable while the disease runs its course, whereas antibiotic therapy is often indicated for bacterial infections which are most often secondary to pulp disease or periodontal disease. Systemic reactions of an inflammatory nature are frequently the result of a dermatologic disease or allergy. In the case of systemic reactions manifesting themselves in the mouth, consultation with a physician for systemic therapy may be indicated. When oral allergic reactions are the result of systemic drug therapy prescribed by a physician, it may become necessary to request the physician to use an alternate drug.

The treatment of diseases of the teeth is the forte of general dental practice and the full responsibility for planning treatment lies in the realm of general dentistry, within the limits of the technical ability of the individual dentist.

The treatment of dental caries is dependent on the amount of carious destruction already evident, the rate at which the carious activity is progressing, the age of the patient, and the condition of the supporting structures of the teeth. As already stated, treatment of dental caries should include an evaluation of the caries rate. Rapid destruction of teeth by caries which has extensively involved many teeth may call for a treatment plan which includes complete extraction and complete dentures. Whenever possible, dietary control of dental caries should be attempted. Prevention of loss of teeth in young individuals is extremely important in the prevention of periodontal disease in later life.

The rate at which the carious process is progressing may be a deciding factor in the type of restoration and type of restorative material to be used. In some cases the coverage of all caries-susceptible surfaces of the tooth with gold is the treatment of choice where it is felt that caries is a major consideration in planning treatment. This may be especially true in preparing bridge and partial denture abutments.

Treatment of traumatized teeth is often an emergency procedure. Root fractures, dislodged teeth, and fractured incisors are common problems which require careful treatment planning. Reimplantation of a tooth requires special planning and follow-up. Periodic observation of a traumatized or fractured tooth to determine vitality of the pulp should be planned on a definite schedule.

The area of developmental disturbances of teeth is a fertile field for dental treatment planning. The severe disturbances such as dentinogenesis imperfecta and amelogenesis imperfecta require careful planning to ensure longevity of the teeth and maximum esthetics. Minor disturbances are often esthetic problems which require correction. The dental stigma of congenital syphilis may be partially erased by a few well-planned anterior restorations.

Modification of the Treatment Plan.—Treatment planning should always be done with an ideal objective in mind. While it is not always possible to attain the ideal objective because of mechanical or financial problems, such an objective serves to guide the treatment planning in a direction which will provide the patient with the most desirable form of treatment.

The ideal plan offers the patient the greatest perfection attainable by means of specialized forms of treatment and by use of the finest restorative methods and materials. Ideal treatment may be quite simple or very complex. Whether simple or complex, the plan should be made known to the patient for his acceptance or rejection.

Since the ideal treatment plan may be rejected by the patient, the dentist should prepare an alternate plan. The alternate plan may contain one or more variations from the ideal plan, and it is usually presented because the patient is unable to assume the expense entailed by the ideal plan. It should be kept in mind that alternate treatment plans are not poorer forms of dental treatment, but rather forms of treatment which come as close to the ideal as possible.

Presentation of the Treatment Plan to the Patient.—The presentation of the treatment plan to the patient must be made in an atmosphere of confidence and in the spirit of willingness to provide good dental treatment. It should never be in terms of how much it will cost but rather in terms of what treatment is necessary to attain good oral health.

If the presentation of the plan has been preceded by a careful collection of diagnostic information and a carefully studied diagnosis and if the plan has been intelligently prepared, the patient will find the plan of treatment a desirable procedure. However, if the examination is hasty and incomplete, the explanation of the oral condition vague, the treatment plan presented with uncertainty, and the prognosis indefinite, the patient will find it difficult to accept the treatment plan with confidence.

The dentist should make use of his diagnostic aids in presenting treatment plans. The patient is usually extremely interested in the radiographs and models because they represent his problem. The models and radiographs can be used to point out areas of both health and disease and the areas in need of special attention. The use of models to show the patient what the various types of restorations will look like when completed may be an important deciding factor in acceptance of the plan when anterior teeth are involved or when a removable prosthesis is contemplated.

A frank discussion of fees is in order when the treatment plan is presented. The patient should know the expense involved before he is allowed to accept a treatment plan; otherwise in the middle of treatment he may decide he is unable to meet the expense. With the payment plans available today for dental treatment, ideal dental therapy is within the reach of much of the population.

· · ·

In the last analysis a diagnosis is but one of the components in an evaluation of a case. A diagnosis is only as accurate as the steps leading up to it. In dentistry the use of the term diagnosis may be used to indicate the recognition of a single disease or the result of an appraisal and summary of all the abnormalities concerning a patient. In the latter all the significant abnormal findings should be summarized. It is this summary, termed the diagnosis, that is the basis for treatment planning. The following illustrative case is presented to show how a case should be evaluated.

ILLUSTRATIVE CASE (FIGS. 244 to 246)

The patient is a female, 52 years of age.

Chief Complaint (C. C.)

"I have a sore place on my gums."[1]

Present Illness (P. I.)

The patient had no complaints[2] about her mouth until about three weeks ago[3] when a very painful, tender, swollen area occurred overnight on the gingival tissues adjacent to the lower lateral incisor.[4] It was intensely painful, especially during eating.[5] The pain was continuous, throbbing, and burning and radiated over the lower jaw; it was not related in any way to recumbency or exertion,[6] nor did it keep the patient awake or prevent her from eating. The tooth was not particularly sensitive to touch, but the gingiva was very tender.[7] After a day or so there was a remission of the acute pain, but a continuous feeling of discomfort persisted. The remission was associated with a decrease in the size of the swelling and the occurrence of a bad taste in the mouth.[8] The patient noted some mobility of the tooth but no fever, malaise, lethargy, or swelling under the chin or neck.[9] She did not recall having eaten any pop corn, nut meats, or food containing seeds, nor had she noted that her toothbrush was losing bristles prior to the onset of her complaint.[10] She had noticed that food frequently caught between the teeth in the area of the lower central incisors and there that had been a recession of the gum for the past several months.[11] She did not consult a dentist but treated herself by placing aspirin directly on the swelling for relief of the pain. She also thought this medication would kill infection.[12]

The patient states that she has tried to go to the dentist once a year. On her present visit to the dental clinic she expected to "get her teeth cleaned, gone over, and fillings checked."

---

[1]This is the patient's chief complaint in her own words.

[2]It is apparent that the onset of this condition was abrupt. A statement of prior health is helpful in determining the type of onset. It also indicates the patient's attitude toward her oral health prior to the time of her chief complaint.

[3]This statement begins the chronology of the primary symptoms.

[4]This statement gives the location of the complaint and some associated symptoms.

[5]It is significant that the character of the symptom should change with a specific activity. It directs attention toward factors present during eating which could be contributing to the cause of the symptoms.

[6]This is negative correlative data and points out to some extent that the condition is not due to pulpal disease.

[7]This serves also as a negative correlative fact to further emphasize that this is probably not pulpal disease.

[8]The sudden decrease in symptoms with an associated "bad taste" suggests the possibility of a draining abscess.

[9]The fact that there were no constitutional symptoms is significant and aids in determining the severity of the disease process. The presence of tooth mobility tends to point to the possibility of periodontal disease. The lack of swelling in the neck suggests the absence of lymph node involvement.

[10]These are the factors which may be the initiating causes of periodontal abscess, especially in the presence of periodontal disease with periodontal pockets.

[11]Food impaction and gingival recession in the area of the chief complaint prior to the onset of the chief complaint are positive correlative data pertaining to the possibility of periodontal abscess.

[12]It is important to know what the patient did for treatment and what she expected of her treatment. It is obvious in this case that her treatment was incorrect, and her premise as to the effect of the drug was wrong. In this particular case, we may know on later physical examination that there is a good possibility of an aspirin burn.

She is concerned about her teeth because her husband recently had immediate dentures made and is experiencing difficulty with them.[13]

The patient complains of a pain in her back that has been present for some time—"possibly to the time of hysterectomy" that was done about three years ago. She also thinks that possibly her "bad teeth may be poisoning her system." The pain is localized to the neck and shoulders and is dull in character.[14] On further questioning she believes that the pain in her neck and shoulders might be associated with "overwork" since she is no longer able to do things she likes—like being out of doors, gathering wood, etc.[15] She has a lump in her throat when her back aches.[16]

The patient consulted a chiropractor who indicated that she had "overdone" since her son had been in the Army. She commented that the chiropractor said she had a "tricky back" and she believes he is the only one that can put it back.[17] She believes she is developing a case of arthritis or something.[18]

She has recently gained eight pounds which she attributes to eating too much. She has had no fever and complains of some fatigue associated with "overdoing."[19]

Past History (P. H.)

The patient had "severe" measles, with a temperature of "105.5°," at about 18 or 19 years of age. She lost most of her hair at the time but does not remember any other complications. She does not remember having had any other childhood diseases[20] nor any severe toothaches or premature losses of primary dentition.[21] The patient denies any history of typhoid fever, malaria, asthma, eczema, pneumonia, or pleurisy. She has a "little hay fever and cannot take aspirin."[22]

There is no history of tuberculosis, weak heart, nervous breakdowns, stomach ulcers, anemia, or kidney trouble,[23] nor a history of herpetic gingivostomatitis.[24] The patient states that her upper right and left third molars were extracted because of discomfort associated with

---

[13]This suggests that the patient's primary concern is not so much the pain but the thought of losing her teeth and the necessity for replacement with complete dentures which she believes would probably be unsuccessful since her husband's were not successful.

[14]In discussing her general health and its relation to her teeth, the patient has assumed that poisons from her teeth may be responsible for the neck and shoulder pain. The duration and character of the pain and the fact that she can sleep at night gives some estimate of the actual severity of the complaint. One might wonder at this time if the hysterectomy has any connection with this complaint; since it is not logical to assume teeth have anything to do with complaints relative to the neck and shoulders aside from possible muscle tensions, it becomes necessary to consider the reason for the hysterectomy and, if it were for a neoplastic disease, whether or not the presence of these associated symptoms might be referable to metastatic lesions.

[15]An associated complaint suggests that she might have some limitation of former capacity.

[16]This associated symptom gives the impression of being psychogenic in origin rather than organic.

[17]In questioning the patient as to her last visit to her physician she disclosed she has seen a chiropractor in addition to her family physician. This is significant since her physician has not considered her complaints organically important.

[18]It is well established what the patient believes the cause of her complaint to be. Upon inquiry as to why she thought she was getting arthritis, she gave very vague answers which strongly imply that she has a desire to get some argument for her diagnosis.

[19]The patient has given what she considers to be a true answer, and without further contributory evidence to the contrary it must be accepted. However, further questioning relative to possible causes are in order at this time.

[20]While the patient seems to have had severe measles, there does not appear to be any contributory history in reply to questions concerning possible sequelae.

[21]In relation to childhood diseases, the premature loss of deciduous dentition is of significance in the development of malocclusion. There appears to be no contributory evidence here.

[22]No doubt this is based upon her experience of using aspirin locally on her gums; in any event do not prescribe aspirin.

[23]These are additional illnesses with possible associated sequelae that are significant to dental procedures.

[24]This may at times be confused with Vincent's disease, and detailed questioning may be needed to bring out the differences.

their eruption. Her "lower stomach teeth" were extracted "many years ago." She had never been injured.[25] She had her tonsils removed fifteen years ago because of frequent sore throats. None of these episodes were severe enough to confine her to bed.[26] A mastectomy was done when she was 38 years of age and a hysterectomy when she was 46 years of age because of neoplastic disease.[27] No complications have been recognized, and she last saw her physician about six months ago.[28]

Family History (F. H.)

The patient's mother and father are deceased. Her father died at the age of 73 as a result of cardiovascular disease and her mother at the age of 73 as a result of postoperative complications following gall bladder removal.[29] The patient does not recall any history of diabetes, cancer, tuberculosis, allergy, or nervous or mental disease in her immediate family.[30] She does not remember any significant information regarding the status of her parents' dentition.[31]

Personal and Social History

The patient is happily married and has one living child. She lost a set of twins during the first pregnancy but does not remember the cause.[32] She is a housewife, and her duties are fairly light. Her son is in the Army in Korea and this has been of considerable concern. While the family income seems to be adequate, it is not so good as it could be because her husband has not been able to work because of glaucoma.[33] She appears to be apprehensive about her condition but not overly so. She does not use tobacco in any form but likes "to eat, especially candy."

Systems Review[34]

Head.—The patient does not have headaches.

Eyes.—She wears spectacles because of failing vision. She has not noticed any changes in vision recently, and there is no history of pain, inflammation, burning, or diplopia.

Ears.—Hearing is good. There is no history of deafness, discharge, vertigo, or tinnitus.

Nose.—No history of epistaxis. The patient has frequent colds and is bothered with hay fever and "sinus trouble." She states that she has no difficulty in breathing through her nose.

---

[25]This category is not limited to major injuries. All injuries should be noted. Patients tend to forget small insignificant injuries.

[26]This gives an estimate of how severe "sore throats" may have been. It is well to determine where possible why the tonsils were removed. The patient should be questioned regarding the possibility of an association with rheumatic fever.

[27]The time of occurrence and reason for operations should be listed. The patient's operations are significant because they indicate the possibility of further neoplastic disease by metastases.

[28]The patient should be questioned at this time to explore the possibility of recurrence of disease by asking about her last visit to her physician and about what he had to say concerning her present status. Associated complaints indicated the necessity for eliminating possibility of metastases.

[29]By inference this may suggest the possibility of gall bladder disease; however, the patient was able to state that her physician had already eliminated this possibility.

[30]The patient was not positive in her knowledge, so under such circumstances it is best to state that she does not recall any history of these diseases.

[31]Even though a patient may remember this information, the correlation between a patient's condition and that of the parents is no greater than the correlation in most other diseases except in malocclusion, where there seems to be a somewhat higher rate of correlation. It must be remembered also that histories are for the collection of data for the study of such problems.

[32]It is important to know about recent severe illnesses during pregnancy because they may have a direct reflection on the care and conditions of the gingival tissues.

[33]Financial status of the patient indicates that she may be unable to assume the expense of ideal treatment if too extensive in nature.

[34]The systems review may be carried out at a later date if necessary, and at times it is well to obtain this part of the history at a later appointment since many times a patient may recall some of the information desired after the initial reminder and can give a better account at the next appointment.

Throat.—Tonsils were removed fifteen years ago as indicated under past history.[35] She has a "lump in her throat" when she has neck and back pain.[36]

Cardiorespiratory.—The patient complains of shortness of breath[37] when she is nervous, and her heart "pounds" at such times. She has not noticed any recent change in her ability to climb stairs or any undue shortness of breath.[38] "I have pressure on the heart sometimes and can't take a deep breath and I believe indigestion causes it."[39] The patient complains of pain in the substernal and epigastric regions.[40] This pain is related to the time she experiences pressure on the heart and not to exercise. She complains of edema of her lower extremities on standing and walking and attributes this to tight shoes. She does not think the swelling is very noticeable. She has night sweats that occur fairly frequently, but they are not drenching in character.[41] She does not give a history of cough or hemoptysis.

Gastrointestinal.—The patient complains of "gas" on her stomach and also of constipation. Her appetite is good. Up to four or five months ago she complained of pain in the epigastric region that frequently lasted about two hours. It did not seem to be associated with eating or exercise. The patient got some relief from nausea by "stretching out on her stomach."[42]

A gastrointestinal series was done recently with no significant findings, and the patient's physician ruled out gall bladder disease.[43] She was treated twenty-five years ago for "very, very red, inflamed, and sore gums that felt like they were drawing up."[44] She was treated three times with a "greenlike solution that seemed to shrink the gums."[45] This took place during her first pregnancy. Two of her lower "stomach teeth" were extracted at about the age of 16 years because of abscesses.[46] No excessive hemorrhage occurred with the extractions.

Neuromuscular.—The patient complains of insomnia and nervousness and sometimes uses phenobarbital to sleep. Her hands and fingers are frequently "asleep" in the morning irrespective of her sleeping position.[47] She has pain in the back as described under present illness.

---

[35]It is permissible to refer to items previously reviewed. History of sore throat, dysphagia, hoarseness, and other symptoms should be reviewed to remind the patient of any symptoms missed previously.

[36]There seems to be no indication that the associating complaint is organic in nature.

[37]This is an important complaint and should be given considered attention in the clinical examination.

[38]This information serves to give some quantitative evaluation to her complaint of shortness of breath.

[39]This information seems to indicate that her complaint of shortness of breath may be referable to cardiorespiratory disease.

[40]Complaints of substernal pain and pain in the epigastric region are significant. Substernal pain should be evaluated in relationship to the patient's complaint of shortness of breath, and the epigastric pain should be evaluated in reference to her examination by her physician for gall bladder disease. It is also possible that her complaints may be poorly localized and due to flatulence.

[41]The description of the night sweats and the lack of associated symptoms suggest that the patient does not have tuberculosis. The possibility of other diseases should also be ruled out. Those diseases in which night sweats occur should be remembered and their symptoms reviewed.

[42]In many instances methods of gaining relief and whether or not the relief is gained are of significance in evaluations of a complaint.

[43]The suggestion that the patient may be suffering from gall bladder disease has been ruled out by her physician. The information that she had a "G.I. series" indicates that she has been examined for these complaints by her physician. This serves to relieve the dentist of any responsibility for further evaluation of this phase of the patient's health status.

[44]This description is highly suggestive of Vincent's infection. It is of considerable significance in reviewing the oral health and the etiology of her present condition.

[45]The medication used is helpful in establishing the disease. This is positive correlative data for establishing a history of Vincent's infection.

[46]The reasons for dates of extractions are important because of their relation to the etiology of oral conditions. At times it is important to determine the contributing factor in subacute bacterial endocarditis, actinomycosis, abscesses, etc.

[47]Anesthesia of the hands may be seen in many diseases. While it is not uncommon for it to occur in one extremity as a result of sleeping on that extremity, it is uncommon for it to occur bilaterally and so regularly.

There is no history of syncope, convulsions, paralysis, or ataxia and no mental confusion.[48] The patient has had some changes of temperament; she is more irritable lately. She has no particular loss of memory except that it "does not seem to be as good as it used to be."

Bone and Joint.—The patient complains of pain along the right and left sides since her hysterectomy. She had pain and swelling of one knee joint during her second pregnancy. Otherwise there is no past history of pain, limitation of motion, or swelling of any joints, including the temporomandibular joint; lately, however, she has had some stiffness of the finger joints.

Genitourinary.—The patient has no history of hematuria, dysuria, or nocturia and urinates with a normal frequency of three or four times per day.

Catamenia.—The patient complains of "hot flushes," palpitation of the heart, flatulence, some nausea, constipation, and occasionally dizziness. The "hot flushes" are localized over the upper portion of the body and produce a sensation of warmth. This patient is in menopause.[49]

Clinical Physical Examination (P. E.)

The patient is a well-developed, heavy set, white female weighing 150 pounds, of about her stated age, and appears to be in good health.

Head.—The external features of the cranium are normal.

Skin.—The hair shows greying commensurate with the patient's age.[50] The texture and quantity of the hair are normal. An increased amount of hair on the upper lip has forced the patient to shave.[51] The skin is of normal consistency for her age. There is no evidence of drying, pigmentation, or discoloration. There is no evidence of flushing.[52] The lips are of normal color and are not chapped or fissured. The nails appear to have good care, and the hands are normal.

Eyes.—The patient has difficulty seeing anything close up without her spectacles, and she does not have photophobia. Both accommodation and light reflection appear to be normal. There is no discharge, inflammation, or restriction in the movements of the eyeballs.

Nose.—The patient has a postnasal drip, and there is no obvious sign of obstruction of the nose nor inability to breathe through the nose.

Neck.—Palpation of the thyroid gland does not indicate any obvious abnormality as to its size, shape, or attachment. There appears to be no apparent enlargement of the lymph nodes in the neck and preauricular region. The salivary glands appear to be of normal size and consistency. The veins of the neck do not show any distention or pulsation when the patient is seated in the dental chair.[53]

Mouth.—The transition between the skin and the oral mucosa is fairly uniform with the exception of a few ectopic sebaceous glands on the inner aspects of the lips near the commissure. The mucous glands on the inner surface of the lower lip are fairly prominent but of normal consistency. The labial frenulum is attached high on the gingiva and is red. It is attached in an area of inflammation associated with the periodontal pocket and gingival recession.[54]

The buccal mucosa has no scarring and is not particularly prominent. The orifices of the

---

[48]This is a minimum review of this system. Other history should be listed when indicated.

[49]This should be suspected in view of her hysterectomy. The menopause must be proved in this particular case by the symptoms since no menstrual bleeding is possible. In view of the fact that this patient is in the menopause, all of her many symptoms must be evaluated in light of this.

[50]Greying of the hair in older people is of little significance but may be of considerable importance in younger age groups.

[51]This may well relate to symptoms of menopause and can be considered as positive correlative data to this effect.

[52]While this may be negative correlative data regarding the menopause, "flushing" may not be a consistent finding or occur at the time of the examination.

[53]This is negative correlative data regarding cardiac insufficiency but does not rule out cardiac disease.

[54]The labial frenulum may contribute to the maintenance of a periodontal pocket when the attachment is high on the gingiva and the free margin of the gingiva is low on the tooth.

Fig. 244. *Illustrative case.*

parotid duct are prominent but show no inflammation.[55] The mucosa is pink and shows no obvious pigmentation. The vestibular fornix is shallow in the posterior region and in the lower anterior region.[56] There is no evidence of abnormality except in the area of "aspirin burn" adjacent to the lower right incisors. There is a change in the normal red coloration of the mucosa in the fornix and of the pink color of the attached gingiva in the region of the lower right lateral incisor. The latter is associated with the area of swelling of the patient's chief complaint. The hard palate is pale pink from the rugae to the junction of the hard and soft palates. In the anterior region the rugae adjacent to the teeth are red, swollen, and spongy. There are no changes in the orifices of the mucous glands of the palate. The soft palate is reddish in color and shows no evidence of any inflammation, lesions, or induration on inspection and palpation. The tongue is coated. The circumvallate papillae are not particularly prominent. The filiform papillae are not atrophic, and the fungiform papillae are normal. There are no lesions on the dorsal or inferior surfaces of the tongue. There is no prominent fissuring of the tongue, and the median rhomboid area is not conspicuous. The orifices of the glands in the floor of the mouth are normal.

The color of the gingival margin is bluish-pink in all areas except adjacent to the mandibular right central and lateral incisors. The rest of the gingiva is bright red. The attached gingiva is bluish-pink but does not have the same intensity of blue that the free gingival margin does. The attached gingiva in the area of the mandibular lateral incisor is bright red, with a central area of white discoloration extending to the labial vestibule and labial mucosa.

---

[55]Large parotid papillae are not uncommon and are usually of no clinical significance.

[56]This is of importance in determining periodontal therapy, toothbrushing instruction, and placing of prosthetic appliances.

Fig. 245. *Illustrative case.*

The form of the free gingiva is abnormal. The margin is blunted and rolled in all areas and is nowhere closely adapted to the surfaces of the teeth. The interdental papillae do not fill the interproximal areas, and in some areas they are bulbous and have no functional contour. There is no stippling of the free or attached gingiva. The density of the papillae and free gingiva is characterized by being soft, spongy, and flabby. The attached gingiva is soft and is not firm or dense.

The depth of the gingival crevice is everywhere more than 3 mm.[57] The level of attachment is nowhere on the enamel, and the lowering of the attachment measures from 5 to 9 mm.[58] There is a swelling and light discoloration on the labial gingiva of the mandibular right lateral incisor. Pus may be expressed from the crevicular area adjacent to the swelling. The area is painful to touch. There are distal trifurcation exposures of the maxillary left first and second molars and a bifurcation exposure on the lingual side of the mandibular left second molar.[59]

There are considerable supragingival and subgingival calculus deposits in all areas of the

[57]Any crevice over 2 mm. in depth can be considered as abnormal.

[58]This information is also placed on the periodontal chart.

[59]The treatment plan is dependent to a large extent on the status of these areas. The fact that these areas are involved with disease is an indication for removal of the teeth so involved.

mouth. Pockets of 8 to 9 mm. in depth are present on the distal side of the maxillary lateral incisors and on the mesial side of the mandibular right cuspid.

During swallowing, the floor of the mouth adjacent to the alveolar ridge containing the sublingual gland rises to a level higher than the height of the crest of the alveolar process at the site of the extraction of the lower permanent molars.[60]

Radiographic Examination

There is a discontinuity of the lamina dura at the alveolar crest between all the teeth.[61] There is extensive loss of 7 to 8 mm. of bone support between the upper right and left lateral incisors and the cuspids.[62] There is a widened periodontal space about the upper left second bicuspid as well as an irregular lamina dura.[63] There is an extensive loss of bone on the mesial side of the lower left and right tipped permanent second molars.[64] The loss of bone support ranges from one-third to one-half the length of the root, and in some instances (lateral incisors and lower right cuspids) there is a greater loss of bone support.[65]

In those areas of interradicular bone loss, there is a loss of lingual and labial cortical plate bone, but this is not extensive. There are overhanging margins present on the mesial surface of the maxillary right and left bicuspids. The lamina dura is continuous about the apex of the roots of all teeth. The upper right second molar has a root canal filling present.

Examination of the Teeth

The teeth show spacing due to loss of teeth, extrusion, and occlusal changes. There are areas of pronounced occlusal wear, and some teeth are without centric stops or functional contacts. There are many restorations; some have faulty margins and overhangs and have become broken. There is evidence of dental decay throughout the mouth, and there are a few instances of cervical decay.[66] There is No. 2 to 3 mobility of the upper right and lateral incisors and No. 3 to 4 mobility of the lower left and right second bicuspids. There is No. 1 to 2 mobility of the lower right second and third molars but not so pronounced as in the other teeth mentioned.[67] There is a discrepancy between centric relation and centric occlusion.[68] The patient has limited functional efficiency because of loss of teeth and loss of occlusal contact. The

---

[60]This is of considerable importance in the placing of partial or full dentures since this mass of tissue tends to displace the denture saddles.

[61]This gives some indication as to the severity of the condition and is helpful in calling attention to particular areas that may occur as in traumatic occlusion, apical abscesses, and overhanging margins.

[62]This points out particular areas of bone loss and should call attention to possible causes such as food impaction, occlusal trauma, malposition of teeth, and inadequate toothbrushing technic.

[63]The width of the periodontal space is some indication of the amount of function of the tooth. Very narrow width indicates a loss of function, whereas wide periodontal membrane spaces indicate heavy function. If the function exceeds the physiologic limit of the teeth or a sustained orthodontic type of force is placed upon the tooth, there may be a crushing of the periodontal membrane between the tooth and the bone so that there is a very narrow periodontal membrane space. Where there is any irregularity of the width of the periodontal membrane space, the possibility of occlusal trauma should be evaluated.

[64]Loss of first molars has contributed to this area of disease.

[65]The loss of bone as evidenced by radiographs does not necessarily indicate that there is a pocket of the same depth present. This should be correlated with actual measurements of the pockets with a thin probe. The measurements should be recorded on a periodontal chart.

[66]Cervical decay makes periodontal therapy difficult. The presence of unrestored cervical cavities makes it difficult to decrease gingivitis. When gingivectomy is anticipated in the presence of cervical decay, the possibility of rapid decay of the exposed surfaces of the roots should be taken into consideration. A lactobacilli count is indicated under these circumstances.

[67]Mobility may be indicated in terms of relative movement such as No. 1, 2, 3, 4 or in terms of millimeters and is incorporated in the periodontal charting.

[68]This is a slide in centric relation and is an important factor in occlusal trauma. When possible, gross premature contacts should be indicated and an estimate of the functional efficiency in lateral excursions should also be made. The presence of balancing interferences should be recorded.

Fig. 246. *Illustrative case.* Periodontal charting completed; see Fig. 137 for meaning of symbols.

patient has an abnormal pattern of mastication characterized by anterior chewing and chopping action. There are balancing interferences in both right and left working excursions of the mandible. The interocclusal space is about 4 mm. when the patient is at tonus or rest position.

Diagnosis

This patient has extensive periodontal disease involving supporting structures of all the teeth. She has an *acute periodontal abscess associated with periodontitis.*[69] She appears to be in the climacterium.[70] Most of her complaints appear to be referable to this or to her concern over her son being in the Army. There appears to be no real evidence of heart disease or other systemic disease.

Significance of the Diagnosis.—The patient has mentioned that she expects to see her physician in the near future. Because of previous neoplastic disease, her complaints referable

---

[69]This is the diagnosis of the chief complaint referable to the oral cavity.

[70]This is the impression obtained from the complaints referable to her status of health.

to her back, etc., should be evaluated for the presence of metastatic lesions. In view of the appraisal of her medical status, a report from her physician should be requested.[71]

The presence of deep periodontal pockets with the entrapment of bacteria and debris has led to the formation of an abscess on the labial aspect of the mandibular right lateral incisor.

The patient's oral condition is the result of poor oral hygiene, migration of teeth, occlusal trauma, loss of teeth, faulty restorations, previous gingival disease, and chronic inflammation. The menopause factor (less inclination for home care) could only add to the already present local factors sufficient in themselves to produce the present condition. This condition has been present many years and was present before the onset of the menopause. Scientific evidence available at this time precludes the possibility that the patient's teeth per se or the complaint per se is responsible for her arthritis or neck and back complaints.

Prognosis

The prognosis depends to a large extent upon her ability and desire to cooperate in home care. While her temperament is not the best at present, it may be assumed that it will be better when the menopausal symptoms have subsided. Her son's arrival home in May of this year should also contribute to her well-being. Her husband's attitude regarding dental service may be a handicap; however, her cooperation is expected in view of her concern over losing any teeth.

In view of the patient's previous neoplastic disease, it is well to consider the prognosis of this disease. The undertaking of extensive rehabilitation in the presence of metastatic neoplasm is contraindicated. Medical consultation is indicated here before any extensive therapy is considered.

The quantity of restorative dentistry necessary and the number of periodontal treatments necessary indicate that the time required for treatment will be extensive. Patient cooperation and tissue response cannot be fully evaluated at this time. The completed treatment should present a favorable term of service provided adequate maintenance is carried out. Certain deviations from the ideal treatment plan may have to be carried out for economic reasons.

Treatment Plan

The following treatment plan has been suggested for this patient in view of the diagnosis and significance of the diagnosis. It is not to be considered as a completed or detailed treatment plan nor a final treatment plan. Modifications may be instituted as response of the patient and the tissues is evaluated.

    I. Systemic treatment
        A. A consideration of the patient's constitutional status relative to nutrition, metabolism, and hormonal balance indicates that she has a hormonal imbalance related to menopause.
        B. A review of the patient's health history indicates the possibility of the presence of neoplastic disease metastases; consultation with her physician should be requested.[72] If the disease is present, the periodontal therapy plan outlined here should be modified.
    II. Preparatory treatment
        A. Treatment of periodontal abscess[73]

---

[71]The information gained from the case history and clinical examination makes possible an intelligent request for a medical consultation that is based on sound principles. It indicates that there are no outstanding contraindications to dental therapy in this patient. However, it does indicate the possibility of systemic disease of importance to the patient. In the event that the patient is in menopause, certain factors such as temperament complaints and inadequate cooperation should be carefully weighed.

[72]Referral of a patient or a request for information relative to a patient should be by written inquiry with patient's permission.

[73]Treatment of periodontal abscess should be carried out as soon as a preliminary examination has been made. Sufficient history should be acquired to determine whether or not there are contraindications for this form of therapy.

      1. Establish drainage
      2. Scale the teeth
      3. Irrigate with iodine lotion
      4. Place Terramycin paste in the periodontal pocket
  B. Scaling and polishing of all teeth
  C. Home-care instructions[74]
  D. Removal of overhangs[75]
  E. Extractions of teeth 18, 15, and 31[76]
  F. Observation of tooth 14; observation of patient cooperation and tissue response
III. Corrective treatment
  A. Occlusal adjustment and reduction of the lingual cusp of tooth 14 for occlusion with lower fixed prosthesis[77]
  B. Gingivectomy and gingivoplasty[78]
      1. Subgingival curettage of upper lateral incisors
      2. Combined subgingival curettage and gingivectomy of the lower anteriors
      3. Gingivectomy of bicuspids and molar region
  C. Operative dentistry
  D. Prosthetic dentistry
      1. Splinting of teeth 20 and 21 with attachment to tooth 17, replacing teeth 18 and 19
      2. Splinting of teeth 28 and 29 with attachment to tooth 32, replacing teeth 30 and 31
IV. Maintenance phase

At the completion of the corrective phase of treatment, periodontal tissues should be in a physiologic state of health which can be maintained by adequate home care. The patient should be instructed to return for periodic prophylaxis as needed. This will be determined at the time of each visit and will be based upon the patient's oral hygiene. The patient should be examined at least two or three times a year to evaluate the condition of her oral hygiene. A thorough examination of her mouth, including oral hygiene, dental caries, and dental appliances, should be carried out often enough to prevent further disease.

If it is determined that this patient is in the final phases of metastatic carcinoma, only limited and palliative periodontal therapy should be considered. While it is recognized that only complete dental service and periodontal therapy can prevent the progressive loss of her teeth, palliative therapy may be the treatment of choice.

---

[74]Home-care instructions should be given the patient regarding irrigation with warm saline solution at time of treatment of the abscess.

[75]This includes the removal of gross overhangs. In some instances replacement of the restoration may be necessary. However, as much as possible of the overhang must be removed at this time for the most effective results of the scaling and polishing procedures.

[76]Extraction of tooth 15 is necessary because of trifurcation involvement and extraction of tooth 31 because there is a bifurcation involvement. Removal of tooth 15 should only be done prior to the placing of the lower fixed appliance because of the possibility of extrusion of the opposing teeth.

[77]There is a beginning distal trifurcation involvement of tooth 14. Because of this position and the possibility of treatment by gingivectomy, this tooth will be treated and observed since its removal does not basically alter the treatment plan at this time.

[78]Because of the irregularity of loss of supporting structures in the lower anterior region (area of periodontal abscess), elimination of the residual pocket must be modified in order to establish a more favorable gingival contour of this area. Subgingival curettage is carried out at the time of gingivectomy. In this instance the surgical removal of the gingiva does not extend to the complete depth of the periodontal pocket. In this manner, part of the pocket is removed by gingivectomy and part by an attempt at reattachment through subgingival curettage.

Index

A

Abrasion, 256, 257
Abscess, alveolar (periapical), 117, 173
    periodontal (pericemental), 222, 364, 436
Accretions, teeth, 235-237
Acromegaly, 126
Actinomycosis, 131, 136
Addison's pigmentation, 205
Adenoma, sebaceous, 137
   thyroid, 153
Allergy, 91-95
Alveolar crest, 325, 350
Amelogenesis imperfecta, 252, 253
Amyloidosis, 179
Anaphylactic shock, 92
Anemia, 46
Angina pectoris, 44
Anhidrotic ectodermal dysplasia, 255
Anorexia, 102
Arthritis, rheumatoid, 111
Asthma, 40
Auscultation, 118, 158

B

Bacteriology studies, 366
Biopsy, 383
Bleeding, 59
   gingiva, 43
Blood dyscrasia, 30
    produced by drugs, 95
   pressure, 39
    high, 58
   studies, 370
    in anemia, 371
    in bleeding, 372
    in chemotherapy, 377, 378
    in leukemia, 376
    in polycythemia, 371
Bones and joints, 110
Breath, 161
Bullae, 63

C

Calculus, 235, 237
   location, 352

Calculus—cont'd
   x-ray appearance, 332
Cancer, alveolar ridge, 305
   face, 141
   lip, 169, 170
   palate, 190
   tongue, 204, 206
Canker sore, 43
Carcinoma (*see* Cancer)
Caries, dental, 258, 259
    cervical, 251
    location, 352
    x-ray appearance, 331
Catamenia, 106
Cementoma, multiple, 345, 348
Charting, gingiva, 238, 240
   teeth, 266
Cherubism, 127
Chickenpox, 138
Chief complaint, 78, 79
Chronic atrophic gingivitis, 233
Cleft palate, 193
Cleidocranial dysostosis, 255
Climacteric, 107
Cold sore, 43
Conjunctivitis, 94
Constipation, 103
Contact areas of teeth, 264
Coronary thrombosis, 88
Cough, 44
Cretinism, 128
Crusts, 70, 72
Cyanosis, 141
Cyst, incisive papilla, 191

D

Dentin dysplasia, 254
Dentinogenesis imperfecta, 254
Dentition, analysis, mixed, 278, 280, 281
    primary, 277
    secondary, 284
Denture complaints, 305
Desquamation, 70, 72
Diabetes, 38, 90, 427

Diagnosis, concept of, 17
  differential, 415
  method for, 416
  of neoplasms, 423
Diarrhea, 103
Dilaceration, 335
Dilantin gingivitis, 231
Disclosing solution, 412
Disease, cardinal manifestations, 50
  childhood, 86
  gastrointestinal, 100
  venereal, 39
Drugs, 30, 31
  allergy to, 40, 91
Dysphagia, 102
Dyspnea, 57

E

Epidermolysis bollosum, 136
Epithelial attachment, 227
Erosion, 66, 256
Erythema multiforme bullosum, 68
Eschars, 69, 71
Examination, buccal mucosa, 171
  edentulous mouth, 299
  emergency, 33
  eyes, 132
  floor of mouth, 160, 196
  general, 119
  gingiva, 160, 211
  head, 124
  hygienist's role in, 28
  instruments and materials, 162
  lips, 159, 163
  mouth, 160
  nails, 144
  neck, 145
  nose, 134
  occlusion, 160, 269, 287
  oropharynx, 160, 194
  partially edentulous mouth, 306
  periodic health, 21
  radiographic, 313
  screening, 22
  skin, 135
  skull, 125
  teeth, 160, 245
  temporomandibular joints, 289
  tongue, 160, 245
  types, 21
  value of hygienists, 32
Exfoliative cytology, 389
Exophthalmos, 133
Exostosis, 226

F

Facial form, analysis, 271, 272, 275
  profile, 130
    asymmetry, 130, 131
Facies, 126
Fibroma, traumatic, 222
Fingernails, 144, 145

Fissures, 67, 168
Fluorosis (mottled enamel), 250, 251
Fordyce spots, 176
Frankfurt plane, 273
Frenula, 174, 183, 184, 301
Furrowed tongue, 203
Fusion, 248

G

Gait, 121
Gastrointestinal system, 100
Genitourinary system, 106
Geographic tongue, 210
Gingiva, changes in color, 217
  in density, 225
  in form, 221, 222
  in sulcus depth, 227
  in texture, 225
  examination of, 235, 237-241
  in anemia, 218
  in leukemia, 218
  in pregnancy, 232
  McCall's festoons, 223, 224
  normal, 213, 214, 216
  pigmentation of, 212
  recession of, 224
  retrocuspid papilla, 215
Gingival bleeding, 43
Gingivitis, 229, 230
  atrophic, 235
  chronic atrophic senile, 233
    desquamative, 233, 241
  Dilantin, 231
  hereditary gingival fibromatosis, 230
  herpetic, 230
  hormonal, 233
  leukemic, 232
  necrotizing ulcerative, 220
Goiter, 146
Granuloma gravidarum, 222

H

Hair, 144
Hairy tongue, 211
Hay fever, 40
Headaches, 41, 56, 97
Health questionnaire, 24, 25, 29
  significance of, 36
Heart attack, 39
  failure, 89
  murmur, 39
Hemangioma, 142, 177
Hemophilia, 30
Hemoptysis, 44
Hereditary brown teeth, 253
  gingival fibromatosis, 230
Herpes simplex, 170
  zoster, 140
Herpetic gingivostomatitis, 230
History, case, 75
  dental, 84
  family, 78

History—cont'd
  medical, 86
  outline of, 77
  past, 78
  personal, 78, 96
  plan, 77
Hodgkin's disease, 146, 147
Hutchinson's incisors, 250, 252
Hygroma colli, 149
Hypercementosis, 334
Hyperemia, palate, 190
Hypertension, 58, 89
Hypoplasia, enamel, 249

I

Illness, present, 78, 83
  serious, 88
Illustrative case, 436
Injury, 90
Inspection, 114
Irradiation, 91
  effects of, 141

J

Jaundice, 38, 89, 104,142

K

Keratosis, 65

L

Lamina dura, 320, 321, 323, 350
Lesions, primary, 60
  secondary, 66
Leukemia, gingiva in, 232
Linea alba, 176
Lipoma, 131
Lupus erythematosus, 135
Lymph glands, 151
  nodes, 147
Lymphadenopathy, 146, 147, 148
  tuberculosis, 146

M

Macules, 61
McCall's festoons, 223, 224
Median rhomboid glossitis, 203
Melanin, 143
Melanosis, gingival, 211, 212
  oral, 205
  skin, 143
Menopause, 107
Mongolism, 128
Mottled enamel, 250
Movements, mandibular, 293, 295
Mucocele, 181
Mulberry molar, 252

N

Neck, 145, 146, 153
Necrotizing ulcerative gingivitis, 220, 224, 229
Neoplasms, radiographic appearance of, 347

Neuralgia, 55
Neuromuscular system, 108
Nevi, 143
Nicotine stomatitis, 67, 189
Nodules, 62
Nosebleeds, 42

O

Occlusion, 269
  balancing position, 294
  centric position, 292
    relation, 292
  functional analysis, 287
  protrusive position, 294, 295
  rest position of mandible, 296
  slide in centric, 290
  vertical dimension, 297
  working position, 294
Odontogenic tumors, 344
Operations, 90
Oral diagnosis, practical approach to, 35
  scope of, 17
Osseous lesions, 336
  combined radiolucencies and opacities, 346
  cysts, 339
  osteolytic, 338
  radiolucencies, 337
  radiopacities, 343

P

Paget's disease, 125, 380
Pain, 51-56
Palatal papillomatosis, 192
Pallor, 138, 180
Palpation, 58, 114, 115, 154, 155, 156, 157, 173, 177, 198, 199
Papillae, circumvallate, 200, 202
  foliate, 200, 202
  fungiform, 200, 202
  interdental, hyperplastic, 222
Papilloma, 65
Papules, 62
Parotid glands, 150
Pellagra, 209
Percussion, 116, 117
Periapical radiolucency, 328
Periodontal disease, classification, 229
  pockets, 242
  space, 324
Periodontitis, 234, 235
Pernicious anemia, 209
Pigmentation, gingiva, 212
  oral, 144, 180
  skin, 143
Porphyrinemia, teeth in, 247
Pregnancy, 46
  gingivitis, 232
  tumor, 222
Prognathism, 130
Pseudomembrane, 69
Pubertal gingivitis, 231

Pulp stones, 330
    testers, 394
    tests, 391
        considerations in, 398
        interpretation of, 401
        thermal, 400
Pulpal calcification, 329, 352
Pulse, 122
Pupil, Argyll Robertson, 133
Purpura, 181
Pustules, 63

Q
Questionnaire, health, 25, 26

R
Radiation hazards, 41, 356
Radiographs, children's, 356
    complete mouth, 320
    interpretation of, 314, 359
    landmarks, 315, 318, 319
    posterior bite-wing, 350, 360
    supplemental, 353, 354, 355
    temporomandibular joint, 355
Ranula, 199
Resorption, 333
    external, 333, 334
    internal, 333, 334
Retrocuspid papillae, 196, 215
Rheumatic fever, 38
    heart disease, 427

S
Saddle nose, 134
Sclera, 133
Scleroderma, 139
Serologic tests, 378
Sialorrhea, 182
Signs, Chvostek's, 118
Skeletal system, 110
Skin, 135
    color, 137
    texture, 136
Smoker's patch, 169
Solar cheilitis, 68, 165
Stains, 246
    black, 236
    green, 236
    tobacco, 236
Stillman's clefts, 223
Stroke, 39, 89, 109
Study casts, 403
    articulation of, 403
Subacute bacterial endocarditis, 87
    prevention of, 30
Supernumerary teeth, 255, 349
Surveyor, 411
Symptoms, objective, 49
    subjective, 49
Syncope, 109
Syndrome, Cushing's, 129

Syphilis, tongue, 206, 207
Systems, gastrointestinal, 100
    genitourinary, 106
    neuromuscular, 108
    review, 78, 96
    skeletal, 110

T
Teeth, abrasion of, 256
    amelogenesis imperfecta, 252
    anhidrotic ectodermal dysplasia, 255
    anodontia, 255
    caries of, 258
    dentin dysplasia, 254
    dentinogenesis imperfecta, 254
    discoloration of, 246, 247
    erosion of, 256
    examination of, 262
    fluorosis of, 250
    form, 248
    fusion of, 248
    Hutchinson's, 250
    hyperplasia, 249
    in porphyrinemia, 247
    mobility of, 228, 244
    mottled enamel in, 250
    number of, 248
    sensitivity of, 42
    size of, 248
    structure of, 248
    supernumerary, 255
    tetracycline, 247
    Turner's, 248
    vitality of, 258
Temporomandibular joint, 110, 289
    arthritis, 290
Tests, laboratory, 363
    antibiotic sensitivity, 366
    bacteriologic, 366
    blood chemistry (biochemical), 379
    caries activity, 368
    contact sensitivity, 383
    hematologic, 370
    root canal, 368
    serologic, 378
    urinalysis, 382
    pulp, 391
Tetracycline pigmentation, 247
Thrombocytopenic purpura, 181
Tongue, benign migratory glossitis, 210
    carcinoma, 206
    furrowed, 203
    geographic, 210
    hairy, 211
    median rhomboid glossitis, 203
    papillae, 202
    pellagra, 209
    pernicious anemia, 209
    syphilis, 206, 207
    thrust, 195
    tuberculosis, 207
    vitamin B deficiency, 209

Tonsils, 194
Treatment planning, 425
    outline of, 426
    principles of, 432
Tuberculosis, 39
  lypmph node, 146
  ulcer, 207
Tumor, 64
Turner's teeth, 248

U

Ulcer, 67, 69
Urine studies, 382
Urticaria, 93

V

Varicosities, 202

Venereal disease, 39
Vesicles, 63
Vincent's infection (*see* necrotizing ulcera-
    tive gingivitis)
Virus infections, examples of, 73
Vitamin B deficiency, 209
Vomiting, 101

W

Weakness, 56
Weight, changes in, 59

X

Xanthoma, 137
Xerostomia, 182